DOCTORED

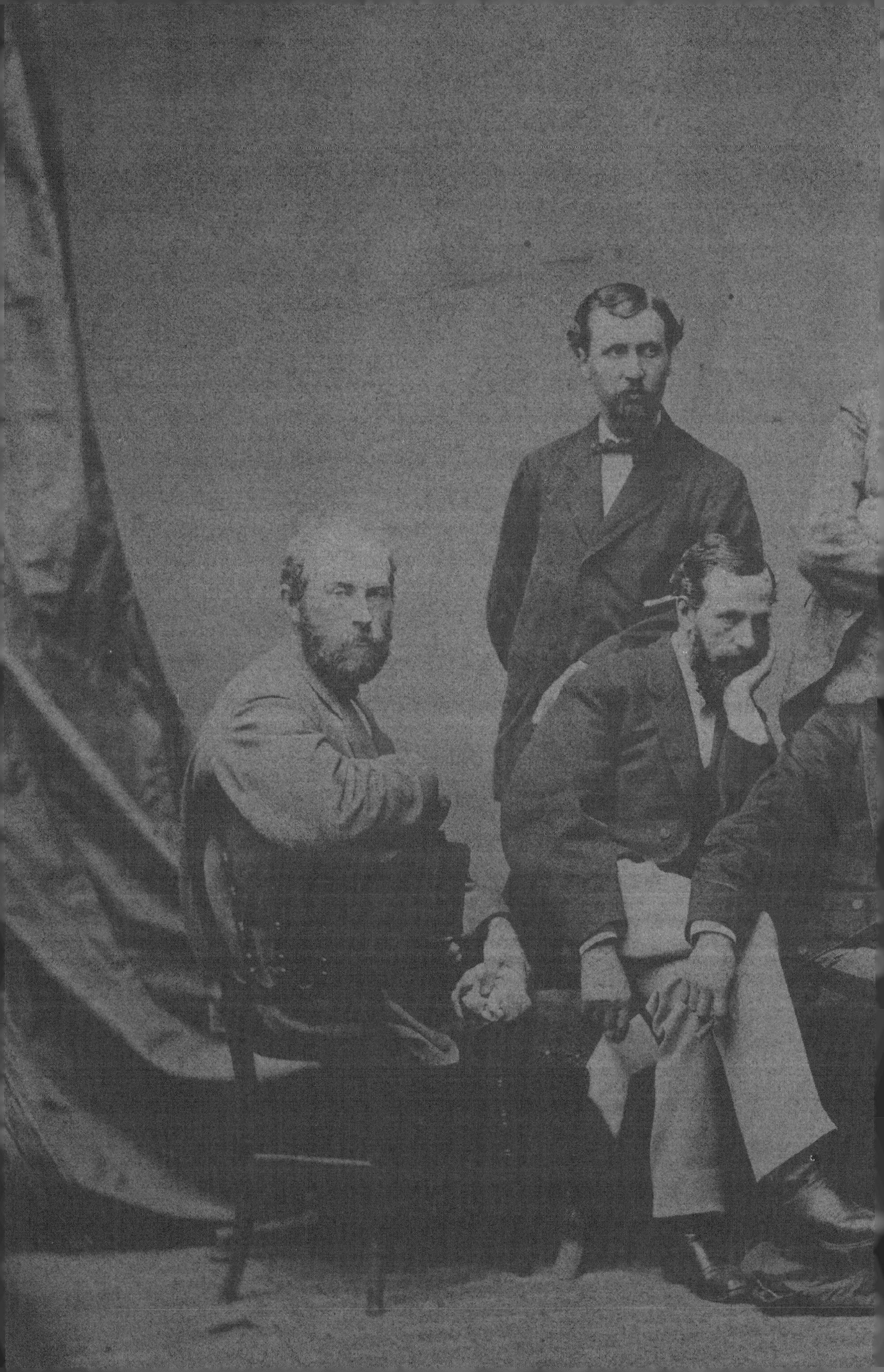

DOCTORED

The Medicine of Photography in Nineteenth-Century America

Tanya Sheehan

The Pennsylvania State University Press | University Park, Pennsylvania

Library of Congress Cataloging-in-Publication Data

Sheehan, Tanya, 1976– .
    Doctored : the medicine of photography in nineteenth-century
America / Tanya Sheehan.
          p.   cm.
Medicine of photography in nineteenth-century America
Includes bibliographical references and index.
Summary: "Examines the relationship between photography and
medicine in American culture. Focuses on the American Civil War
and postbellum Philadelphia to explore how medical models and
metaphors helped establish the professional legitimacy of commer-
cial photography while promoting belief in the rehabilitative powers
of studio portraiture"—Provided by publisher.
ISBN 978-0-271-03792-9 (cloth : alk. paper)
ISBN 978-0-271-03793-6 (pbk. : alk. paper)
1. Medical photography—United States—History—19th century.
2. Photography—United States—History—19th century.
I. Title.
II. Title: Medicine of photography in nineteenth-century America.

[DNLM: 1. History of Medicine—United States. 2. History, 19th
Century—United States. 3. Photography—history—United States.
4. Portraits as Topic—history—United States. WZ 70 AA1]

TR708.S535 2011
770.2'461—dc22
2010041914

for K. S. C.

CONTENTS

List of Illustrations   ix
Acknowledgments   xiii

INTRODUCTION   1

1   EDUCATING "DOCTORS OF PHOTOGRAPHY"
Medical Models and the Institutionalization of Photographic Knowledge   26

2   MAKING FACES AND TAKING OFF HEADS
The Operations of Photography and Medicine   48

3   "PANES CURING PAINS"
Light as Medicine in the Photographic Studio   81

4   A MATTER OF PUBLIC HEALTH
Photographic Chemistry and the (Re)production of Healthy Bodies   106

5   PHOTO DOCTORS AND PIXEL SURGEONS
The Medicine of Photography in the Digital Age   132

Appendix: Philadelphia Photographic Periodicals, 1864–1890   151
Notes   155
Selected Bibliography   182
Index   196

ILLUSTRATIONS

Fig. 1   C. Cohill, *Root Gallery, Fifth and Chestnut Streets, Philadelphia*, 1866. Albumen print. The Historical Society of Pennsylvania, Philadelphia.   5

Fig. 2   Joseph Keppler, *Death's-Head Doctors.—Many Paths to the Grave*, 1881. Color lithograph. From *Puck* 9, no. 230 (August 3, 1881): 372–73. Courtesy of Dartmouth College Library, Hanover, N.H.   7

Fig. 3   Thomas Nast, *Doctor Lincoln's New Elixir of Life*, 1862. Lithograph. From *New-York Illustrated News*, April 12, 1862, 368. The Library Company of Philadelphia.   13

Fig. 4   Map of Philadelphia, 1869. Color lithograph by James McGuigan. The Library Company of Philadelphia.   15

Fig. 5   DeWitt Clinton Baxter, *Chestnut Street from Seventh to Eighth (South Side)*, 1859. Color wood engraving with letterpress. From *Baxter's Panoramic Business Directory of Philadelphia* (Philadelphia: D. W. C. Baxter and Co., 1859). Courtesy of George Eastman House, International Museum of Photography and Film, Rochester, N.Y.   16

Fig. 6   Robert Newell, *Interior View of "Union Avenue" at the Great Central Sanitary Fair, Logan Square, Philadelphia*, 1864. Albumen print. From the *Philadelphia Photographer* 1, no. 10 (October 1864). Brown University Library, Providence, R.I.   20

Fig. 7   Frederick DeBourg Richards, *Charter Members of the National Photographic Association*, 1868. Salted paper print. Courtesy of George Eastman House, International Museum of Photography and Film, Rochester, N.Y.   31

Fig. 8   Frederick Gutekunst, *Group Portrait of Pennsylvania General Hospital Resident Physicians*, 1867. Albumen print. Courtesy of the Library of the College of Physicians of Philadelphia.   32

Fig. 9   Thomas Eakins, *The Gross Clinic*, 1875. Oil on canvas. Courtesy of the Pennsylvania Academy of the Fine Arts, Philadelphia, and the Philadelphia Museum of Art. Gift of the Alumni Association to Jefferson Medical College in 1878 and purchased by the Pennsylvania Academy of the Fine Arts and the Philadelphia Museum of Art in 2007 with the generous support of more than 3,400 donors.   39

Fig. 10   Charles H. Stephens, *Anatomical Lecture by Dr. William Williams Keen*, 1879. Oil on cardboard. Courtesy of the Pennsylvania Academy of the Fine Arts, Philadelphia.   41

Fig. 11   Frederick Gutekunst, *Interior of the Philadelphia School of Anatomy*, ca. 1870s. Albumen print on stereograph mount. Courtesy of the Library of the College of Physicians of Philadelphia.   43

Fig. 12   *Sitting for a Daguerreotype*, ca. 1849. Wood engraving. From *Arthur's Home Magazine* 3, no. 3 (February 1854). Brown University Library, Providence, R.I.   49

Fig. 13   Harrison posing apparatus, ca. 1868. Wood engraving. From "Improved Photographic Rest," *Philadelphia Photographer* 5, no. 51 (March 1868): 74. The Library Company of Philadelphia.   52

Fig. 14 Rhoads' New Photograph Gallery, *Portrait of an Unidentified Boy*, ca. 1860s. Albumen print on *carte de visite* mount. The Library Company of Philadelphia. 56

Fig. 15 Henszey & Co., portrait of an unidentified woman, ca. 1860s. Albumen print on *carte de visite* mount. Private collection. 57

Fig. 16a–b James McClees, *The Children of the Battle-Field*, ca. 1864. Albumen print on *carte de visite* mount (recto and verso). Collection of Mark H. Dunkelman. 61

Fig. 17a Unidentified photographer, *Case of Cheiloplasty (Private Rowland Ward, Co. E, 4th New York Heavy Artillery)*, ca. 1864. Albumen print. National Museum of Health and Medicine. From Army Medical Museum, *Photographs of Surgical Cases and Specimens*, vol. 4, SP186. 63

Fig. 17b Unidentified photographer, *Case of Cheiloplasty (Private Rowland Ward, Co. E, 4th New York Heavy Artillery)*, ca. 1865. Albumen print. National Museum of Health and Medicine. From Army Medical Museum, *Photographs of Surgical Cases and Specimens*, vol. 4, SP168. 64

Fig. 17c Unidentified photographer, *Case of Cheiloplasty (Private Rowland Ward, Co. E, 4th New York Heavy Artillery)*, ca. 1865. Albumen print. National Museum of Health and Medicine. From Army Medical Museum, *Photographs of Surgical Cases and Specimens*, vol. 4, SP169. 65

Fig. 18 Frederick Gutekunst, *Portrait of an Unidentified Soldier*, ca. 1860s. Albumen print on *carte de visite* mount. The Library Company of Philadelphia. 66

Fig. 19 Frederick Gutekunst, *Portrait of an Unidentified Man*, ca. 1860s. Albumen print on *carte de visite* mount. The Library Company of Philadelphia. 67

Fig. 20 Retouching frame, ca. 1870. Wood engraving. From "Our Picture," *Philadelphia Photographer* 7, no. 75 (March 1870): 92. Brown University Library, Providence, R.I. 69

Fig. 21 Portrait of Mlle. Artot, untouched and retouched, ca. 1875. Albumen print. From Hermann Vogel, *The Chemistry of Light and Photography* (New York: D. Appleton and Co., 1875), 245. 70

Fig. 22 Anatomical diagram of the face, ca. 1876. Lithograph. From J. P. Ourdan, *The Art of Retouching* (New York: E. & H. T. Anthony, 1880), plate 2. 71

Fig. 23 *Sketch of Gen. A. J. Pleasonton's Grapery, in the 24th Ward of the City of Philadelphia, Displaying the Arrangement of Blue and Transparent Glasses*, ca. 1876. Color lithograph. From Augustus J. Pleasonton, *The Influence of the Blue Ray of the Sunlight and of the Blue Color of the Sky. . . .* (Philadelphia: Claxton, Remsen and Haffelfinger, 1876), frontispiece. 82

Fig. 24 *Application of Blue Light, Full Bath*, ca. 1877. Color lithograph. From Seth Pancoast, *Blue and Red Light, or Light and Its Rays as Medicine. . . .* (Philadelphia: J. M. Stoddard and Co., 1877). 83

Fig. 25 Unidentified photographer, *Markoe House, 919 Chestnut Street, Philadelphia*, ca. 1875. Albumen print mounted on cardboard. The Historical Society of Pennsylvania, Philadelphia. 84

Fig. 26 The glass-house of Henszey & Co., 812 Arch Street, Philadelphia, ca. 1865. Wood engraving. From "The Glass-House," *Philadelphia Photographer* 3, no. 30 (June 1866): 162. The Library Company of Philadelphia. 86

Fig. 27 Thomas Worth, *Honey, Does Yer See How's I'se Bleachin' Under de Blue Glass?* 1877. Lithograph. From John Carboy [John A. Harrington], *Blue Glass, a Sure Cure for the Blues* (New York: J. B. Collin, 1877), 32. Reproduced by permission of The Huntington Library, San Marino, Calif. 94

Fig. 28 Unidentified photographer, *Portrait of William I. Lancaster*, ca. 1865. Albumen print mounted on cardboard. From *Portrait Album of Well Known Nineteenth Century African American Men of Philadelphia, 1865–1885*. The Library Company of Philadelphia. 98

Fig. 29   William C. Withers, portrait of an African American man, ca. 1890s. Albumen print on cabinet card mount. Private collection.   99

Fig. 30   James Cremer, portrait of the Arms family, ca. 1865. Albumen print on *carte de visite* mount. Private collection.   100

Fig. 31   W. L. Germon, portrait of a servant with baby, ca. 1865. Albumen print on *carte de visite* mount. Private collection.   101

Fig. 32a–b   Draper & Husted, portrait of a baby, ca. 1865. Albumen print on *carte de visite* mount (recto and verso). Private collection.   102

Fig. 33   Fowler Studio, portrait of a family with baby, ca. 1892. Albumen print on cabinet card mount. Private collection.   103

Fig. 34   Interior of darkroom, ca. 1874. Wood engraving. From Edward L. Wilson, *Wilson's Photographics; A Series of Lessons, Accompanied by Notes, on All the Processes Which Are Needful in the Art of Photography* (Philadelphia: Edward L. Wilson, 1881), 91, fig. 34. Brown University Library, Providence, R.I.   107

Fig. 35   *The American Emigrant Car*, ca. 1882. Wood engraving. From *Puck* 11, no. 277 (June 28, 1882): 271. Courtesy of Beinecke Rare Book and Manuscript Library, Yale University, New Haven, Conn.   116

Fig. 36   Advertisement for W. A. Wetherbee, M.D., and Taylor & Wetherbee, Analytical, Pharmaceutical, and Photographical Chemists. From M. P. Simons, *Photography in a Nutshell, or The Experience of an Artist in Photography* (Philadelphia: King and Baird, 1858). The Library Company of Philadelphia.   126

Fig. 37   Wenderoth, Taylor & Brown, advertisement for James F. Magee & Co., Manufacturers of Pure Photographic Chemicals, 1871. Albumen print mounted on cardboard. From *The Gallery of Arts and Manufacturers Album*. The Library Company of Philadelphia.   128

Fig. 38   *Instinct*, ca. 1910. Wood engraving. From *Puck* 67, no. 1742 (July 20, 1910): 5. Courtesy of Beinecke Rare Book and Manuscript Library, Yale University, New Haven, Conn.   136

Fig. 39   Tim Daly and David Asch, *Digital Photo Doctor: Simple Steps to Diagnose, Rescue, and Enhance Your Images* (Pleasantville, N.Y.: Reader's Digest Association, 2006), cover. Courtesy of The ILEX Press, Ltd., Lewes, East Sussex, U.K.   138

Fig. 40   Barry Jackson, *Photoshop Cosmetic Surgery: A Comprehensive Guide to Portrait Retouching and Body Transforming* (New York: Lark Books, 2006), cover.   139

Fig. 41   Allen Showalter as "The Photo Doctor" on WHSV-TV, Harrisonburg, Va. Online at http://www.king1hourphoto.com (accessed January 15, 2010).   141

Fig. 42a–c   Screen shots from *Nip/Tuck*, season 2, episode 29 (originally aired October 5, 2004, on FX).   149

ACKNOWLEDGMENTS

I owe a great debt to the many institutions that have supported this project financially. They include the Department of History of Art and Architecture at Brown University, the College of Physicians of Philadelphia, the Chemical Heritage Foundation, the Society for the History of Technology, The Library Company of Philadelphia, and the Historical Society of Pennsylvania. A publication subvention grant from the Research Council at Rutgers, The State University of New Jersey, helped defray the cost of producing a book rich in visual material.

Special thanks go to Sarah Weatherwax and Connie King at The Library Company as well as to Ann Dodge, Andy Moul, and the staff at the John Hay Library, Brown University; together they pulled thousands of objects from their collections, displaying infinite patience for the often confounding research methods of an interdisciplinary cultural historian. At the George Eastman House, Joe Struble guided me through the Louis Walton Sipley Collection and fielded my many questions about its contents. The late Gretchen Worden offered me unfettered access to the clinical photographs at the Mütter Museum and imparted her deep knowledge of Philadelphia's medical past. Shortly before this book was completed, Mark H. Dunkelman kindly invited me into his Providence home to peruse his extraordinary collection of Civil War *cartes de visite,* while Michael Rhode at the Otis Historical Archives generously shared his research on the photographs produced by and for the Army Medical Museum.

In its initial stages of development, this book benefited from the intellectual support of K. Dian Kriz, Mary Ann Doane, and Kermit Swiler Champa at Brown University. Although Professor Champa passed away before seeing his commitment to the project bear fruit, memories of my conversations with him have remained close to me over the years, shaping the direction of my thinking in many ways; it is to him that *Doctored* is dedicated. The book was further enriched by my participation in the 2001–2 Pembroke Seminar "Technology and Representation" and the 2004–5 Mellon Graduate Workshop "Science and Technology Studies." I would like to thank the members of these seminars—especially Anne Fausto-Sterling, Mary Ann Doane, Evelyn Lincoln, Tess Takahashi, Charlotte Biltekoff, Heather Fielding, and Lisa Brocklebank—for creating spaces in which to conduct challenging, cross-disciplinary dialogues.

More recently, the ideas in these pages have been shaped by exchanges with Geoffrey Batchen, Martin Berger, Rachael Ziady DeLue, Elizabeth Hutchinson, Susan Sidlauskas, Shawn Michelle Smith, Jennifer Tucker, Andrea Volpe, and Andrés Zervigón.

My collaborations with faculty and students through the Center for Cultural Analysis at Rutgers have also provided invaluable opportunities for me to rethink the relationship between photography and medicine. Thankfully, my colleagues in the 2008–9 CCA seminar "New Media Literacies: Gutenberg to Google" helped me build the tools I needed to reflect on the evolution of that relationship in the digital age. I would further single out the projects that Andrés Zervigón and I have undertaken for The Developing Room, a photography working group we co-founded at the CCA, and particularly the fall 2009 symposium "Photography and Medicine: Critical and Creative Perspectives." Those who contributed intellectually to that event—Ana Blohm, Robin Glazer, Eric Gottesman, Julie Livingston, and Susan Sidlauskas—inspired me to push an old subject (to my mind) in new directions.

I would be remiss not to mention the unwavering support that this book has received from the Pennsylvania State University Press. I cannot thank my editor, Ellie Goodman, enough for the enthusiasm she has demonstrated for the project and for her choice of two extraordinary reviewers, whose insights vastly improved my manuscript. Thanks also to editorial assistant Danny Bellet, the production staff at the Press, and my copyeditor, Suzanne Wolk, whose diligence made the experience of publishing *Doctored* a pleasurable one.

Finally, I am extremely grateful for the support of those closest to me, for they have put up with a lot and have even more to look forward to. My former peer and closest friend, Hope Saska, has remained a well of kindness and good humor over the decade I have known her. While my son, Hayden Sheehan Harkett, did nothing to hasten my writing, I appreciate his willingness to "assist" me on my frequent trips to the photocopier, the stacks, and the café of the Brown University Library. I leave these last words of acknowledgment for Daniel Harkett, whose uncompromising faith in me has led to the completion of this book and all of the moments in my life that make sense.

Boys, come in and take your first medicine of photography.

—"The Humor of It," *Wilson's Photographic Magazine* (January 18, 1890)

In 1871, Henry Hunt Snelling made one of his first and most eccentric contributions to America's premier photographic journal, the *Philadelphia Photographer*. Snelling explained that he had suffered from a persistent toothache for years, having undergone several unsuccessful dental operations and tried all of the available remedies. Then one afternoon, while he was working in his darkroom, a "good little invisible sprite" named "Doctor Photo" told him to put together a chemical prescription. This medicine, which relieved his pain completely, contained ether, iodide of potassium, bromide, and gun cotton—a combination that was "almost identical with the photographic collodion formulas of the present day."[1] After further experiment and a second visit from Doctor Photo, Snelling discovered that photography was in fact "the special physician" for a range of debilitating and seemingly incurable diseases that ravaged the bodies of photographers as well as the American public. The photographer, moreover, functioned as a "medium" whose divination of medical knowledge lent him the power to drive out the "evil" spirits of toothache, rheumatism, and neuralgia.

That Snelling had practiced photography for decades, written one of the earliest practical manuals on daguerreotypy, and edited two widely read photographic journals meant that readers of the *Philadelphia Photographer,* many of them commercial photographers, would have recognized him as an aging but reputable authority on photography.[2] They were therefore prepared to read Snelling's story not as the musings of a madman prone to hallucinations in his darkroom but as yet another of his serious meditations on the state of photography as a practice and profession. The story with which Snelling introduces his article encouraged such a reading, specifically by setting up Doctor Photo as an embodiment of commercial photographers' aspirations for themselves and their work. Artists, he recalls, once "turned up their noses" at the idea that photography could rival painting, but now they "throw aside their prejudice, and choke down their pride, and seek the aid of the camera" in demonstrating to the public that their painted representations are artistic and true to nature; scientific investigations of nature have likewise been greatly aided by photography, proving that it is equally and intimately connected to "legitimate" sciences. What we find in Doctor Photo, Snelling concludes, is an entirely new social function for the medium, or what he calls the beginnings of "a phase . . . of photography not hitherto touched upon" that would radically redefine its relationship to art and science and transform the social identities of those who practiced it. Within this new phase of "photography as a physician," the precarious health of Americans would come "entirely under the control of photography," allowing the photographic profession, like Doctor Photo himself, to operate as a single body with potentially unrivaled authority.[3]

As fantastic as Snelling's argument may seem to modern readers, the relationship between photography and medicine that his article proposes was by no means uncommon in nineteenth-century America. As photography was becoming increasingly popular in American cities at midcentury, commercial portrait photographers began constructing medical metaphors to describe the space of the urban photographic studio, the materials central to studio practices, and the physical and social effects of photographic operations. This practice became so pervasive in early photographic literature, in fact, that one rarely finds an issue of a trade journal without references to the photographer as "doctor," his apparatus as "surgical," or his chemicals as "diseased" patients. Portrait photographers also looked to medicine as a model for their institutional structures and their interactions with the studio public, which suggests to the cultural historian further similarities between doctors' and photographers' ways of knowing the body, the social value they attached to such knowledge, and the authority they sought to gain from it.

This book explores the ways in which these medical metaphors and models helped shape the social identities of urban studio photographers and the cultural identity of portrait photography between the late 1850s and circa 1890. By analyzing the trade and popular literature of photography and medicine alongside their visual and material culture, *Doctored* shows how the language and idea of "medicine" worked to strengthen the

professional legitimacy of the commercial photographic community at a time when it
was not well established. While photographers disagreed about what it meant to be part
of a "profession," many of their patrons assumed that they were "merely" mechanical
laborers and that photography was a strange, and at times terrifying, technology. Faced
with such internal and external challenges, those who took portraits for a living sought
to become part of a cohesive group with a collective commitment, as one of them put
it, to "elevating the character of the profession in the eyes of the public."[4] They found
in their conception of medicine a means of representing themselves as professionals
worthy of public respect and even social dependence.

The incorporation of medical metaphors and models into early photographic
discourse did much more than promote the professionalization of commercial photographers, however. It lent them a specific kind of knowledge and authority—namely,
the authority to manipulate, diagnose, treat, and ultimately heal the body—at the same
time that it defined their field of operations, and that of photography itself, as the physical and social health of America's urban public. Although the diverse social groups that
inhabited America's cities saw their bodies as vulnerable to physical disease, moral cor-
ruption, and various forms of social contamination throughout the nineteenth century,
cultural historians have demonstrated that those perceptions were heightened during
the period of this study, as Americans responded to regular epidemics of disease, vastly
accelerated industrialization, steady waves of immigration and the racial and ethnic
conflicts they fueled, as well as the carnage and consequences of civil war. While many
cultural institutions, social reformers, and commercial entrepreneurs promised to foster
a nation of healthy bodies that conformed to the ideals of whiteness and respectability,
urban studio photographers, through their persistent relationship to medicine, portrayed themselves and their practices as both technically and socially suited to rehabilitating the "disordered" and "diseased." Calls for photographers to study anatomy
or to keep their studios clean, for instance, shaped their public image as educated and
scientifically trained professionals who produced pleasing portraits of healthy subjects.
Descriptions of the camera as scalpel and photographic chemicals as therapeutic drugs
defined photography's rehabilitative powers in terms of its unique ability to touch, penetrate, and even become the bodies of its subjects.

RETHINKING PHOTOGRAPHIC AUTHORITY

For more than a century, historians of American photography have represented its
first fifty years as a period when the fledgling medium strove to become a legitimate
art. Their narrative begins with the 1840s, when photography's first critics labeled it a
mechanical process that did not require in its practitioners the intellect and imagination of fine artists. Determined to earn public recognition as legitimate producers of
"high" culture, commercial photographers fought back in the decades that followed by
increasingly incorporating the rhetoric and aesthetic conventions of the fine arts into
their practices and establishing institutional structures based on artistic models, including photographic exhibitions, societies, and periodicals. They also made every effort to

distinguish themselves from the hordes of amateur photographers who appeared on the American scene at midcentury, since amateur work, while generally respectful of aesthetic principles, threatened the legitimacy of photography as a serious artistic practice.[5] After decades of struggle, the narrative concludes, American photographers ultimately won their battle. In the hands of full-fledged artists, photography entered the twentieth century as a widely recognized independent art form.

This story of the legitimization of photography as art began to take shape as early as the 1860s, when the preeminent Philadelphia daguerreotypist Marcus Aurelius Root proposed its trajectory in *The Camera and the Pencil, or The Heliographic Art* (1864).[6] Root intended his book to provide practical instruction to his fellow commercial photographers, reflect on the status of photography in its first quarter-century, and outline his aspirations for the medium in the decades to come.[7] Its use of the terms "heliography" (sun painting) and "solar pencil," discussion of painterly concepts such as "expression" and "harmony of color," and frequent quotation of such canonical painters as Raphael and Reynolds are a few of the ways in which Root emphasized the aesthetic character of the photographic medium and the artistic skills required of those who practiced it. His promotion of photography as a fine art was also supported by the commercial studios that bore his name (fig. 1). According to the photographs and prints of the Root Gallery that were made around the time *The Camera and the Pencil* was published, Philadelphians who rounded the southeast corner of Fifth and Chestnut streets would have seen the book's claims confirmed in the form of a veritable "art gallery" whose second-floor windows were lined with reproductions of finely painted portraits that depicted equally fine ladies and gentleman.

Root's artistic bias, which he shared with many of his contemporaries, articulated an important element of early portrait photographers' aspirations for themselves and their work in the decades after photography's invention. It continued to dominate historical surveys and practices of American photography into the twentieth century, from the writing of critics Charles Caffin and Sadakichi Hartmann and the pictorialist aesthetic they championed to the later modernist art histories of Beaumont Newhall and John Szarkowski, which celebrated the "art" of Alfred Stieglitz and his circle.[8] Although these authors replaced the object of Root's self-interest (commercial portraiture) with that of their own circles (landscape, amateur, and self-proclaimed "art" photography), they retained the daguerreotypist's commitment to narrating the history of photography in terms of its development as a fine art. Early commercial photographs and their "artists" have once again become important subjects of critical analysis in recent decades, demonstrating that the historiography of American photography has yet to experience a sea change that would allow for other narratives of legitimization to structure the history of the medium.[9] As *Doctored* demonstrates, however, a competing narrative did unfold in American photographic literature and defined urban studio practices in the second half of the nineteenth century. The portrait photographers who contributed to and consumed this literature became the architects and objects of a pervasive discourse aimed at legitimizing photography not exclusively as art but as a science of the body.

Examining the centrality of medicine to this discourse introduces new ways of thinking about the sources of and challenges to photographic authority in the period of

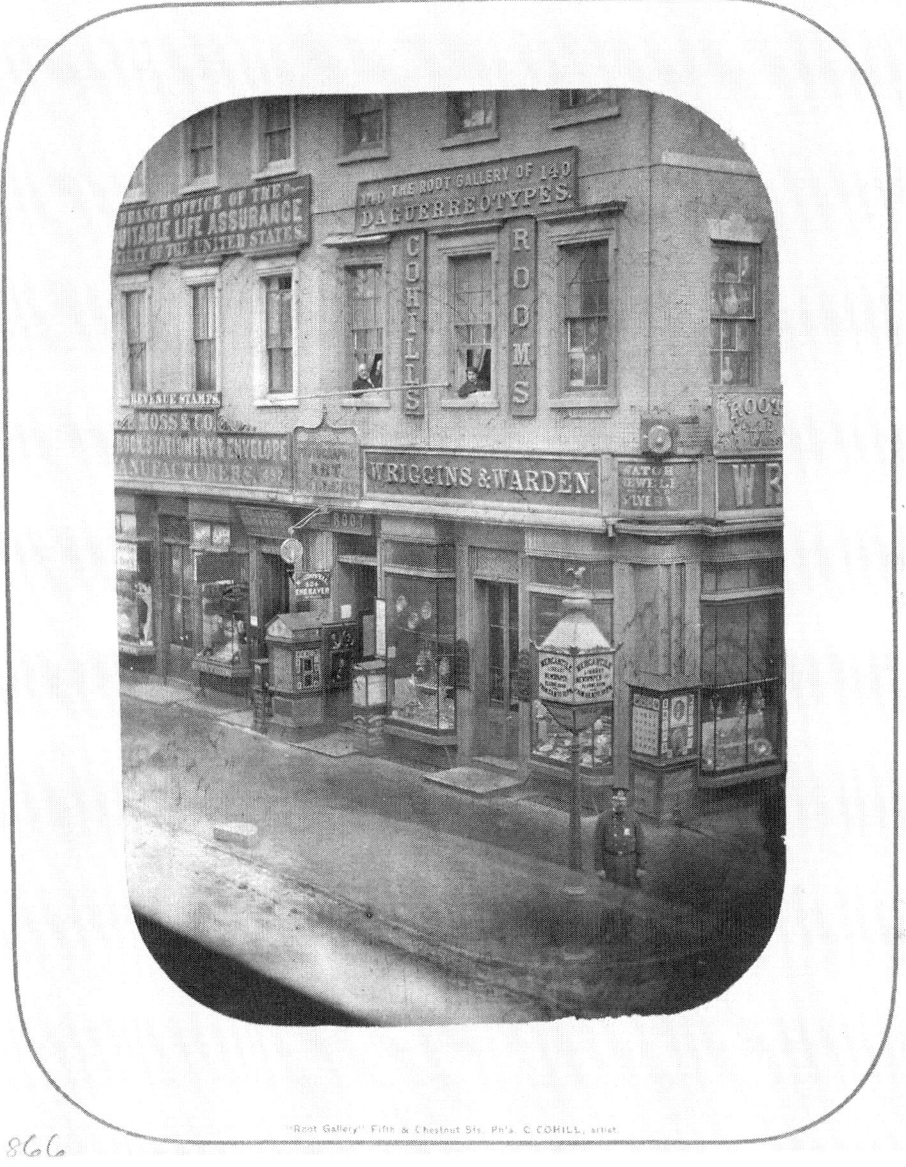

FIGURE 1 C. Cohill, *Root Gallery, Fifth and Chestnut Streets, Philadelphia*, 1866. Albumen print.
The Historical Society of Pennsylvania, Philadelphia.

its initial formation. I speak here of two kinds of photographic authority: professional,
which is closely tied to the body of the photographer, and representational, which impli-
cates the body of the sitter. To do so is itself to challenge several widely held assumptions in the critical historiography and theory of photography, including the notion that
neither a sociological nor a historical analysis of photographic authority is possible. As
Allan Sekula and John Tagg proposed in the 1980s, portrait photography's character
has been (re)produced through the historically specific institutions, discourses, and
practices in which the technology has been embedded.[10] The idea that a photograph
is existentially bound to its referent and thus a marker of the real is, as a result, not an

essential characteristic of the photographic medium; rather, it is a cultural belief constructed in a particular time and place that powerfully effaces the work that has brought it into being.[11] Adopting this methodological position, *Doctored* assumes that a consideration of social and historical phenomena—from the rise of a new professional and consumer culture to the redefinition of citizenship that took place during the Civil War and Reconstruction periods—is inseparable from any critical history of photography. Building upon recent scholarship on early commercial photography in the field of American studies, this book sets out to show how these changes to the American cultural landscape informed studio photographers' use of medical metaphors and models while contributing to the larger analogies between portrait photography and medicine that emerged from them.[12]

Doctored also challenges a tendency among historians of photography, even those attentive to social context, to define photographic authority exclusively as the so-called objectivity of the photographic image. This book demonstrates that in nineteenth-century America the perceived rehabilitative powers of portrait photography were just as important as its "reality" when it came to defining the medium. Public perceptions of those powers, moreover, depended as much on the appearance, knowledge, language, and skills of portrait photographers as they did on photography's apparent ability to heal the body; as a result, analyzing photographers' bodily performances and professional discourse becomes crucial to understanding the authority of their visual practices.[13] To that end, *Doctored* focuses on photographers' actions and statements within commercial photographic literature and the urban portrait studio. It shows how medical metaphors and models encouraged studio patrons to trust "doctors of photography," and the character of their portraits, in a period when middle-class Americans wanted to see doctors as honorable gentlemen whose manipulations and treatment of the body could remedy their perceived ills.

It is important to recognize, however, that not all doctors conformed to this ideal type in the nineteenth century, when American medicine was regularly challenged as a profession and ineffective as a practice. These historical facts alone called into question the power of all medical references when they were most prolific in photographic discourse, or at least rendered that power ambivalent in certain contexts; what is more, the specific types of medicine to which studio photographers compared their practices were very often the objects of popular criticism. In fact, a satirical print published in the American comic magazine *Puck* in 1881, titled *Death's-Head Doctors.—Many Paths to the Grave* (fig. 2), includes in its illustration of quackery the medical models most commonly invoked in early photographic literature, the same models that are examined in this book: operative medicine (in the form of surgical amputation), phototherapy (General Pleasonton's blue-glass cure), and pharmacy and therapeutics (a variety of pills and potions). Many of photographers' business practices, moreover, associated them less with orthodox or "regular" physicians than with "irregulars"—those who, in the world of *Puck,* promoted homeopathy, hydrotherapy, folk remedies, magnetic cures, and patent medicines. Like these popular practitioners of alternative medicine in nineteenth-century America, few portrait photographers spent enough time with a "patient" to establish an ongoing relationship or history; photographers were also excellent salesmen who promised miraculous and pain-free results, generally believed that newer materials were necessarily more effective than old ones, made an elaborate show of their credentials, and relied on the authority of others for their credibility.[14]

Photographers certainly ran the risk of representing their operations as socially destabilizing and even life-threatening by explicitly or implicitly associating them with irregular medicine, much of which the professional medical community of the period deemed quackery. *Doctored* argues that the massive popularity of these popular remedies among the American middle class nevertheless had the potential to provide studio photographers with the kind of authority they sought. In a period when American medicine was undergoing a widespread professional crisis, what mattered was that photographers' medical models incorporated the appearance and rhetoric of science while satisfying middle-class desires for easily accessible, allegedly fast-acting, and relatively inexpensive rehabilitations of the body. It was this same social group that eagerly consumed and put stock in alternative medicines—the group, in other words, that photographers were most concerned to attract to their studios and hoped would believe in the rehabilitative powers of their practices.

Informing these explorations of photographic authority is another important intervention in the historiography of photography, one that recasts the relationship between photographic portraiture and medicine in nineteenth-century America as mutually constructive. Focusing on clinical photographs of doctors and their patients, previous

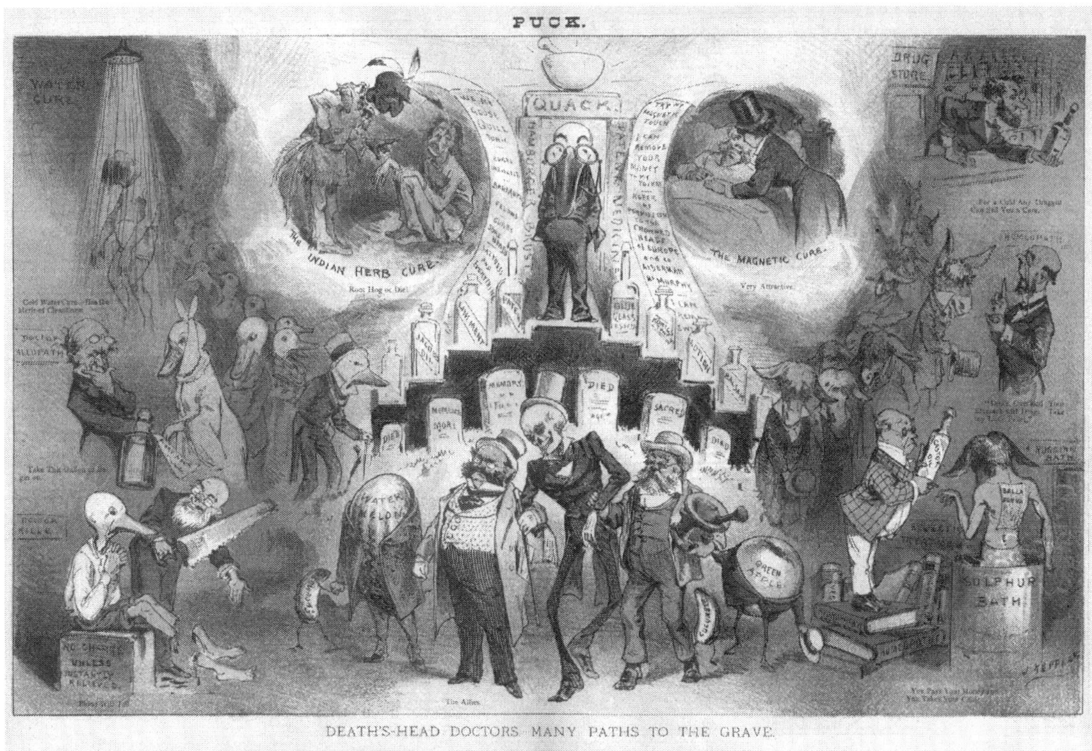

FIGURE 2 Joseph Keppler, *Death's-Head Doctors.—Many Paths to the Grave*, 1881. Color lithograph. From *Puck* 9, no. 230 (August 3, 1881): 372–73.

scholarship has represented photography as instrumental to medicine, particularly to medicine's emergence in the modern period as an authoritative epistemology and practice, which was tied to the development of its professional and scientific character.[15] *Doctored* revises, and in a sense reverses, this order of things by understanding medicine as central to the "marketplace strategies" of commercial portrait photography—strategies that medical historian John Harley Warner has described as directed toward the acquisition of "cultural authority and professional success."[16] While Warner and others have represented American doctors in the mid- to late nineteenth century as attempting to buttress the authority of their unstable profession through their use of photography, this book shows how studio photographers' reliance on medical discourse worked to bail them out of a similar professional crisis; this, in turn, helped stabilize the authority of medicine as well as shape the scientific character of the photographic medium, which medical historians have argued made it such an attractive tool for nineteenth-century doctors.[17] Professional borrowings, such as those between portrait photography and medicine, therefore had doubly creative potential, in that complex negotiations gave shape to both sides of the relationship.

Just as important as the instrumental character of that relationship, which is embodied by the genre of clinical photography, is the presence of the "medical" in *all* forms of commercial portrait photography in the nineteenth century. As several theoretically informed histories of medical imaging have proposed, a genealogical relationship existed between self-consciously medical and vernacular portraiture as well as between photographic technologies and medical practices, which accounts for their similar ways of representing the body as diseased and hence as an object to manipulate, analyze, and control.[18] *Doctored* takes these observations as a starting point, extending their implications to the historically and culturally specific study of studio photography in American cities. At stake in its mobilization of the history of medicine and critical theories of the photographic image is a new understanding of photography's "medical" roots as constructed in a particular time and place and operating outside, but always in relation to, the spaces, apparatuses, and procedures of modern medicine.

THE WORK OF MEDICAL METAPHOR

In its close readings of early photographic literature, *Doctored* assumes that medical metaphors represent more than a creative use of language and actually serve as a means of structuring thought and action. George Lakoff and Mark Johnson advanced this view in their highly influential study *Metaphors We Live By* (1980), which argues that the "primary function of metaphor is to provide a partial understanding of one kind of experience in terms of another kind of experience." That is to say, while *portrait photography* and *medicine* refer to different "experiences," in the second half of the nineteenth century the former was "partially structured, understood, performed, and talked about" in terms of the latter. When we speak of the *medicine of photography,* moreover, we are referring not only to a particular linguistic expression but to an ontological and epistemological mapping from the "conceptual domain" of medicine to the "target domain" of photography.[19] This restructuring could be expressed in many varieties of figurative language, and indeed it was in the historical period *Doctored* examines, most often taking the form of traditional metaphors, similes, analogies, and personifications.[20]

Important to my analysis of these forms is Lakoff and Johnson's claim that metaphorical concepts are only ever partial—that is, they highlight selected aspects of an experience or concept and hide others—since it accounts for the coexistence of the multiple metaphors for photography observed by its historians; each of these brought to light different characteristics of the medium that spoke to competing, culturally specific ideas about what it could be and do. As Geoffrey Batchen demonstrates in his survey of the labored efforts to name photography before 1839, its inventors constructed a "mass of metaphor" before settling on the albeit uneasy combination of "light" and "writing" that foregrounds the medium's simultaneous connection to nature and manual production.[21] Alan Trachtenberg has similarly approached the figurative language in early critical responses to the daguerreotype in the United States, observing that the common notion of the "photograph-as-mirror" articulated the daguerreotype's affinity with the black arts as well as its capacity to stand for both "truth and deception." [22] My own work points to the ways in which the *medicine of photography* largely downplayed the medium's connections to natural forms, fine-artistic practices, and magic while emphasizing others that resonated with the desires and anxieties of those who produced and consumed it between the late 1850s and circa 1890. This metaphor specifically implied a vision of photography as a technology or material that operates within the field of the body by acting directly upon bodies; it further assumed an investment on the part of photography and its practitioners in the eradication of disease and the promotion of health.

Contemporary theories of metaphor also have much to offer in understanding how and why particular figurative conceptions of photography come into being. The idea that metaphors are not arbitrary but are grounded in physical experience, for example, has led scholars to observe their basis in material fact; the daguerreotype is a mirrorlike reflective surface that reverses the image it represents, just as the proliferation of "light" metaphors in writing on photography continues to be based on the medium's means of production.[23] The primary texts discussed in this book likewise identify basic points of connection between the material practices of commercial portrait photography, which involved dressing, posing, and lighting bodies in the studio, and the wide range of corporeal manipulations associated with medicine, from administering oral, topical, and indeed light treatments to bandaging wounds and amputating diseased limbs. These preexisting connections provided the motivation and groundwork for the emergence of the *medicine of photography,* which in turn created new relationships between portrait photography and medicine that affected how the former was perceived, talked about, and practiced in nineteenth-century American cities. Cast in Lakoff and Johnson's terms, medical metaphor had a hand in defining photography as a coherent idea and in shaping the "realities" of photographic experience by guiding the thoughts and actions of studio photographers and their patrons in both conscious and unconscious ways.[24]

Doctored further draws upon scholarship that recognizes the important contributions metaphorical concepts can make at key moments in the history of a technology.

Reflecting on changes in the medium of film at the turn of the twentieth century, for example, Tom Gunning has observed that the "introduction of new technology in the modern era employs a number of rhetorical tropes and discursive practices that constitute our richest source for excavating what the newness of technology entailed."[25] Attending to the figurative language associated with the advent or redefinition of a new medium, in other words, enables the historian to see what was novel, surprising, and even strange about it. Gunning's observation also suggests that the timing of medical metaphors for photography was anything but random; indeed, seen from a technological perspective, they first emerged in commercial photographic discourse precisely as new formats like the *carte de visite* and the tintype were making studio portrait photography increasingly available to a broad American urban public, and when that social group was struggling to make sense of the medium's aesthetic conventions and effects on the body. While photographers' investment in the photographic marketplace differed substantially from that of studio patrons, in the decades after the medium's invention they, too, disclosed the strangeness of their practices through metaphor, often in the form of medical humor; the epigraph with which this introduction begins is one of many such examples that the reader will encounter in the pages that follow.

Building upon anthropological and sociological studies of metaphor, *Doctored* acknowledges a degree of self-interestedness on the part of commercial portrait photographers in the construction of *photography as medicine.* Their expressions of this metaphorical concept, in other words, constituted creative acts typical of a social group that desires power, specifically one seeking to establish its professional legitimacy and incorporate its practices into a well-defined system of knowledge with widely recognized social value. Within this scenario, the commercial photographic community attempted to further its professionalization by aligning itself with a social structure that dominant culture deemed "natural" and granted considerable authority; analogies facilitated this process by transferring aspects of the preexisting group onto the burgeoning group and proposing a resemblance between the two.[26] The primary objects of analogy for many aspiring professions in modern America were, in fact, the social relations they associated with medicine, relations that doctors worked hard to naturalize through a similar set of procedures throughout the nineteenth century. JoAnne Brown speaks of this trend in *The Definition of a Profession* (1992) by observing that social workers, engineers, and psychoanalysts have all practiced what she calls a "linguistic mimicry and modeling" of medicine during their respective periods of professionalization. The subjects of her case study, American psychologists of the early twentieth century, "compared themselves to medical doctors, mental and social problems to bodily disease, and their methods, such as the 'IQ' test, to diagnostic instruments like the thermometer, the x-ray, and the blood count."[27] Viewed in this context, commercial photographers can be seen as participating in a widespread professional practice in modern America by adopting language ordinarily associated with medical men.

While acknowledging that many groups found in medicine a language in which to articulate and promote their social aspirations, *Doctored* is also concerned to elucidate the peculiar character of medical metaphor making in the history of photography. One aspect of this character has already been touched upon—namely, the fact that photographers compared their practices to both orthodox and alternative forms of medicine, including popular treatments that the American medical profession, then and now, would consider quackery. As the chapters in this book argue, different forms of medicine became associated with different kinds of work in early portrait studios—manipulating bodies, operating the camera, adjusting the lighting conditions under the skylight, retouching negatives, developing prints—and thus enabled the construction of different kinds of photographic authority. In addition, unlike the actors in Brown's case study, both studio photographers *and* their patrons regularly challenged the apparent dissimilarities on which their metaphors were based. Unsurprisingly, photographers' representation of photographic knowledge and operations as more like those of doctors than not functioned as a powerful professional strategy. The public's interpretation of the *medicine of photography* as a literal comparison between two identical objects, by contrast, tended to emphasize the absurdity of this concept, threatening to undo the positive work it could perform for the commercial photographic community. The construction of photographic authority thus involved a continuous (re)invention of the basis of medical metaphors and careful management of their complex and multifarious meanings—a difficult if not impossible task.

In addition to collecting and characterizing the many explicit metaphors made by those who encountered photography in nineteenth-century America, I see the job of the cultural historian as seeking out the deep structural similarities between different cultural practices within a given historical period, constructing a shared group of rules that orders their subjects (a discourse), and defining the system that enables and governs the particular set of relations between their distinct elements and statements (a unity of discourse).[28] As Michel Foucault argued in *The Order of Things,* these similarities are "hidden" from historical actors not because of their intellectual inability to perceive them but because analogies have been crucial to the establishment of systems of knowledge and representations of the social order throughout the modern period; this work was necessarily unconscious at the time of their production—or, if conscious, the awareness was "superficial, limited, and almost fanciful." Adopting this Foucauldian paradigm, *Doctored* proposes figurative relations of its own to demonstrate that studio photographers and medical doctors in the nineteenth century often "employed the same rules to define the objects proper to their own study, to form their concepts, to build their theories."[29] These points of connection, I argue, helped establish photography as a discrete concept and institution while contributing to the formation of a cultural discourse on the diseased and disordered body in urban America.

One important analogy that this book proposes between portrait photography and medicine concerns the ways in which these technologies continually negotiated what anthropologist Mary Douglas has described as "two kinds of bodily experience": the physical and the social. In Douglas's terms, we can say that the human body in commercial photographic and medical discourses functioned similarly as "an image of society," such that its physical boundaries, potential, and weaknesses corresponded to ideas about social boundaries, potential, and weaknesses on both an individual and a collective level.[30] Or, to return to Foucault's model of cultural history, we can see photographers' and doctors' struggles to control the bodies in their care—to ensure that they realized their maximum potential, maintained their health, shored up their boundaries, and ultimately remade their appearances—as expressions of social control and commentaries on the social order.[31] Bringing these paradigms into dialogue with each other, *Doctored* interprets the representations of sitters' bodies in early photographic discourse as vulnerable, unruly, and in need of rehabilitation in relation to a disordered public body during and after the American Civil War. Efforts to control bodies in urban portrait studios through specific rhetorical and mechanical means, moreover, attempted to remake individuals, the city, and the nation, and to establish a professional body of photographers as a powerful agent of social change.

This connection between physical and social health brings portrait photography into dialogue with American political discourse, which has long been rich in medical metaphor. In the years during and immediately after the American Revolution, political leaders and theorists such as Thomas Jefferson, John Adams, Alexander Hamilton, Benjamin Franklin, James Madison, and Thomas Paine frequently portrayed American society, and particularly its system of government, as a body prone to illness that could benefit from the therapeutic effects of the war, the subsequent creation of the American Republic, and the maintenance of a strong Constitution. According to the historian Martha Banta, these representations can be divided into two categories, "that of infections requiring quarantine to check their spread and that of therapies based either on heroic methods of interference or on devices that credit the self-limiting nature of disease."[32] They are common, moreover, in the political writings and speeches that Banta surveys as well as in the visual culture of the period. So we find that in 1774 Paul Revere famously distributed a British etching titled *The Able Doctor, or America Swallowing the Bitter Draught*, which depicts a British minister forcing the tea tax down the throat of a half-naked, female America, while less than a decade later Thomas Jefferson compared the "mobs of great cities" to "sores" that weaken the human body because of their lack of support for "pure government"; "degeneracy" in the "manners and spirit of a people," Jefferson added, "is a canker which soon eats to the heart of [a republic's] laws and constitution."[33] Such references remained popular in the nineteenth century, especially at the time of the Civil War, when Abraham Lincoln compared slavery to a cancer on the nation that had to be excised with extreme care, lest the afflicted patient bleed to death under the "surgeon's knife."[34] Picking up on Lincoln's fondness for medical metaphor, the American editorial cartoonist Thomas Nast published in an 1862 issue of the *New-York Illustrated News* his visual commentary on the socially therapeutic benefits of the president's proposal for a gradual and voluntary emancipation of black slaves in the southern states (fig. 3). Depicting Lincoln holding a cup to the mouth of an African American in his sickbed, *Doctor Lincoln's New Elixir of Life* suggests that the "elixir" of emancipation would bring social healing to the South and its black population, and ultimately to the national body.

It was at the same moment that Lincoln and Nast were reinvigorating the tradition of imag(in)ing America as an ailing body that urban portrait photographers were increasing their trade in medical metaphors, portraying their profession, their patrons, and even their materials as "bodies" in urgent need of "medical" care. In strikingly similar ways, "photographic" and "political" communities in the Civil War and postbellum periods envisioned an intimate relationship between the individual and the collective, such that the health of a photographer, middle-class sitter, politician, or American citizen was shaped by and contributed to that of the photographic profession, the middle class, the political process, and the nation itself, respectively. In addition to noting photographers' explicit references to the war and other threats to the U.S. government in their trade literature, *Doctored* sets out to demonstrate that much of their medically inflected writings were deeply political, in the sense that they reinforced dominant contemporary constructions of class, race, and nation.

PHILADELPHIA: A MIDDLE-CLASS CITY

Doctored reconstructs the historical and cultural foundations of the *medicine of photography* within the specific context of mid- to late nineteenth-century Philadelphia. Along with Boston and New York, Philadelphia in this period was home to the country's

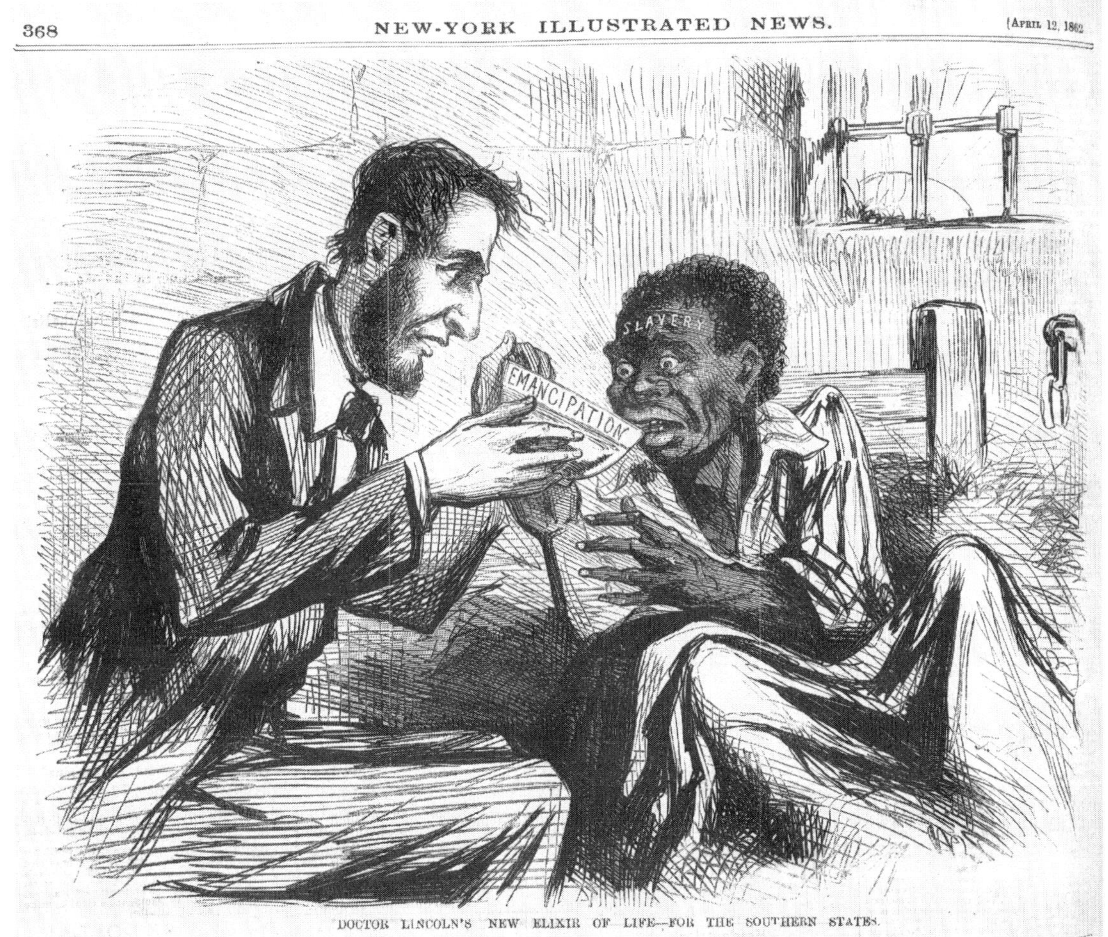

FIGURE 3 Thomas Nast, *Doctor Lincoln's New Elixir of Life*, 1862. Lithograph. Reproduced in *New-York Illustrated News*, April 12, 1862, 368.

preeminent medical institutions.[35] In the field of American medicine, however, it had long been a city of firsts: most notably, the Pennsylvania Hospital was the nation's first hospital (1751); the University of Pennsylvania School of Medicine (1765) and Jefferson Medical College (1824) were its first and second medical schools, respectively; the College of Physicians of Philadelphia (1767) is its oldest professional medical organization; the Philadelphia College of Pharmacy (1821) was the first American institution to offer a professional pharmaceutical education; and the American Medical Association, founded in Philadelphia in 1847, was the country's first national medical society.[36] These institutions both attracted and fostered some of the most celebrated figures in modern American medicine, including Benjamin Rush, Philip Syng Physick, Samuel Gross, David Hayes Agnew, William W. Keen, S. Weir Mitchell, and many others, who together made invaluable contributions to every branch of medicine.

In the words of one of American photography's earliest historians, Julius F. Sachse, Philadelphia was also "the birthplace of photographic portraiture as well as the mother city of modern photography."[37] Most histories of the technology's development credit Philadelphians with making the first American daguerreotype in October 1839 (Joseph Saxton), inventing the bromide process that made daguerreotype portraiture possible (Paul Beck Goddard), and shortly thereafter producing the world's first (surviving) photographic portrait (Robert Cornelius). Philadelphia photographers also opened the first photographic studio in America, and perhaps in the world, in 1840 (Cornelius again) and established one of the earliest photographic societies in 1860 (the Photographic Society of Philadelphia), in addition to publishing the first historical account of the medium in the United States in 1864 (Marcus Aurelius Root), and the country's most widely read photographic journals before the turn of the century (Edward L. Wilson).[38] That the city was unique in witnessing the technical development of both medicine and portrait photography in the nineteenth century, along with the professional advancement of doctors and studio photographers, makes Philadelphia and its institutions an ideal site of investigation for this study.

Much of *Doctored* focuses on the geographical, commercial, and cultural heart of Philadelphia, now known as Center City, which is bounded by Vine Street to the north, South Street to the south, the Delaware River to the east, and the Schuylkill to the west (see wards 5 through 10 in fig. 4). During the period it considers, this area contained businesses and private residences primarily in three- and four-story brick row houses situated on a rigorously ordered grid of horizontal and vertical streets. An engraving of Chestnut Street published in *Baxter's Panoramic Business Directory of Philadelphia* (fig. 5) shows us just how many photographers operated on a single block of one of the most fashionable commercial streets in Center City in 1859. Amid shops that sold gas fixtures and housewares, a gentleman's clothing store, importers of women's hats and dresses, a manufacturer of spectacles, and a commercial penmanship service, Philadelphians encountered as many as four portrait studios: (from left to right) Germon's; the firm of Fredericks, Penabert and Germon; Spieler's; and Dinmore's. Many of the city's best-known and most respected portrait photographers established their businesses elsewhere on Chestnut, among them Marcus Aurelius Root, the Langenheim and McAllister brothers, Samuel Broadbent, Montgomery P. Simons, James McClees, and

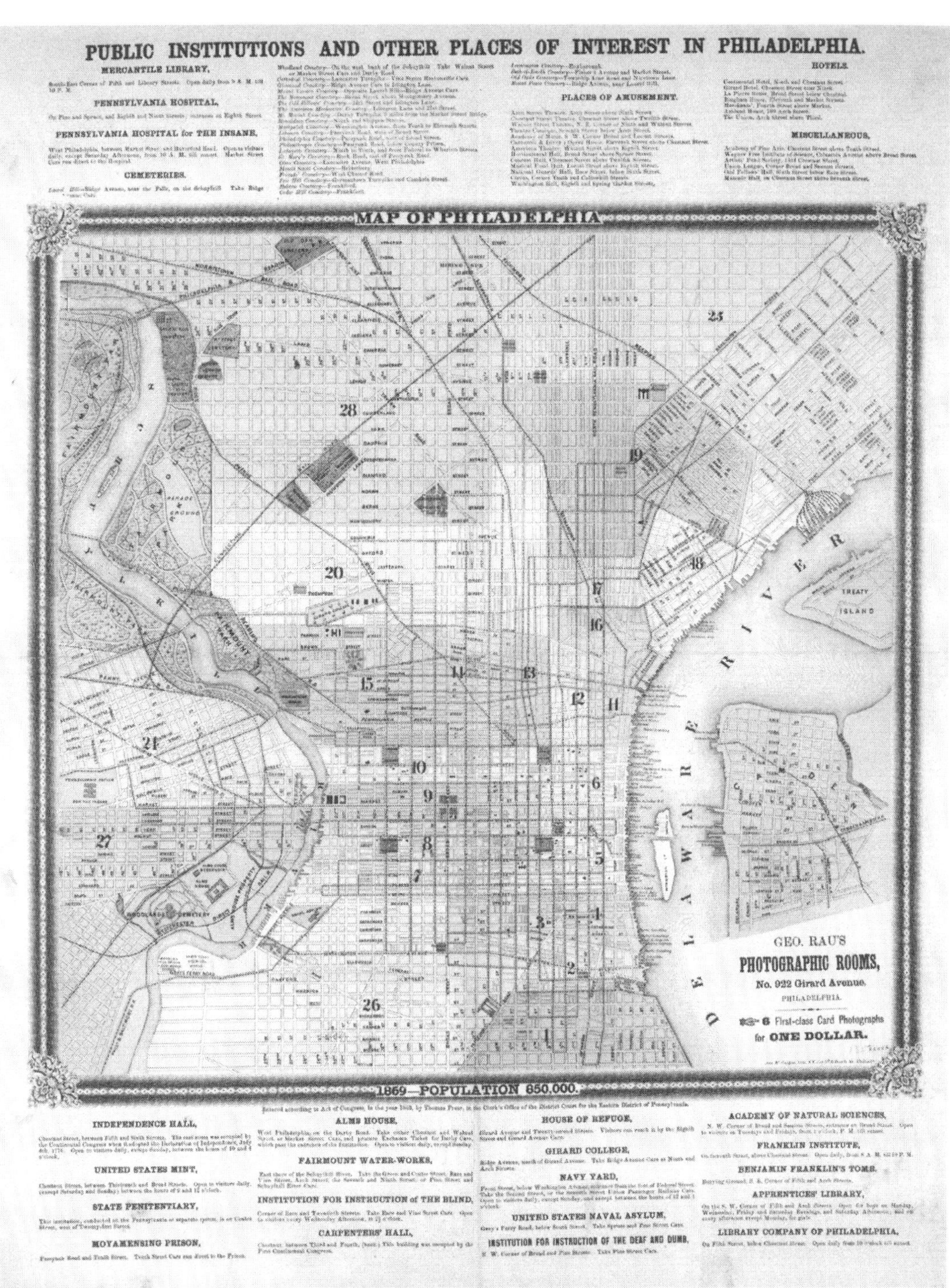

FIGURE 4 Map of Philadelphia, 1869. Color lithograph by James McGuigan. The Library Company of Philadelphia.

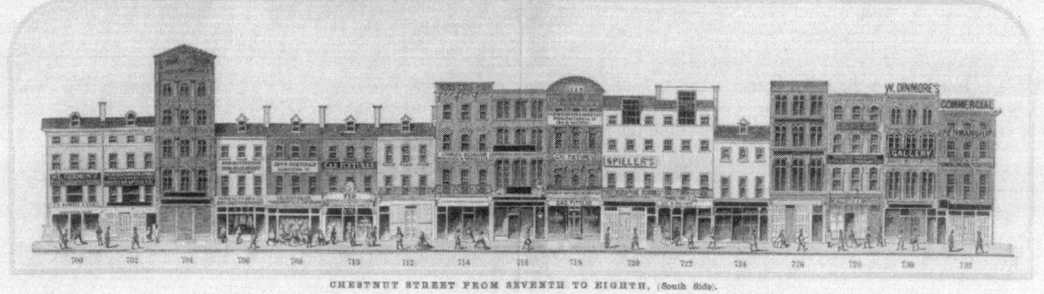

FIGURE 5 DeWitt Clinton Baxter, *Chestnut Street from Seventh to Eighth (South Side)*, 1859. Color wood engraving with letterpress. From *Baxter's Panoramic Business Directory of Philadelphia* (Philadelphia: D. W. C. Baxter and Co., 1859).

F. A. Wenderoth; other high-profile photographers, such as W. L. Germon and Frederick Gutekunst, operated on nearby Arch Street, while clusters of both large and small-scale studios could be found on Market, Walnut, Vine, Eighth, and Ninth. In addition to signaling the vigor with which Philadelphia photographers promoted their work, the advertisement for George Rau's Photographic Rooms printed on the map in figure 4 reminds us that portrait photography was also flourishing in the districts, boroughs, and townships just outside Center City; situated at 922 Girard Avenue in the Penn district (ward 20), Rau's studio was perhaps the most prominent photographic establishment to serve this busy commercial street. In 1854, when the Act of Consolidation incorporated the Penn district, along with twenty-eight other wards, into the boundaries of the "city," bringing them under the control of a centralized government, more than three hundred photographers worked in Philadelphia, most of them commercial daguerreotypists; by 1890 approximately 120 photographic studios were in operation, most with multiple employees, producing portraits in a wide variety of formats.[39]

Crucial to my understanding of the photographic profession, its public, and its material and rhetorical practices is the social fabric of the city. Although intended to facilitate the enforcement of law and order, the consolidation of Philadelphia in 1854 brought social tensions to a city already troubled by economic depression and labor strikes as well as racial and ethnic conflicts. In the 1840s Philadelphia had experienced a massive population increase due to the immigration of rural Americans from Pennsylvania and the mid-Atlantic states, runaway slaves and free blacks, and poor immigrants from Ireland, Germany, and other European countries who settled in the city and county of Philadelphia. The strain this increase placed on Philadelphia's resources and the clash of social identities and values that it produced encouraged the city's "native" white Protestants to assert their dominance over "nonnative" groups through legislation, public protests, and a series of violent race riots. Their efforts to preserve the racial and economic homogeneity of "the birthplace of America" were largely unsuccessful, however, as "nonnative" immigrant groups continued to be attracted to, and to help shape, the rapid urbanization and industrialization of Philadelphia in the middle decades of the nineteenth century. It was out of these patterns of social movement and conflict that

Philadelphia became the world's fourth-largest city in this period, experiencing a seven-fold increase in its population that can be accounted for only in part by the act of 1854. Before the turn of the century, Philadelphia's population doubled again, exceeding one million.[40]

For the majority of "native" Philadelphians, the consolidation of the city that took place in the period of this study meant joining together its separate parts with very little possibility of constructing a unified organic whole. They envisioned a solidification and strengthening of the city, and by extension of the nation, that involved excising parts they deemed weak or unwanted and reorganizing those that remained. Behind this vision stood a fantasy of respectability that was synonymous with whiteness and health and that informed every aspect of the dominant culture and public life in Philadelphia, as it did in many other large American cities of the period. The visual representations of Philadelphia's commercial district in directories like *Baxter's* are only one means by which desires for social "sanitization" found popular and insidious expression; one cannot help but marvel at the armies of uniformly white, top-hatted, and petticoated bodies in these images, given the mix of social types that historically occupied the homes, businesses, and streets of the great American metropolis. One of the goals of this book is to present commercial portrait photography as a rising profession and practice that gave material form to this vision of the city and its people as ideally white and middle class, in part through its sustained dialogue with medical discourse.

Social historians, from Stuart Blumin to John Hepp IV, have portrayed Philadelphia not only as a typical "middle-class city" but as one that exemplified middle-class urban culture in modern America.[41] This is not to say that the city's many lower-class and elite inhabitants did not significantly shape its rich history and culture, but rather that life in Center City was organized in the nineteenth century around the values and desires, as well as the daily routines and social networks, of the middle class. According to Blumin, a "relatively coherent and ascending middle class," a distinct social position between the "poor and 'inferior' inhabitants of the city" and the "members of the mercantile elite," began to take shape in the early nineteenth century and was fostered by decades of industrialization, urbanization, and institutionalization. In Philadelphia and other large northeastern cities, Blumin explains, membership in this growing middle class depended both on one's economic wealth and on the nature of one's work, given that a social stigma was associated with even the most skilled forms of manual labor. Like other categories of identity, of course, class was also socially constructed and publicly performed through one's daily interactions in the theater of the city; it both defined and was defined by "a specific set of experiences, a specific style of living, and a specific social identity."[42]

The urban portrait studio was one social space in which Philadelphians could participate in the construction of their own gendered and raced class identities in relation to the ideal norms of the dominant social group. In part, their participation was conscious, in the sense that many commercial photographers and their patrons were keenly aware that their work habits, social interactions, and physical appearance called perceptions of their identity into question. Photographers acted upon this knowledge by taking measures to professionalize their work and self-image, linking the elevation of their social

status with that of idealized medical men; sitters, in turn, trusted these would-be professionals to portray their bodies and "selves" as legibly respectable and, in most cases,
visibly white. Returning to the engraving in *Baxter's,* one might argue that every shop-
keeper on that stretch of Chestnut Street was in this business of self-(re)making. While
most provided clothing and home furnishings suitable for men and women of proper
social standing, commercial portrait photographers manipulated lighting and exposure,
prop and pose, offering Philadelphians of all economic and ethnic backgrounds seemingly truthful, permanent, and circulatable visual records of their "white middle-class"
selves. How conventional studio portraits in the nineteenth century, from daguerreotypes to cabinet cards, helped construct the social identities of their sitters is a question
that historians of early American photography have recently been keen to explore.[43] Their
responses have invigorated new interest in commercial photography and its practitioners, photographers' trade literature, and the material practices of the portrait studio,
at the same time that they have laid the groundwork for new areas of inquiry. Stepping
into this space, *Doctored* asks how photographers were implicated in and affected by
the processes of identity formation that scholars have associated with the production of
commercial photographic portraiture. How were photographers and sitters able, both in
their own ways, to manipulate those processes to promote their own social elevation (or
not)? Further, how was the identity of the photographic medium itself constructed as a
result and in relation to other technologies of the body that functioned as instruments
of physical and social rehabilitation in modern American culture?

THE NATIONAL CITY AND THE CIVIL WAR

The preoccupation with rehabilitation that runs through this book and the commercial
photographic discourse it explores speaks directly to the vital role that Philadelphia
played in the Civil War. As J. Matthew Gallman recounts in his in-depth social history of
wartime Philadelphia, the city was the Union's second-largest and a major contributor
of men, materials, and other much-needed support. Most "able" Philadelphians who
were white, male, and between the ages of eighteen and forty-five—between eighty and
a hundred thousand out of a total 138,000 men in this group—served in the Union
army.[44] Many who did not enlist, including a significant group of white middle-class
women, participated in the war effort by raising funds through the city's many volunteer
societies. Their largest project, in terms of physical and economic scale, took the form
of the Great Central Fair in June 1864, which aimed to assist the United States Sanitary
Commission (USSC) in its mission to provide supplies for and oversee the proper care
of Union soldiers. Held in a temporary exhibition space in Logan Square—"constructed
and decorated," art historian Elizabeth Milroy has observed, "to elicit patriotic fervor
and national pride"—this event attracted more than four hundred thousand visitors
to its display of domestic and manufactured goods, military and farm equipment,
artworks, and curiosities donated by the residents of the Delaware Valley.[45] In addition to raising more than a million dollars for the USSC, the Great Central Fair created
a utopian national space—literally bedecked in red, white, and blue—in which every

Philadelphian (who could afford the not insignificant price of admission) imagined that he or she was contributing to a northern victory through material production and consumption (fig. 6).

Despite the fact that a battle never took place on city soil, Union troops were continuously present there, many of them in desperate need of medical care. Early in the war, the U.S. government had designated Philadelphia as a primary site at which it would treat the sick and wounded owing to its size, its geographical location on the Union's southern border, and its major port and railroad lines. As the president of the USSC proclaimed before a large audience of Philadelphians in 1863, no city in the country had "been nearer to the seat of the war, and more directly in contact with the great highway to the army. Every soldier almost who has been to the war, at least in the Eastern Department, has been obliged to cross your threshold." The welcome and care that each received there, he continued, left "the stamp of this city on his heart," thanks to the efforts of volunteers who provided hundreds of thousands of soldiers in transit with meals, clothes, beds, and bathing facilities in refreshment saloons as well as in shops and taverns converted into temporary medical facilities.[46] When these facilities were unable to accommodate the injured pouring into the city from the battlefield, a network of military hospitals was created. The largest of its institutions, Mower General Hospital, was built across from the Reading railroad depot in Chestnut Hill, eclipsing the already sizable Satterlee General Hospital, located in West Philadelphia. By the end of the war in 1865, Philadelphia's nearly two dozen military hospitals had offered six thousand beds to the 157,000 soldiers who received medical treatment in the city.[47]

The regular sight of wounded, disfigured, and otherwise ailing bodies in virtually every corner of Philadelphia during and after the Civil War had an enormous impact on its citizens, institutions, and cultural practices. Historians have examined this impact by pointing to the preoccupation with corporeal disorder in medical and popular literature of the period, which imagined an intimate relationship between physical, psychological, and national disease.[48] Many of these scholars have pointed to the intimate relationship between these types of disease in the writings of S. Weir Mitchell, who performed surgical operations during the war at Philadelphia's Filbert Street Hospital before devoting himself to the study of postoperative nerve diseases at Turner's Lane General Hospital. In "The Case of George Dedlow," a fictional first-person narrative based on Mitchell's experiences in these institutions, the title character reflects upon his experience of losing his limbs to gunshot wounds and gangrene, which lands him in Philadelphia's "Stump Hospital" on South Street. Through the eyes of a quadruple amputee who imagines that he is nothing more than "a useless torso, more like some strange larval creature than anything of human shape," Mitchell observed the "horrible variety of suffering" that the battlefield inflicted upon Union soldiers, their families, and the national body they fought to preserve.[49]

Commercial photographers also responded to this widespread perception of bodies in pieces during and after the war, taking as their aim not only the depiction of the wounded but the restoration of physical and national health. As Alan Trachtenberg and Joan Burbick have argued, publicly exhibited battlefield photographs representing the "mutilated remains" of fallen heroes forced the middle-class Americans who viewed

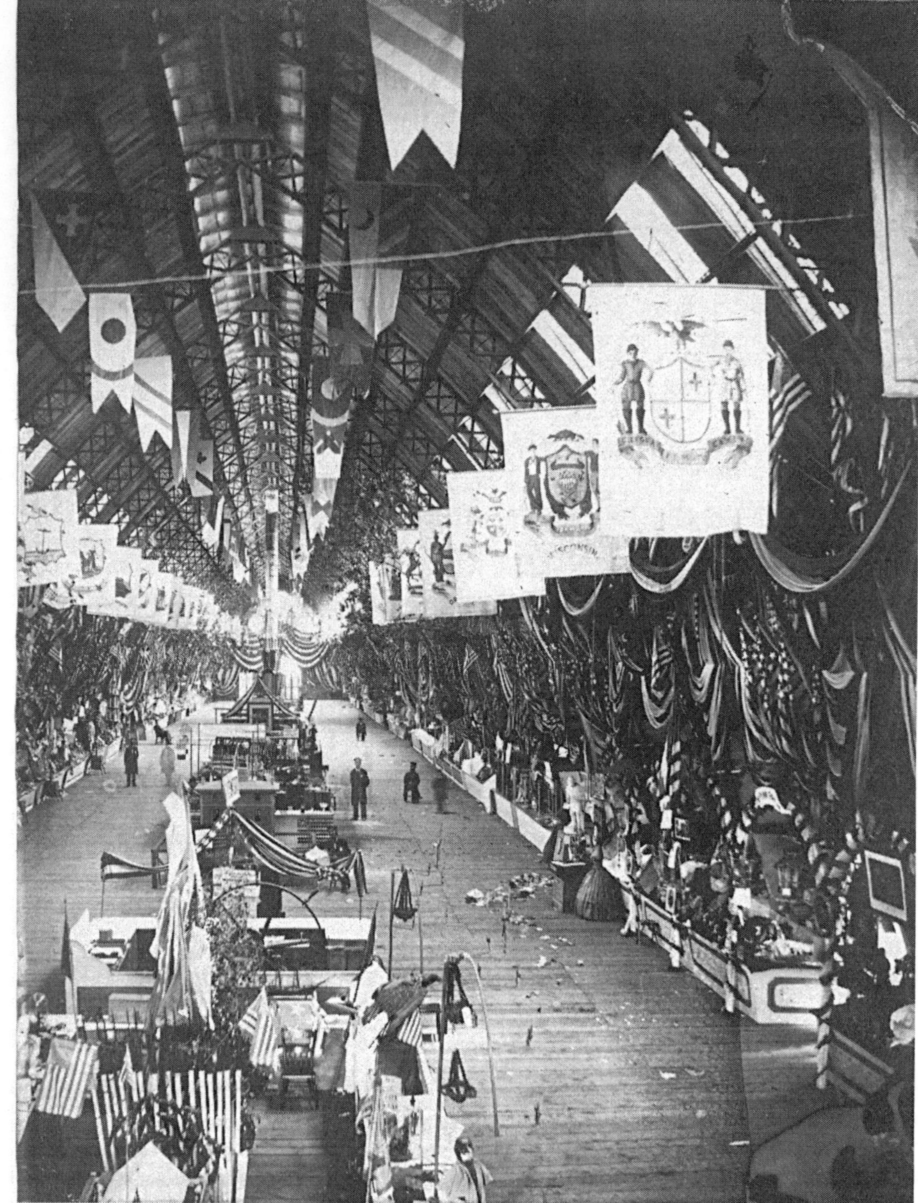

FIGURE 6 Robert Newell, *Interior View of "Union Avenue" at the Great Central Sanitary Fair, Logan Square, Philadelphia*, 1864. Albumen print. From the *Philadelphia Photographer* 1, no. 10 (October 1864).

them to confront the corporeal realities of the conflict and imagine the redemption of a dismembered United States. Reflecting upon Matthew Brady's Antietam photographs in 1863, the physician-photographer Oliver Wendell Holmes saw in these images a powerful means of representing war as "repulsive, brutal, sickening, [and] hideous" that pointed to both the cause of and treatment for America's ills. "Where is the American, worthy of his privileges," he wrote in the *Atlantic Monthly*, "who does not now recognize the fact, if never until now, that the disease of our nation was organic, not functional,

calling for the knife, and not for washes and anodynes?"[50] Clinical photographs of
soldiers who survived the conflict—the victims of fractured and shattered bones,
disfigured flesh, and infected tissues—similarly performed a dual documentary and
therapeutic function. Portraying grotesquely injured soldiers before and after medical intervention, the photographic studies undertaken for the Army Medical Museum,
considered in chapter 2, demonstrated that debilitated military bodies, along with the
nation they both symbolized and served, could return to a state of health.[51]

What *Doctored* adds to existing scholarship on Civil War photography that takes
such images as its subject is a fuller understanding of the ways in which the "everyday"
practices of urban commercial portraiture aimed to contribute to the national project
of rehabilitation. At the broadest level, the chapters that follow reframe the boom in the
commercial photographic industry that took place in Philadelphia between 1860 and
1866—a staggering 450 percent increase in the total manufacturing output for photographs and materials—as connected to the contributions photographers and their
patrons imagined photography could make to the war.[52] More specifically, they interpret
the commonly acknowledged relationship between medical and vernacular studio portraiture in the 1860s and '70s as much more than a matter of shared aesthetic conventions by observing that their points of connection stem from a similar way of envision-
ing bodies—as diseased, disordered, but essentially operable—that would dominate
the cultural imagination of the postbellum city.

BODIES OF LITERATURE

The primary evidence that *Doctored* mobilizes to this end consists of a vast yet under-
studied body of photographic literature produced and/or consumed by Philadelphians
in the second half of the nineteenth century. Because they constitute the most widely
read texts on the subject of American photography at the time, I focus on the photographic trade journals founded and edited by Edward L. Wilson (1838–1903). Wilson
began his work in the field of photography in the early 1860s, when he assisted Frederick Gutekunst in his internationally known Philadelphia studio; he went on to make
enormous contributions to the professionalization of photography in the United States
by co-founding the largest publisher of texts for the American photographic community,
organizing the National Photographic Association in 1868, overseeing the production
and display of photography at the Centennial Exhibition in 1876, and writing several
important photographic manuals between 1881 and 1893.[53] During this time Wilson was
able to exert perhaps his greatest influence on the development of the photographic
profession in his role as editor of the *Philadelphia Photographer,* the two periodicals it
absorbed (the *Photographic World* and the *Photographer's Friend*), its annual review (*Photographic Mosaics*), and its successor (*Wilson's Photographic Magazine*).

Described in the appendix to this book, Wilson's journals were published for most
of their existence in Philadelphia and were read by a great many of the city's practicing
photographers. The *Philadelphia Photographer* in particular also had a large circulation within other urban photographic centers in the United States, such as New York,

Boston, Chicago, and St. Louis, whose photographic societies published reports of their activities in its issues. Like Wilson's other publications, the journal additionally printed international photographic news contributed by foreign correspondents. To speak of the "Philadelphia photographic community" that Wilson helped construct in the second half of the nineteenth century is to speak of a nearly all-white and all-male fraternity of photographic studio owners and operators, instructors and students, as well as suppliers and buyers who lived and worked within and beyond the boundaries of consolidated Philadelphia. The individual photographers and studios named in *Doctored* therefore have ties to a variety of geographical locations but share a common connection to Philadelphia through their consumption of and contributions to the city's photographic literature.

It should come as no surprise that relatively little attention has been paid to this body of writing in the histories of photography, given that scholars have long privileged self-consciously artistic over commercial photographic production. As Steve Edwards explains in his recent study of the relationship between art and industry in English photographic discourse, moreover, the "strange, hybrid literature" that includes Wilson's journals can be "difficult to unpack," given that it often articulates competing positions and interests and juxtaposes artistic theories with what modern readers might see as banal and technical minutiae.[54] Published anonymously or under pseudonyms and generally lacking "critical moments of rupture," articles in these journals also deny scholars the opportunity to attribute eloquent, paradigm-shifting statements to individual authors whose names can be found on (or easily added to) the growing list of "master" photographers that has constituted the (art) history of photography since the early twentieth century.

Like Edwards, I aim to construct a different kind of photographic history, one that privileges the "incessant, everyday speech of photographers" articulated in their trade literature.[55] The chapters that follow read texts in this genre as one might critically interpret works of fiction—that is, by offering close readings of their narrative structures, points of view, themes, characters, style, and figurative devices. To read photographic literature as fiction, in other words, does not involve denying its basis in "reality" or its importance in disseminating factual information about the practice of photography, whether that information concerns cyanide poisonings in the darkroom or the technical difficulties that photographers faced when lighting dark-complexioned sitters. Rather, it involves asking, how were these "facts" constructed through any number of literary elements in the text? And how can such formal analysis inform, while being informed by, an understanding of the social and historical contexts in which the text was conceived, published, and consumed?

Because *Doctored* situates portrait photography in relation to other technologies and discourses, literatures other than "photographic" serve as valuable objects of analysis. This is especially the case for Philadelphia's medical literature, which is as eclectic as the medical metaphors and models through which nineteenth-century portrait photographers and their patrons imagined photographic practices. The examples discussed in the following chapters range from journals such as the *Philadelphia Medical Times,* which circulated widely among members of the American medical profession, to clinical handbooks for surgeons and medical students that were published in the city, to advertisements for locally produced pharmaceuticals, to treatises on alternative and home remedies written by well-known Philadelphians. The city's popular literary and domestic magazines, notably *Arthur's Home Magazine* (1852–87) and *Lippincott's Magazine* (1868–1915), also contain discussions of both portrait studio and medical practices that speak to the social values and experiences of their predominantly urban, white, middle-class readers.

As a book focused primarily on figurative relationships between photography and medicine expressed in written texts, *Doctored* reproduces an admittedly unusual collection of images; many of these belong to the category of commercial visual culture, and some fall outside the traditional category of "photography." It reads, for instance, the engraved illustrations that fill Philadelphia's photographic literature in the second half of the nineteenth century as important evidence of the material culture of the city's early portrait studios. While such images, like the written descriptions that accompany them, can provide valuable information about the physical objects and experiences in photographic studios, they are, of course, themselves complex texts that require interpretation. When published in the context of a photographic journal or textbook, an engraving of an operating room or darkroom can express an idealized vision of the work and bodies it depicts and hence compete with other, at times satirical representations of studio interiors that appeared in the popular press. Studying the space of the early portrait studio thus requires a critical navigation of re-presentations that can only ever produce a highly mediated "reality" of that environment.

Although it is attentive to "photographic culture" in a variety of forms and contexts, *Doctored* remains fundamentally interested in the enormous number of photographic portraits produced by Philadelphia studios between roughly 1860 and 1890. In making such a claim I do not intend to mislead the reader, who might expect to find copious reproductions and formal analyses of these portraits in a book where relatively few are to be found. Rather, I mean to suggest that *all* of the written and visual texts I examine tell us something about what studio portraits could mean to photographers and sitters who persistently compared studio portraiture and medicine. The albumen portraits that do appear in the book, moreover, are interpreted as the visual products of such modeling and metaphor making. And so a group portrait of the National Photographic Association's founding members speaks to the medical roots of photographers' professional self-image, a *carte de visite* of a young boy held stiffly erect by a posing stand tells us about the complex surgical connotations of the photographic "operation," and a cabinet card depicting a family of three shows us how white skin functioned in both photographic and medical discourses as a sign of good health.

OUTLINE OF THE BOOK

Doctored begins by investigating the ways in which early portrait photographers, concerned about their precarious social status, turned to American medicine as a professional and epistemological model beginning in the 1860s. Chapter 1 shows how this model informed the structure of photographers' trade literature, the aims and practices of their first national union, and proposals for schools to train young men to enter the burgeoning profession. By exploring the specifically medical roots of photographers' institutionalization strategies, this chapter emphasizes the centrality of science and the field of the body to establishing portrait photography's cultural identity and authority. At the same time, it acknowledges that photography's relationship to medicine was a matter of much debate through the 1880s, as the leaders of the Philadelphia photographic community vigorously explored its nature and limits.

This discussion sets the stage for an analysis of the medical foundations of photographers' material practices in the portrait studio. Chapter 2 looks at the many resemblances between photography and "operative medicine" that took shape around the time of the Civil War. Perceptions of these similarities resulted in part from the bodily discomfort studio patrons associated with photographic "operations." While sitters often likened the posing stand to dental instruments, in expressing apprehension about their painful effects on the body and threats to bourgeois respectability, photographers portrayed their operations as relying upon a diagnostic way of seeing that was associated with surgical practices of the period. Adopting the guise of surgeons, photographers imagined that they could penetrate deeply into the body, distinguishing the normal from the pathological, with the aim of physically and socially remaking their subjects. Additional analogies between photography and anesthesia, which were as much assertions of photographers' professional character as comments on the physical experience of posing in the portrait studio, rationalized photographers' power to radically reconstruct the "face" of the American public.

The book goes on to examine how photographers adopted the values of public health reform in an effort to further their professionalization and contribute to the postbellum project of restoring national fitness. Chapter 3 considers how portrait photography's reliance upon light lent the technology significant therapeutic potential at a time when many middle-class Philadelphians believed that bathing in a combination of blue light and sunlight could cure everything from hair loss to nervousness. At the height of the blue-glass craze, which coincided with the end of Reconstruction, the standard use of blue glazing in photographers' skylights motivated the idea that a visit to the portrait studio could be a similarly healthful and restorative experience, one that potentially rid sitters' bodies of any deviations from the ideal of whiteness. The chapter's discussion of phototherapeutics, both in and out of the studio, is fundamentally concerned with perceptions of race as an unstable social category in the decades after the war. Technologies of light were ravenously consumed at the same time that they were satirized and discredited in this period, I argue, because they promised a mass "whitening" of the nation's urban population.

Unlike the operation room (or glass house) of the commercial portrait studio, which was generally modeled on an ideal domestic interior, the photographic laboratory was widely viewed as a bustling, unhealthy space of labor and production. To ensure its physical and social well-being, the commercial photographic community had to carefully manage the interactions among the chemical operations performed in that environment, the toxic substances employed, and the bodies that occupied the portrait studio. Chapter 4 explores how these perceptions of the photographic laboratory took shape after the war, specifically in relation to measures to sanitize American cities and treat urban epidemics. Not only were photographers trained by their trade literature to perform emergency and preventive medicine in response to the perilous effects of darkroom work, but, as Snelling's "Doctor Photo" reminds us, those texts also ironically transformed the serious health risks associated with photographic chemistry into an occasion for praising the unparalleled healing powers of photographers and their materials. In these ways, photographers could be seen as gentlemen of science and major actors in public health reform throughout the postbellum period, while photography could function as a technology whose unmediated access to the body allowed it to cure the seemingly incurable.

The final chapter enlarges the book's historical and geographical focus to discuss the recent reemergence of medical models and metaphors in digital photographic discourse. Since the 1980s, digital camera technologies and image manipulation software have revolutionized the art of "doctoring" photographs for fine artists, commercial operators, and amateur snapshooters. These groups, moreover, have frequently portrayed themselves as "photo doctors" and "pixel surgeons" who perform a set of virtual medical procedures on the bodies of their subjects. Taking these representations as its subject, chapter 5 reframes the discussion of Philadelphia's commercial photographic community in *Doctored* as a prehistory of the medicalization of digital photography in our contemporary "makeover culture," revealing how "old" cultural practices continue to shape conceptions of "new" media in the twenty-first century.

EDUCATING "DOCTORS OF PHOTOGRAPHY"
Medical Models and the Institutionalization of Photographic Knowledge

In his sociological study *Photography: A Middle-Brow Art* (1965), Pierre Bourdieu portrays photography as engaged in a process of legitimization that preoccupied its practitioners from the first decades of the twentieth century through the 1960s. Defining its primary social function as the integration of the family and class delineation, Bourdieu observes that the medium existed outside the sphere of cultural legitimacy occupied by the "fully consecrated arts such as theatre, painting, sculpture, literature and classical music." Such practices, he explains, are "organized according to a particular type of system, developed and inculcated by the school, an institution specifically responsible for communicating knowledge, organized into a hierarchy, through a methodical organization of training and practice."[1] During the period of Bourdieu's study—or, as he puts it, "at the very moment when photographic activity is becoming easier and consequently less specific"—amateurs, artists, and commercial photographers all attempted to elevate photography's status within the cultural sphere by organizing themselves into distinct groups in which they could communicate to one another the rules of their activity, or the basis of its knowledge.[2] For those who practiced photography as a profession, this was no easy task. Not only were there significant disparities among photographers with regard to social status, income, business models, and actual practices—the local craftsman toiling in his darkroom, for example, as compared to the orchestrator of a high-fashion photo shoot—but they could not agree on what constituted success in the field of photography. According to Bourdieu's collaborators, Luc Boltanski and Jean-Claude Chambordeon, these realities of the photographic profession stemmed from the fact that formal training was not legally required to gain access to it—neither "the possession of the most basic state diploma . . . nor attendance at a school, nor even apprenticeship with a photographer."[3] This, along with fears of an amateur threat, would become one of the few points of cohesion for the profession as it worked to legitimize its practices.

In the second half of the nineteenth century, or what we might call the initial period of photography's professionalization and institutionalization in the United States, commercial portrait photographers similarly came together around the issue of education. This group faced not only a lack of strictly regulated, state-mandated instruction but quite often an absence of training in studio practices altogether. As the leaders of the Philadelphia photographic community would regularly observe between the 1860s and the 1880s, this state of affairs lay "at the root of all photographic ills."[4] It accounted for perceptions of portrait photographers as "dabsters" and "Cheap Johns," as Henry Snelling once described the untrained men who filled the "photographic ranks," rather than professionals with expert knowledge and specialized skills; it also attracted unrespectable patrons to their studios and thwarted public recognition of photography as a legitimate art or science.[5] Like other tradesmen who sought to improve their public image and acquire cultural legitimacy in nineteenth-century America, commercial photographers thus called for the formalization of their education by means of national and local societies, trade literature, and schools.[6] In this way they made valiant efforts to portray themselves as men of high social standing whose work warranted the rigorous preparation required of well-established professions.

As the few histories of early photographic education have shown, the models of organization and learning developed by American painters and sculptors became instrumental to those efforts as early as the 1840s, and remained so through the early decades of the twentieth century.[7] Within the Philadelphia photographic community, however, comparisons to the institutional practices of the fine arts existed alongside frequent references to the professional activities of medical doctors. Contributing to medicine's appeal for commercial photographers were the general resemblances between the professional histories of medicine and photography. Modern medical historians have consistently portrayed the period between 1830 and 1880 as one of crisis, as American medicine had degenerated into little more than a trade owing to a proliferation of rival sects and inadequate legal regulation of who was authorized to prescribe and heal. The poor state of medical education up to that time made practitioners of regular or "orthodox" medicine even more vulnerable to criticism of their abilities to cure disease and to attacks on their credibility as authorities on the human body. Through a series of educational reforms, doctors met these challenges by pushing for higher admissions standards to medical schools, an increase in the length and number of courses required to earn a medical degree, and the institution of a standardized examination system. Leading these efforts was the American Medical Association (AMA), a national organization established in Philadelphia in 1847, as well as the city's oldest medical institutions, notably the University of Pennsylvania School of Medicine and Jefferson Medical College.[8]

The leaders of the Philadelphia photographic community were certainly aware of the troubled state of the American medical profession, which was often the subject of popular satire and other forms of public criticism that cut across social classes. In its own struggles to reform the training and social status of the men in its ranks, in fact, this group pointed to similar battles fought by doctors. In many cases, this involved idealizing medicine as a highly successful profession structured by powerful institutions and populated by rigorously educated gentlemen. What is more, if photographers imagined that the fight to professionalize medicine had been waged valiantly, they often assumed that the victory, which ideally garnered considerable socioeconomic rewards for the medical community, was well deserved. By portraying medicine and its practitioners as professional models worthy of emulation, in other words, photographers expressed a desire for the cultural authority that urban middle-class Americans believed doctors held symbolically in the nineteenth century, despite their routine failures to heal in practice.

At the same time that they were shaping the professional aims and practices of the photographic community, medical models of education were also at the center of debates about the cultural identity and social value of the photographic medium. While photographers generally agreed between the 1860s and the 1880s that the contributions photography could make to national progress should exceed that of other technologies of representation, their ideas about photography's relationship to medicine in the context of its professionalization and institutionalization reveal internal conflicts about the kind of knowledge it ought to be. Was the work of a national photographic union, based in many respects on that of the AMA, to serve what was essentially the "art" of photography, or would it more beneficially define the medium as a "science"? If portrait photographers could use medical models of teaching and learning to help construct their authority in the field of the body, what would be the epistemological basis of that authority? And how, ultimately, should the fully educated and professionalized photographer expect to relate to the medical men he had envisioned as gatekeepers of that field and guardians of public health: as models or competitors?

LEARNING TO BE PROFESSIONAL

In April 1868, a delegation of photographic studio owners, publishers, and suppliers from cities across the country met at the Cooper Institute in New York City to participate in the first National Photographic Convention. The meeting had initially been called by Abraham Bogardus, Henry T. Anthony, Edward L. Wilson, and other leaders of the commercial photographic community to fight the federal government's renewal of the bromide patent and its taxation of photographs, both of which significantly increased photographers' business expenses. Once they had assembled on an unprecedented mass scale, however, these men saw that mass organization could do much more than solve their financial problems; it would allow working photographers "to resist imposition from all sources, to promote good feeling, to add dignity to our profession," and "to be looked upon as artists, as leaders of public taste, as those who do good and promote the refinement of human nature."[9] Echoing the patriotic rhetoric of the recent war, participants in the convention thus resolved that their "strength" depended on the establishment of America's first permanent and nationwide photographic "union." The wide-reaching benefits of such an institution would continue to be the subject of much discussion within local photographic societies and trade journals until December of that year, when another collection of delegates met in Philadelphia to inaugurate the National Photographic Association of the United States (NPA).

Throughout the eight years of its existence, the NPA modeled its aims and practices on the organizational activities of established professions, hoping that photographers would learn from their successes. The annual exhibitions hosted by the NPA, for instance, which allowed photographers and an interested public to "study the best work that photography can do," were based on precedents in the fine arts and on industrial fairs.[10] The association's regular meetings, by contrast, which brought members into conversation with one another and taught them how to be professional in their operations and discourse, were more closely modeled on the work of the American Medical Association, the first national professional organization for physicians and surgeons. At their initial meeting in Philadelphia in 1847, the leaders of the AMA had acknowledged that "frequent social meetings and regularly organized Societies" were among the "chief means" by which to "sustain the dignity and extend the usefulness of their profession." A union would greatly increase the "influence" of the professional body "for the purpose of common benefit and general good," they argued, using some of the same rhetoric that photographers would invoke decades later; a union would also enable its members to enjoy "a more pleasant and harmonious intercourse, one with another, and an avoidance of many heartburnings and jealousies which originate in misconception . . . of each other's disposition, motives, and conduct."[11] In sum, the founders of the AMA claimed that forming a strong national organization promised the social and moral rehabilitation of its members and would have important implications for the cultural authority of medicine.

The early promoters of the NPA were fond of comparing these anticipated benefits of medical association to those of their own union. As the past editor of *Humphrey's Journal of Photography* and a dean at Geneva Medical College in New York State, Dr. John Towler was especially well positioned to do so.[12] In a lengthy address delivered at the NPA's 1869 convention, he explained that the "value of societies and conventions is well understood by the members of the medical profession, perhaps better than by any other class of men. . . . The benefit to each member, who regularly attends the meetings, is marked on his countenance; he walks, too, with a nobler gait; he speaks a better language, [and] has a more extensive practice than his neighbor." Participation in a professional organization, in other words, inscribed itself on the body and produced what Towler called an "ennobling of the self."[13] Other prominent members of the NPA, like James Ryder of Cleveland, suggested that the union could most effectively promote such an "ennobling" by establishing a *"code of ethics* for the regulation of our conduct with each other and our patrons." Much as the AMA had outlined the proper way for medical men to interact with their peers and patients, Ryder explained to his fellow commercial photographers that "we must improve our manners. We must speak well of our neighbors; we must remember our patrons are entitled to much consideration, and *always* to respectful civility." Only then would it be "possible to improve and dignify our profession *as a profession.*"[14]

In the group portrait of the NPA's founding members, taken by Philadelphia photographer Frederick DeBourg Richards in 1868, we see another means of representing the social effects of a national photographic union in relation to medical models (fig. 7). An inscription on the verso of the albumen print now in the collection of the George Eastman House identifies two of the figures as Abraham Bogardus (standing, center), the highly respected New York studio owner who served as the group's president until 1874, and Edward Wilson (seated, center), its permanent secretary.[15] Although the curtain and side table in the picture could be read as the sitters' occupational tools, on the whole this is not a typical portrait of men who practiced a trade in late nineteenth-century Philadelphia; in the case of studio photographers, such occupational portraits depicted individuals or small groups of men alongside their cameras, posing props, and chemical apparatus. In picturing the NPA, Richards adopted a different pictorial convention, one associated with academic and professional group portraiture of the period, which included institutional images of Philadelphia's medical community.

The formal similarities suggested by Frederick Gutekunst's studio portrait of resident physicians at the Pennsylvania General Hospital (PGH), taken just one year before Richards's photograph, are indeed striking (fig. 8). In each image, the subtly varying poses, gazes, and attire of the nine white men suggest the presence of different personalities that have been brought together by their close physical contact and similar gentlemanly appearance; hands and elbows rest on shoulders, while suits and leather boots proper to professional men in training are sported by all. The central axis is reserved for each fraternity's apparent leader, whose beard and folded arms suggest self-containment and wisdom. The NPA photograph nevertheless subtly challenges the generic conventions of the PGH group portrait, specifically its fondness for stiffly posed bodies, through the figure of the enterprising Wilson, captured in profile, leaning forward with cigarette in hand, top hat on knee, and arm casually draped over his colleague's leg. Taken together, the figures of Bogardus and Wilson in this photograph represent two ways in which the NPA could "ennoble" its members—that is, by producing upright men who gain the respect of the professional community and middle-class public alike, and dynamic leaders who stimulate an exchange of ideas. Invoking medical metaphor, Wilson himself often described these models of professional experience and character as America's first "doctors of photography." He thus implicitly acknowledged that the social advancement of the commercial photographic community depended not only on the inclusion in the NPA of well-respected medical men like Towler; it would also require the cultivation of authorities among those whose livelihood was based on the performance of studio operations.

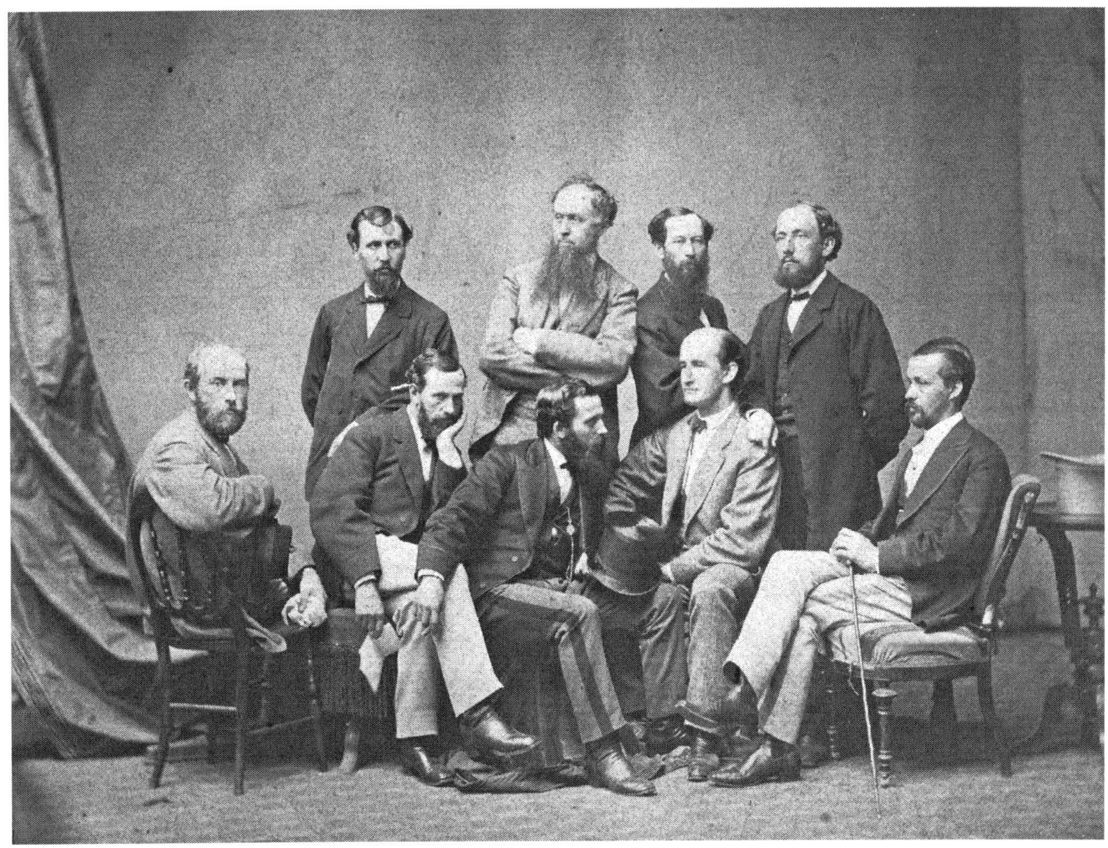

Members of the national medical and photographic associations had remarkably similar ideas about what and who would most hinder such advancement. One of the most troubling internal threats these groups perceived was the proliferation of "immoral" men within their respected practices, men motivated by crude desires for profit rather than a duty to improve themselves and serve their communities; these were the patent owners and sellers of secret formulas who sought to control the distribution of technical knowledge and instrumentation, valuable or otherwise. The AMA and NPA also assumed a defensive posture against apparently external forces, like the public body they served. In vocalizing their support for a national union, photographers routinely complained that studio patrons resisted the acceptance of photography as a profession, refusing to acknowledge its high social value or respect its practitioners. Like doctors and lawyers, who "adhere together with the vital spirit of [a] living organism," they hoped to "sustain each other professionally" in the face of what they took to be a "public invasion or disregard of their rights."[16]

The NPA aimed to combat the external devaluation of photography in part by incorporating guidelines for the proper conduct of sitters in its code of ethics, which were designed to encourage greater deference and respect for studio photographers. Shortly

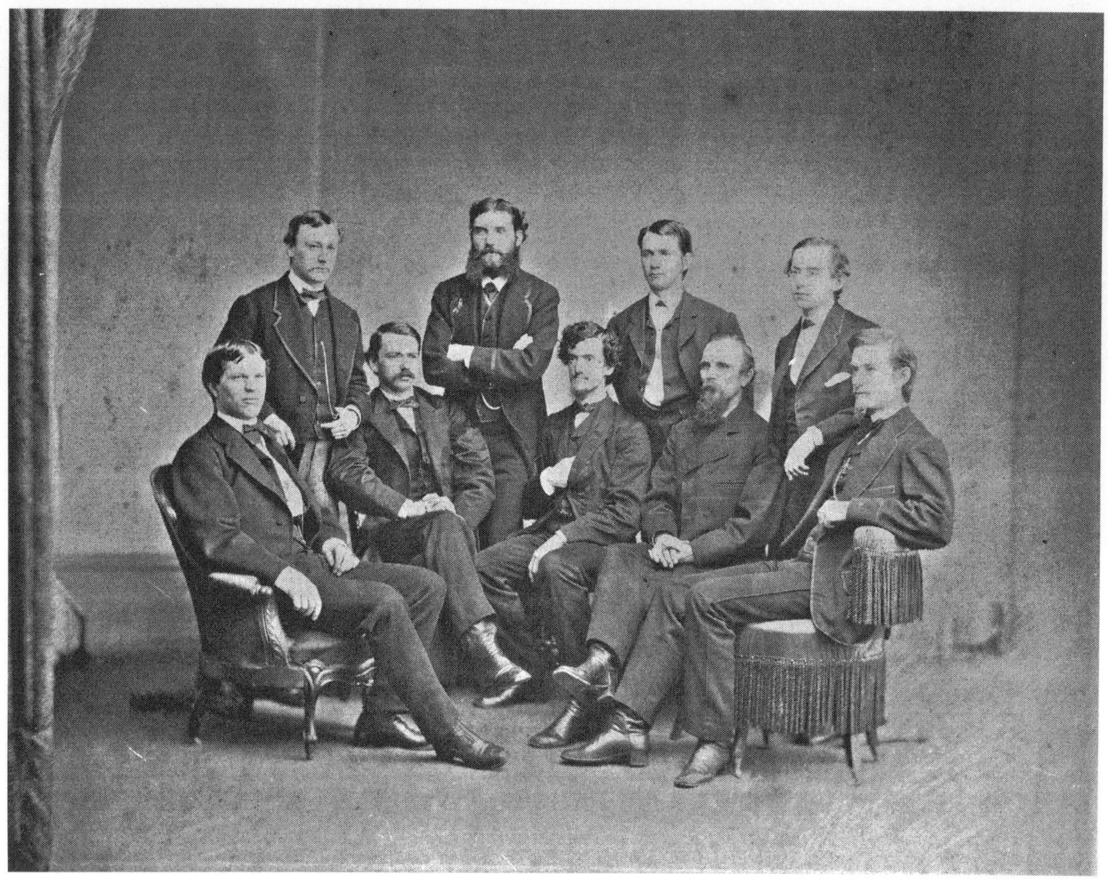

FIGURE 8 Frederick Gutekunst, *Group Portrait of Pennsylvania General Hospital Resident Physicians*, 1867. Albumen print. Courtesy of the Library of the College of Physicians of Philadelphia.

after the union was formed, Edward Wilson defined these rules in a wildly popular pamphlet titled *The Photographer to His Patrons,* which covered a range of topics, from "how to dress" for one's portrait to "how to behave" in the studio. As if anticipating an attack, it opens by asserting that photography "is *not* a branch of mechanics, whereby a quantity of material is thrown into a hopper, and with the grinding of grim, greasy machinery, beautiful portraits may be turned out," but instead "requires skill, good taste, culture, much study and practice," as well as "an expensive outfit and a properly arranged studio," which attest to the medium's relatively high value in the cultural sphere. It is on this basis, Wilson argued, that sitters must acknowledge the authority of the photographer, embodied by the "rules" he established for bodies under the skylight. Turning to a medical model, he instructed the studio patron to be "quite as unwilling to trespass upon such reasonable regulations . . . as you would to apply a fly-blister when your physician orders you to *take* a soothing syrup."[17]

A similar desire to combat the devaluation of photography led Wilson to oversee the establishment of a standard list of prices for photographic work, one that would ensure that they remained sufficiently high that "men of genius, taste, and ambition" would not be undercut by cheap "picture factories."[18] Photographers who placed themselves in the former class admitted that they had much to learn in this matter from members of the medical profession. "What physician ever took a dollar out of Dr. Valentine Mott's, or Dr. Rush's pockets," Henry Snelling once quipped, citing two of the most distinguished medical men in the nation's history, "by underbidding them in a case of surgery, where skill and talent were required for its proper treatment?"[19] The respect that Snelling and many of his colleagues accorded medical models, however, was often accompanied by a growing sense of dissatisfaction with, at times even resentment toward, the idea that regular medicine carried a significantly higher value than photography in the absence of a strong photographic union. In a letter to the *Philadelphia Photographer* on the eve of the NPA's formation, for instance, an aggrieved studio photographer shared his experience of taking a portrait of a physician who, upon hearing that "the price of card-pictures was six dollars per dozen," responded "that that was too much." The author complained that "this veritable physician was charging us HIS fee, five dollars per visit, a price generally adopted by his profession. It takes, I am confident, as much time, patience, expense, and *brains* to make a photographer as it does a physician, and why should not the one be as well paid for services as the other."[20] Appealing to the middle-class American value of common sense, the author urged members of the commercial photographic community to equate the physical, moral, and intellectual investment in their operations with monetary worth, while encouraging the learned, respected men outside their ranks to view portrait photography's socioeconomic value as at least equivalent to that of medicine.

The leaders of the NPA and its successor, the Photographic Association of America (PAA), made repeated comparisons to the medical community in an effort to fetch higher prices for photographs in the 1870s and '80s, acknowledging that success on this front would have social benefits for their members. They nevertheless understood that there were risks in portraying photographers as motivated chiefly by economic interest and a desire for public recognition; such men, after all, were likely to be labeled money-grubbing quacks. Much as nineteenth-century physicians had done in their campaign to rehabilitate their cultural authority, commercial photographers relied on their national union and trade literature to tie their professional aims to a rigorous, and ideally disinterested, search for knowledge.[21] How and what they ought to know was the subject of much debate both at conventions and in the pages of Wilson's journals, but seemingly everyone working in the field of photography could agree that learning to be professional required defining and institutionalizing photographic knowledge with reference to well-established models.

ENVISIONING A PHOTOGRAPHIC SCHOOL

In the 1840s and '50s, young men who were interested in learning how to practice photography in Philadelphia could attend public demonstrations and lectures at venues like the Franklin Institute. There, men of science and inventors, including some of the first American photographers, shared practical knowledge with a reasonably educated public in the hope of promoting the technological development and social advancement of the mechanical arts in the United States.[22] Itinerant photographers, as well as some of the city's studio owners, also accepted students of photography in this period, charging them a fee in return for hands-on training, although the reputation of these instructors and the amount of time they devoted to each pupil varied greatly. For decades afterward, Edward Wilson would announce lectures at the Franklin Institute and other fleeting opportunities to study photography in his trade journals at the same time that he declared his journals "the best and only real practical method of educating photographers."[23] This body of literature was the "great panacea for all photographic difficulties and trials," he reminded his readers in 1879, insofar as it operated as a virtual school for the aspiring professional.[24] In each issue of the *Philadelphia Photographer,* students new and old could learn how to set up the reception and operation room in their portrait studios, pose and light sitters under their skylights, mix their darkroom chemicals, maintain a respectable appearance, and treat customers with respect. Regular instructors in the journal included both nationally and internationally recognized leaders in the field of photography, such as Philadelphia's John L. Gihon, G. Wharton Simpson, and John Towler.[25]

As the photographic portrait industry was experiencing a massive boom in American cities around the time of the Civil War, Wilson and his band of "doctors" began to radically rethink their means of educating commercial photographers. At the center of their efforts were proposals for an institution where both apprenticed photographers and their teachers could receive a formal education in studio practices; this, they argued, was essential to photography's professionalization. One of the earliest proposals to spark lively debate circulated in 1860, when Marcus Aurelius Root announced his desire to establish a "heliographic school" in New York City with the support of the city's photographic society. Root's vision unfolded in a series of letters that he wrote from Philadelphia to the editors of the major New York trade journals: Samuel D. Humphrey (*Humphrey's Journal of Photography*), Charles Seeley (*American Journal of Photography*), and Henry Snelling (*Photographic and Fine Art Journal*).[26] He began by noting that "intelligent, thorough instruction" was required in the "useful arts" practiced by mechanics, who serve as apprentices in order to acquire "mechanical aptitude and skill"; this was also essential to the "Fine Arts" of painting, sculpture, and architecture, in which students are "long and laboriously" schooled so as to cultivate their artistic "genius."[27] Root's primary motive for advocating a school devoted to photography was to better situate the medium in relation to these two varieties of "art" and thus define its relative importance in American culture. With such an institution in place, he predicted, photography would no longer be seen as "a mere *mechanical* process, requiring neither genius nor accomplishment . . . nor [as] one of the fine arts *merely;* but one which, from its peculiarities and the universality of its possible application is likely to render more valuable and desirable services to mankind, than either of the others."[28]

When Root's proposal had still not produced material results a decade later, discussions of photographic education began to focus on the NPA as both a "great educating power" and a powerful body that could oversee its institutionalization.[29] In 1871 the association appointed A. K. P. Trask—the owner of a studio on Chestnut Street, author of a trade manual on ferrotyping, and a frequent contributor to Wilson's journals—to chair a "Committee on Apprenticeship," which recommended that the NPA take over the work of establishing a school for young men seeking to practice photography for a living.[30] Trask's recommendation ultimately led members of the organization to submit a petition to the U.S. Congress in 1873 for the establishment of a national photographic institute in Philadelphia. The "appropriation of $30,000" requested by the NPA—an impressive sum in 1873—attests to the seriousness of its desire to educate commercial photographers and the high value to the nation it attached to the practice of photography. If the bill were to pass, Wilson explained to his readers, it would show those who leveled harsh criticism against photography "what good we can do" and would demonstrate that the medium and its practitioners "will no longer endure it meekly."[31]

It was in designing the curriculum and methodology of these proposed photographic schools that Root, and subsequently the NPA, turned to the most successful models of medical education. Among the many elements of these models that they intended to adopt were mandatory attendance and a required length of study, both of which the AMA continued to work to achieve in medical circles. In a series of articles for the *Philadelphia Photographer* on the subject of "photographic rights," E. K. Hough made what became a common connection between the establishment of compulsory schools and the social elevation of the photographer and his work, announcing in 1875:

> The time is coming when photography will be recognized as a profession . . . , for even now the majority of its practitioners are *compelled* to know nearly as much of general science and its modern developments as half the young lawyers and doctors turned out yearly. Yet we all know that to speak of a young lawyer or doctor would convey a very different idea to a stranger than reference to a young photographer. Primarily, because they are *compelled* [emphasis added] to education at special schools, under legal restrictions, receiving diplomas that give them assured legal and social standing, with well-recognized rights guaranteed to them, both by law and established custom.[32]

Requiring that photographers attend school, Hough reasoned, would help persuade the American public—or, more precisely, the middle-class patrons they hoped to attract to their studios—to see photography as the NPA did: as a medium with high social value whose operations required nothing short of a license to practice. In his articles on photographic instruction that appeared in the *Philadelphia Photographer* in the 1870s, Henry Snelling imagined that compulsory education would bring similar benefits to the commercial photographic community, specifically by preventing members of the lower social classes from entering it. When the men who would "disgrace" the profession were faced with prohibitively high tuition fees, or placed among men with great talent and motivation in photographic schools, he predicted, they would quit photography altogether, "just as we see medical students abandon physic for other business."[33]

Root's proposal went into more detail about the form that photographers' education should take. Writing to the *American Journal of Photography*, he envisioned "a school supplied with proper instruments and appliances," set up in "some heliographic establishment, already in full practice, and in fair repute." It would employ multiple "competent" instructors, each specializing in a different "branch" of photography.[34] In addition to attending lectures and conversing with one another, Root's students would receive their primary training from these instructors according to the following plan:

> Whenever the camera is in operation taking pictures for applicants, let the pupils be on the spot, watching every part of the process, while the operant gives them the reasons for every step he takes; why he stations the sitter *thus* in regard to light; why he selects *this* view of the face; why light and shadow are made to fall *thus and so;* what is the proper height of the camera in relation to the face &c., &c. When the picture passes to the chemical room, let the pupils surround the chemist, see *what* he does, and *how* he does it, and listen to the reasons he assigns for his proceedings. Thus the pupil would get theory and practice together, as medical students do by accompanying their professor, while dealing medicines and performing operations in a Hospital.[35]

In addition to drawing upon existing models of apprenticeship and instruction in the mechanical arts, the teaching method described in this passage mimics what would become an important feature of medical education in late nineteenth-century Philadelphia, when the city's prominent physicians and surgeons sought to involve students more actively in their education.[36] In Philadelphia hospitals, a senior clinician would engage a doctor-in-training in dialogue before a live patient in order to teach the younger members of the institution how to recognize symptoms, diagnose disease, and prescribe a cure. Medical school faculty offered a similar form of instruction to their apprentices. As the renowned surgeon Samuel Gross wrote in his autobiography, he examined his apprentices at Jefferson Medical College "not with book in hand . . . but extemporaneously, often explaining matters in the form of familiar lectures, interspersed with apt questions. . . . The teaching was always conducted in the most systematic manner."[37] In proposing a similar paradigm for photographic education, Root envisioned a specific structure for the dissemination and acquisition of photographic knowledge, one that was concerned as much with the practical (the what and how) as the theoretical (the why), at the same time that he saw its gatekeepers as sagacious "professors," gentlemen with considerable symbolic and socioeconomic capital. In this way the staunch advocate of photography as "one among the noblest of Fine Arts," a man who believed that the genius, honor, and patronage of the photographer should resemble those of "the eminent painter or sculptor," tied a scientific model to his aspirations for the medium.[38]

Although this may strike twenty-first-century readers as paradoxical, in the professional and middle-class cultures of the period, a "scientific" body of knowledge was one that emphasized its practical use, was organized according to a system of clearly defined principles, and was almost invariably used to increase the cultural authority of a given practice.[39] In nineteenth-century Philadelphia, this understanding of science was at the center of the Franklin Institute's mission; it later became instrumental to the professional rehabilitation of the medical community, as we see in Samuel Gross's two-volume *System of Surgery,* now recognized as one of the most important medical textbooks of the nineteenth century, which presents surgery as the rigorously ordered practice of highly skilled gentleman-scientists, not as the unthinking manual work of barbers or butchers.[40] For Philadelphia physicians, incorporating the sciences of experimental physiology, bacteriology, and microscopy into their education and clinical practice also meant adopting a set of specialized tools, which had the benefit of distancing their knowledge from that of the lay public in matters of health.[41] In his effort to incorporate "science" into photographic education, Root thus shared with both mechanics and medical doctors a desire to promote the social advancement of his peers. As his major treatise, *The Camera and the Pencil* (1864), went on to argue in detail, he likewise hoped that placing the "art" of photography in close relation to (but never as one among) the sciences would make it one of the most important discoveries of the modern age.

For decades after Root's letters first circulated in photographic journals, Edward Wilson and many other outspoken proponents of education for the photographer retained the daguerreotypist's aim of promoting photography as a fine art, while "putting more science into those who are, or may come, into our profession."[42] Their debates about teaching and learning in this period nevertheless reveal new ideas about what this might mean, from specifying the content of the ideal photography course of study to describing how to see one's object of representation. Both of these things became important to define as the plans for a national photographic institute were taking shape. In 1875, for example, Wilson shared with readers of the *Philadelphia Photographer* the curricular recommendations of Hermann Vogel, then the German correspondent to the journal and a well-respected "doctor of photography" both in the United States and abroad. Trained as a physicist himself, Vogel believed that students of photography should study chemistry, optics, drawing, art history, and the techniques of negative retouching; a "short course of physiology and anatomy must be added to this," he explained, "to enable the scholar to study the form of the human body."[43] Wilson reported two years later that the "probable" photographic school in Philadelphia would largely adopt Vogel's recommendations, offering lecture courses on "chemistry, physics, artistic anatomy, composition, the education of the eye, and photographic practice in the various branches." It would also provide students with opportunities to work under a large skylight, where they could enhance their technical knowledge, and to study the best "art collections" in America, including the works assembled for the new museum established at the Centennial Exhibition.[44]

The proposed photographic school in Philadelphia had much in common with this new museum, then known as the Pennsylvania Museum and School of Industrial Art, which offered practical training to men seeking to enter the art and textile industries. As Wilson conceived of it in the 1870s, however, the ideal course of study for the young photographer was not equivalent to that of the artisan, who was likely to have studied chemistry or physics along with drawing, modeling, pottery, and metalwork, nor did it closely resemble medical training, where professors lectured on applied sciences in addition to surgery, *materia medica,* and therapeutics. Instead, photographic instruction combined elements of both fine-artistic and medical models of education. The following section suggests one way to explore the benefits and drawbacks of such an epistemological conflation by focusing on the role that anatomical study came to play in teaching commercial photographers how to see the body. Among the many subjects that this group embraced in its pedagogical discourses, anatomy proved to be one of the most crucial in defining portrait photography's relationship to art and science.

ANATOMICAL KNOWLEDGE: BETWEEN ART AND SCIENCE

At the same time that Philadelphia photographers were turning to medicine as a model for a photographic school, the city's most famous artist of the era produced two "surgical" paintings that comment on the practices and education of the realist painter. Like Root's pedagogical proposal, quoted above, Thomas Eakins's *Gross Clinic* (fig. 9) and his later *Agnew Clinic* (1889) depict a form of instruction that an "operator" provides his students as he performs procedures on live bodies.[45] Like the "doctors of photography" that Wilson championed in his journals, moreover, Samuel Gross and David Hayes Agnew are represented in the paintings as gentlemanly authorities on the body. Standing fully erect and bathed in white light from the skylight above—which, perhaps not insignificantly, calls to mind the lighting scheme of the photographic portrait studio—each of these aged professors calmly controls the operation under way as he instructs his assistants and the students in the operating theater. Seated to the right of the tunnel, where he records the scene before him, Eakins included himself among the students in *The Gross Clinic,* as if he were one of the illustrious surgeon's many eager pupils, who lean, crouch, or crane to see, as Root put it, "what he does and how he does it."

Reading the painting's visual signs in relation to Eakins's biography, the art historian Michael Fried has proposed that *The Gross Clinic* is largely metaphorical. As Fried observes, Eakins's action in the scene—"wielding a pencil-like instrument"—is repeated by other figures in the picture: the "recording physician who transcribes the proceedings," "Gross' principal assistant probing the open wound," and Gross himself, whose "right hand hold[s] the scalpel much as one might hold a pencil or pen (or for that matter a paintbrush)." Fried concludes that the close links between the figure of Eakins and the medical personnel in the picture suggest analogies between the operating surgeon and the realist painter, the bloody scalpel and the crimson-coated paintbrush, as well as the patient's body and the painter's canvas, which allow us to read *The Gross Clinic* not only as a "uniquely impressive memorial portrait . . . but also as an indirect or metaphorical representation of the enterprise of painting."[46] While Fried is ultimately concerned with the connections between painting and writing that he believes the image expresses, I am most interested in other connections that stem from Fried's initial comparison of surgery to painting. My aim is not to overburden an image that art historians have already loaded with meanings but to underscore an analogy that shaped the creation of *The Gross Clinic* and the development of photographic education in Philadelphia, one that relates fine-artistic education to medical education and realist representation to a scientific way of seeing the body.

It was impossible for Eakins to have represented an illustrious Philadelphia operator directing a surgical dissection before an audience of medical students without reference to his own pedagogical practices at the time, for it was at the precise moment that

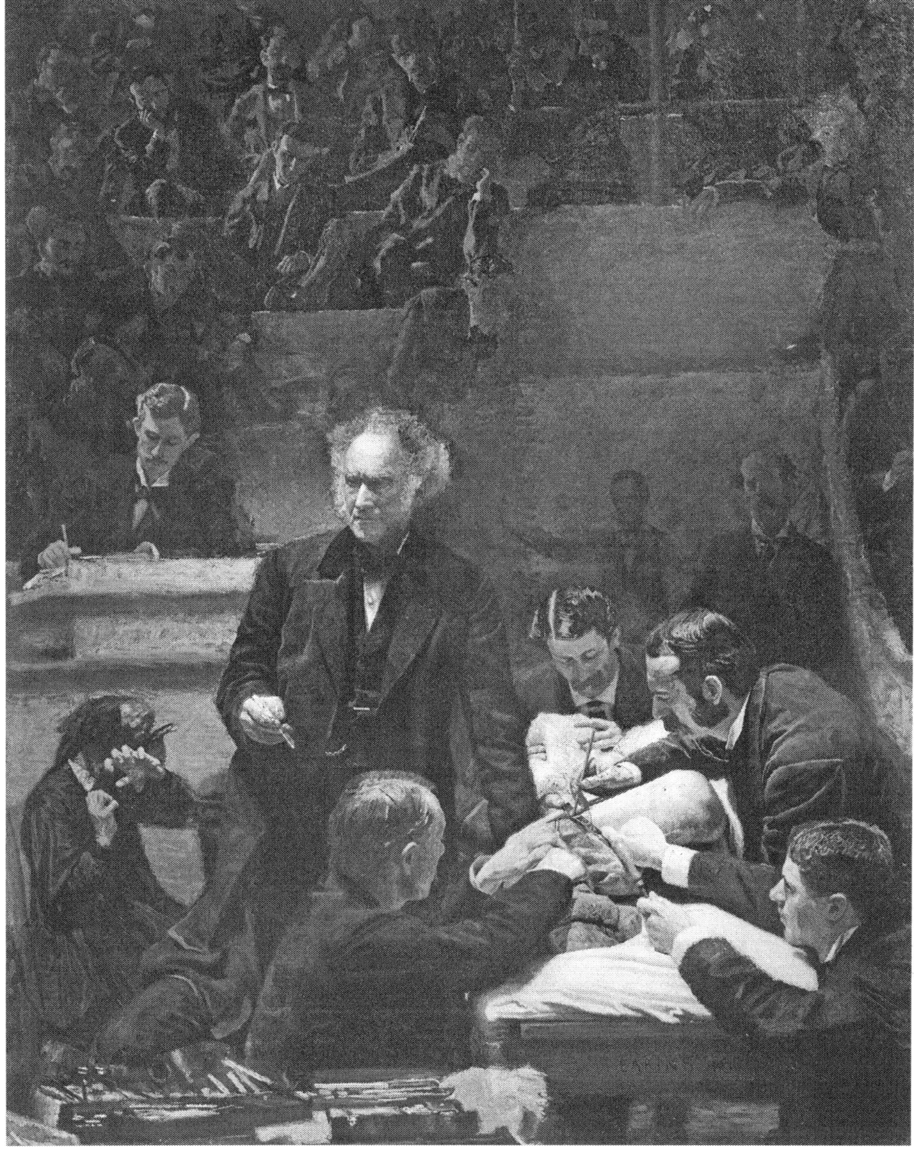

FIGURE 9 Thomas Eakins, *The Gross Clinic*, 1875. Oil on canvas. Courtesy of the Pennsylvania Academy of the Fine Arts, Philadelphia, and the Philadelphia Museum of Art.

Eakins created *The Gross Clinic* that he imagined anatomical knowledge as essential to the practice of painting, developed a curriculum based on that belief that showcased the practice of dissection, and counted the city's most esteemed surgeons and anatomists among his closest colleagues. It is well known that for Eakins and his circle the study of art was tied closely to the study of medicine, particularly anatomy, which then as now has important clinical applications to surgery. Art historians have repeatedly noted that Eakins took courses in human anatomy at Jefferson Medical College between 1861 and 1864 and again in 1874, when he attended surgical lectures and clinics presided over by Professor Gross. Eakins went on to teach anatomy and direct dissections at seven art institutions in Philadelphia and New York, although he is best known for his involvement in the "artistic anatomy" courses offered by Dr. William Williams Keen at the Pennsylvania Academy of the Fine Arts (PAFA). Keen, a prominent Philadelphia doctor who founded the Philadelphia School of Anatomy in 1875 before holding the title of professor of surgery at both Jefferson and the Women's Medical College of Pennsylvania, appointed Eakins prosector to his courses before naming him chief demonstrator of anatomy in PAFA's life classes.[47]

Although anatomy had been studied in American art academies since the early nineteenth century, between 1876 and 1886 Eakins and Keen placed an unprecedented emphasis on it at PAFA, to the extent that it defined the institution's curriculum in that period and indeed the character of artistic instruction in Philadelphia.[48] "What chiefly distinguishes the Philadelphia school" from its New York counterparts, William Brownell explained to the readers of *Scribner's Monthly* in 1879, "is its dissections for advanced pupils" directed by both the "professor of painting" (Eakins) and the "professor of artistic anatomy" (Keen). With more than a hint of cynicism, Brownell described Keen's anatomical course of thirty lectures as "tolerably thorough" and "exhaustive." Required of all of PAFA's advanced students, it consisted of an "introductory lecture upon the relations of anatomy to art, and methods of studying artistic anatomy," followed by eight lectures on the skeleton, twelve on the muscles, discussions and dissections of human and animal heads, four lectures on the "individual features of the face," two lectures on "the skin and its appendages," and four lectures "devoted to the subjects of 'postural expression,' the proportions of the body, and the influence of sex upon physical development."[49]

What Eakins and Keen aimed to cultivate in their art students through these lectures and demonstrations was a "scientific" way of seeing motivated by a desire to penetrate the surface of the body with both the scalpel and the mind's eye so as to observe its structure and mechanism closely. They assumed that in order to produce a realist representation, an artist must perform a physical and mental dissection of his subject through which he brutally divides the body into parts, masters their depths, and creates analogies between their internal functions and external appearances. As Charles H. Stephens expressed in his depiction of an anatomical lecture Keen delivered at PAFA while Stephens was studying there, students were also taught to imagine a direct correspondence between the bodies of their subjects and their visual representations thereof, one that served as an additional prerequisite for artistic realism (fig. 10). In Stephens's grisaille oil sketch, first published in Brownell's article, that correspondence is signaled visually by the artist's modulation of black and white and his spatial arrangement of bodies in the scene. The relative whiteness of the sculpted torso on the left is echoed by that of the cadaver and the bared chest of the male model, uniting these three figures, while pairings within that triad are suggested by the drapery around the torso and cadaver, on the one hand, and the bent left arms of the cadaver and model, on the other. Stephens further positions the cadaver in Keen's lectures as a mediator between the torso and the model on either side of it, suggesting that one can translate the "real" into the "represented" only by way of the dissected body, with the figure of Keen acting as a crucial mediator between the "dissected" and the "live." The viewer's gaze is encouraged to move almost automatically from the shrouded cadaver to Keen's gleaming forehead and then, at the direction of the doctor's pencil-like instrument, to the "subject." In Stephens's visual account of the lecture, Keen's instrument, much like Gross's scalpel, trains artists to see the living model as if they were exploring the depths of the medical body.

With the training of Philadelphia artists in mind, we can now return to the education of portrait photographers in the 1870s and '80s and consider how this group of image makers negotiated its own relationship to anatomical knowledge. In some respects, the Philadelphia photographic community actively forged a direct connection to Eakins and his circle around this subject. While the city's photographic school was still in its planning phase, for example, Wilson made his readers aware of the local institutions where artists in Eakins's circle received instruction from and among medical experts. In the same issue of the *Philadelphia Photographer* in which he published Vogel's recommendations, Wilson encouraged photographers to participate in a course of lectures on artistic anatomy delivered by "one of the most distinguished surgeons of this city"—none other than William Keen. He also urged them to submit examples of their work to the journal

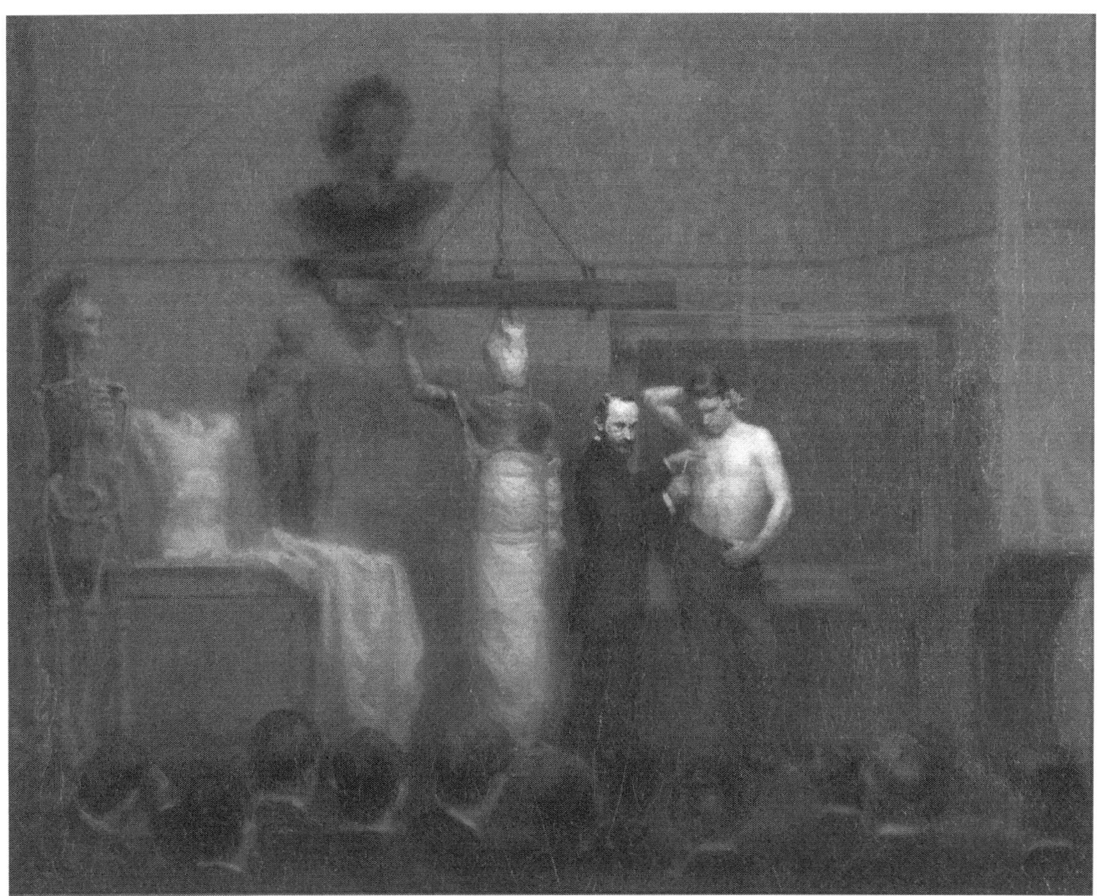

FIGURE 10 Charles H. Stephens, *Anatomical Lecture by Dr. William Williams Keen,* 1879. Oil on cardboard. Courtesy of the Pennsylvania Academy of the Fine Arts, Philadelphia.

for the purpose of illustrating Keen's lectures, particularly photographs of "wrinkled and *contorted,* and *twisted,* and ugly faces" or "anything that will show peculiar expressions, features, noses, eyes, foreheads, and deformities."[50] One month later, in March 1875, Wilson expressed his desire that "*all* photographers have the privilege of attending" Keen's lectures and of learning from his presentation of "charts, photographs, skeletons, and the living and dead body (dissection)."[51] Wilson's promotion of these lectures suggests not only that photography could significantly aid fine artists' understanding of anatomical principles, but that photographers, like young painters, had much to learn from the practice of human dissection.

We know from a rare stereoview of Keen's lecture hall at the Philadelphia School of Anatomy, which Frederick Gutekunst photographed from the perspective of a student in the operating theater in the 1870s, that at least one commercial photographer in Philadelphia accepted (or anticipated) Wilson's invitation (fig. 11). What this view of the uninhabited hall cannot tell us, however, is how many photographers joined Gutekunst in that space and what insights they gained about the photographic body from their encounters with Keen's "artistic anatomy." If his lectures conformed to the epistemology that Stephens's sketch attributed to them, then they would have learned that to know the body was to penetrate it with an anatomical or surgical gaze; photographers would have been trained, in other words, to assume a direct connection between the sitter's body in the studio and his portrait, one maintained by their ability to translate the body's depths into a photographic surface. We will see in the following chapter that, whether or not it could be attributed to Keen, this lesson was well learned by the Philadelphia photographic community, who likened their way of seeing and knowing bodies to that of surgeons.

It is important to compare what the leaders of Philadelphia's art academies, who trained America's finest painters, and the proponents of the nation's first professional photographic schools could have gained from incorporating anatomy into their preliminary education. According to spokesmen for both communities, the benefits to their students were chiefly practical. As Thomas Eakins had explained to William Brownell in 1879, "For anatomy as such, we [at PAFA] care nothing whatever. To draw the human figure it is necessary to know as much as possible about it, about its structure and its movements, its bones and muscles, how they are made, and how they act."[52] Writing for the *Philadelphia Photographer* in 1877, W. H. Tipton, best known for his views of the battlefield at Gettysburg, summarized what portrait photographers could gain from a course in anatomy, similarly representing it as a scientific means to an aesthetic ends:

> Anatomy should be studied by the poser, that he may, by proper lighting and posing, give value to the parts which might seem unimportant, as the bones of the forehead, which form the planes of light and shade; the cheek-bones, which contribute so materially to resemblance, and give character to the face; the jaw, the angles of which can be easily destroyed by inattention; and the bone of the nose, which should be always neatly rendered. An extraordinary development in any part of the anatomy may be subdued by position, as the muscles of the neck, which are sometimes so prominent, if not properly handled. It also teaches us

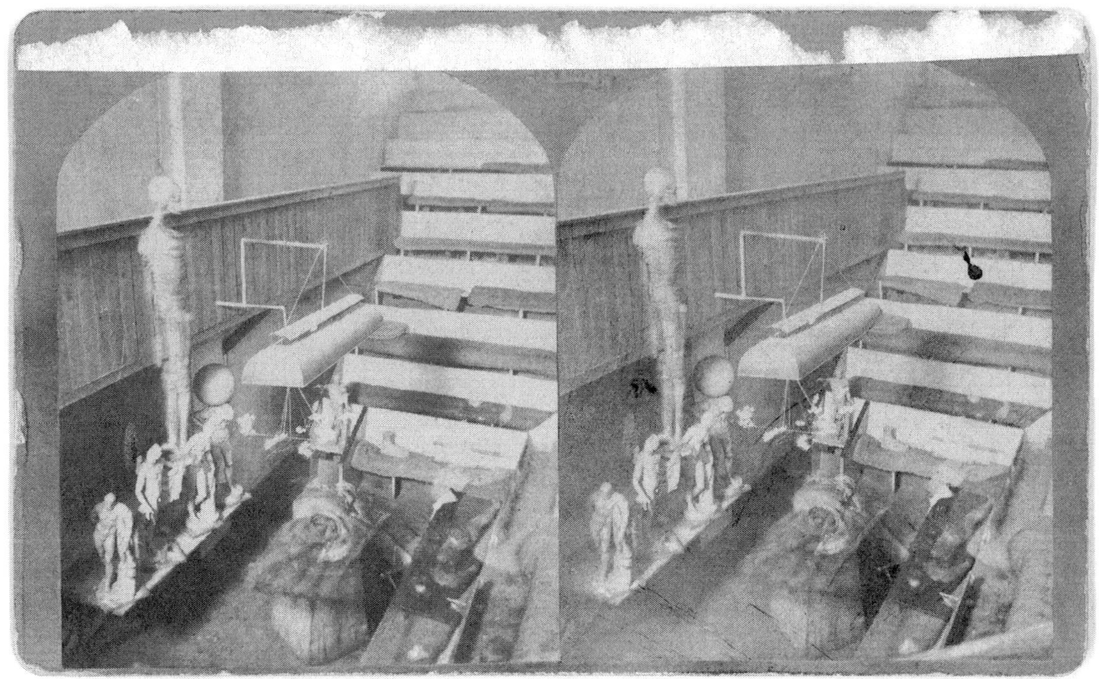

FIGURE 11 Frederick Gutekunst, *Interior of the Philadelphia School of Anatomy*, ca. 1870s. Albumen print on stereograph mount. Courtesy of the Library of the College of Physicians of Philadelphia.

> the natural position of the figure, so that nothing is on a strain, when repose is desired, and the correct form when in action, as we can place a limb in position without the muscles being in action in some cases.[53]

For Tipton, it is through the study of anatomy that the photographer, in posing his sitter, comes to understand the structure of the forehead, cheeks, jaw, and nose, the action of the neck muscles, and the movements of the body's limbs. Such knowledge serves his aim of portraying the "natural position" and "correct form" of the body, which expresses a commitment to pictorial realism that he shared with Eakins.

There were, of course, different implications for Philadelphia's portrait painters and studio photographers who embraced anatomy in the 1870s, given the differences in their professional status and visual practices. Unlike painting, portrait photography had yet to be established as a legitimate profession supported by established institutional structures. Photographers faced heavy criticism as a result, both of themselves and of their practices, against which the association of anatomical with photographic knowledge became an effective defense. As Michael Sappol has argued in his cultural history of anatomy in nineteenth-century America, those who embraced anatomical knowledge could gain a wide range of "social, professional, epistemological, [and] political" benefits. Such had been the case for the practitioners of regular medicine, who promoted the study of anatomy not only as preparation for surgical practice but also as the "essential core of the medical curriculum" in the antebellum period; as such, it played an important role in the formation of medicine's cultural authority.[54] Although the practice of anatomical dissection was fraught with scandal at a time when grave robbing was a common means of acquiring bodies, Sappol argues that the direct knowledge and power that physicians gained from cutting into and exploring the interior of the body "elevate[d] the physician above other healers—and the medical profession above other professions."[55] Requiring anatomical study in professional photographic schools would therefore have tied photography to a "culturally prestigious" branch of science associated with rigorous and in-depth knowledge of bodies, which had the potential to improve photographers' social status in the eyes of the public; it would also have differentiated commercial photographers from the countless amateurs who picked up cameras in the later nineteenth century, thereby mitigating what they actively perceived as amateurs' threat to their serious practice. The instruction one would have received at the Summer School at Mountain Lake Park or the School of Photography at Chautauqua, two popular destinations for amateur photographers in the 1880s, consisted almost exclusively of the "art" of landscape photography, which meant that, for perhaps the first time in the history of American photography, scientific training in the field of portraiture belonged exclusively to professionals.[56] The figure of the "doctor of photography" that commercial photographers hoped to promote through education would likewise be off limits to most amateurs because of their strictly "artistic" knowledge base. Although amateurs were generally middle- and upper-class whites, moreover, this category of photographer included women, who could never conform to the masculine ideal the figure of the "doctor" embodied. The focus on anatomical study in Philadelphia's fine arts academies similarly necessitated the exclusion of women from important elements of their curricula. As Stephens's depiction of the all-male audience at Keen's lectures reminds the viewer, dissection of the body and exploration of its interior were generally considered inappropriate practices for the so-called lesser sex.

Teaching anatomy to commercial photographers would also have specifically combated popular claims that early studio portraiture was mechanical, unflattering, and untruthful. As Tipton represented it to the readers of the *Philadelphia Photographer*, and as the following chapter discusses, anatomical knowledge enabled the photographer to manipulate light and shade at will so as to create a portrait that resembled the sitter, expressed his character, and remedied his physical deformities and defects, or what Tipton tactfully referred to as the sitter's "extraordinary development." The idea that it was possible for a photographer to strike a balance between resemblance and idealization, to produce a "correct" body that also appeared "natural" and true, and to create the appearance of action in spite of the sitter's extraordinary immobilization before the camera suggested that portrait photographers exercised skill and judgment that equaled, if not exceeded, that of painters. Ironically, then, photography's associations with the "science" of anatomy could be used in the late nineteenth century to confirm the artistic, in the sense of inventive, character of photographic work.

Such irony again raises questions concerning the place of "art" and "science" in the theories and practices of image making in Philadelphia. While photographers and painters agreed that scientific knowledge should be an important element in their education, in other words, there was considerable disagreement between and within these groups about its particular relationship to their media of representation. William Brownell's article in *Scribner's Monthly* reminds us of the insecurity that Eakins and Keen were made to experience in placing an enormous emphasis on anatomy in the training of fine artists. In response to Brownell's concerns that his interest in anatomy was becoming too "scientific in its nature" and that the objects and spaces of dissection were themselves "utterly—inartistic," Eakins assured him that "we [at PAFA] turn out no physicians and surgeons," while Keen defensively explained that the goal of his lectures was "not to make anatomists but artists."[57] These responses suggest that American art critics and their readers in 1879 had difficulty imagining an intimate relationship between the "art" of painting and the "science" of anatomy in which the brutality and "hideousness" of the latter did not threaten what they believed to be the former's essential preoccupation with the beauty of the human figure. Although Eakins never desired painting to *become* a science, the stakes were high when it came to preserving the aesthetic principles of the art, so high that *The Gross Clinic* was rejected from the fine arts section of the Centennial Exhibition for which it was intended and was ultimately shown in the U.S. Army Post Hospital exhibit, while Eakins himself was fired by PAFA in 1886, in part because the administration objected to his commitment to scientific principles and practices.

Whether portrait photography was to be viewed and taught as an "art" or a "science" was an open question in this period, much more so than painting in Philadelphia ever had been, and members of the city's photographic community fought relentlessly to find a definitive answer. For men like Marcus Aurelius Root, photography could only ever be counted among the fine arts, but it was the medium's capacity to function as an instrument or "handmaid" of science that would lead to some of its greatest achievements. Other ideas about the nature of photography's interactions with the sciences became popular in the second half of the nineteenth century, however, ideas that did not limit the medium's role to that of a handmaid. In his contributions to Philadelphia's photographic literature in the 1870s and '80s, Henry Snelling argued that photography's "rightful place" was not among the fine arts but instead among the sciences, despite its uses in artistic contexts. Denying the "art" of photography constituted a radical change for the former editor of the *Photographic Art Journal* (later renamed the *Photographic and Fine Art Journal*), who came to believe that the education of studio photographers should not end with the incorporation of scientific subjects into an inherently artistic curriculum. Instead, through his later writings, Snelling trained photographers to acknowledge that they not only deserved the high social standing enjoyed by men of science but also belonged to the same epistemic culture.[58] Debates on these issues, which were waged in the pages of Wilson's journals and at the meetings of photographic societies, thus produced competing ideas of what the ideal student of photography ought to know, while simultaneously exploring the character and limits of photography's interactions with science. Whereas the conflict between Eakins and his critics suggests that the identity of painting as "art" was rigorously policed and therefore never fully open to redefinition, what was always at stake in discussions of photographic education was the kind of knowledge that photography ought to be.

Decades after Root proposed his heliographic school and the NPA petitioned Congress for theirs, questions concerning the cultural identity and social value of photography continued to preoccupy the proponents of photographic education in the United States. How could the institutional models of other professions help transform the commercial photographic community "into a valuable factor in society," as one of the founders of the PAA once put it, that "enriches the world by an example that will be studied and followed"?[59] Would what Snelling called the "extent to which the medium can be carried" be the point at which it achieved a cultural authority equal to that of its models, or could photographers hope to achieve something more?

Regarding photography's interactions with the institutions of medicine in the late 1880s, a pair of international reports published in the *Philadelphia Photographer* offered two common, competing responses. In the first, Wilson celebrated the fact that a "well-known London physician has erected in his waiting-room an excellent photographic apparatus." Dry plates "are taken of his visitors during their time of waiting, are developed by an assistant, and ready to be shown at the next visit of the patient." For Wilson, these "photographic services" demonstrated that the medium improved the relationship between medical men and their patrons just as it did for "barbers and hairdressers" who had "adopted the same plan with their customers in America."[60] Much as Root's *The Camera and the Pencil* had done more than two decades earlier, this report assumed that photography acquired social value through its instrumental relationship to other technologies of the body, particularly those that carried considerable value of their own. In the case of "medical and surgical science," Root argued, photographic representations of disease provided an "advantage" and "incalculable service . . . to practicing physicians and medical students" in their generation and dissemination of scientific knowledge.[61] Wilson's advertisements for clinical photographic studies in the 1870s similarly celebrated them as one of photography's great achievements, insofar as the camera served as "a most efficient helper" to medicine that "enables surgeons to understand disease more easily, and thus human suffering is prevented." It was in the photographic medium's ability to visually document, and thereby authorize, medical knowledge, moreover, that he saw the key to its social elevation. "Were it not for *our* useful art," Wilson explained, "none but those present, when the experiments were made, could see the effect of the treatment, but now any one can see and study them. Thus our art creeps up."[62]

Wilson's second report, which summarized what he called a "curious case," expresses a different understanding of photography's ideal relationship to the institutions of medicine. A London photographer, Wilson wrote, had "complained that a neighboring hospital was a nuisance to his business. The court decided against the hospital, but the case was appealed, resulting, however, in the confirmation of the first decision." Remarkably, the report concluded, the "hospital was moved away from the photographer."[63] Authorized by official court proceedings, the portrait studio was allowed to replace the hospital in the commercial and mass-cultural sphere as the space more essential to the daily operations of the urban public, as if they were in direct competition with each other. Commercial photographers, in other words, no longer functioned as the dutiful servants of medical doctors but instead were granted the jurisdiction over public health these men had once held, if only in the pages of the *Philadelphia Photographer*.

For the modern reader, the improbability of such a competition between medicine and portrait photography playing itself out in practice suggests the overdetermination of photographers' reliance on medical models in their institutionalization strategies. Indeed, in an effort to gain public recognition of their authority, photographers often fantasized that the social contributions of their work were limitless; this led them to exaggerate the foundations of their claims to professional legitimacy and cultural authority, which produced contradictions and absurdities that potentially called both into question. It would be a mistake, however, to dismiss Wilson's "curious case" as a misguided expression of optimism or hubris that ultimately undermined the professionalization and institutionalization of commercial portrait photography. To read the report differently, we can return to Bourdieu's reflections on cultural capital with which this chapter began. In an ongoing effort to increase its economic or cultural capital, Bourdieu reasoned, a social group seeking authority will develop its organizational activities by defining its aims and practices in relation to others that more legitimately occupy the cultural sphere. Its members are also most likely to invest in what they think, consciously or unconsciously, is possible, thereby eliminating themselves from specific fields, or metaphorical spaces in which struggles for legitimacy take place, that are clearly dominated by another group. If we adapt that logic to the early photographic context, we might say that photographers found a way to improve their status within the field of the body in urban American culture at a time when that space was only weakly controlled by doctors and when domination within it was perceived as central to viable claims to cultural authority. The troubled state of the American medical profession, in other words, provided an opportunity for professionalizing groups, like the Philadelphia photographic community, to engage in fantasies of competition with it.[64]

Between the 1860s and the 1880s, commercial portrait photographers increasingly imagined that they were competing with medical men for access to bodies, for intimate knowledge of and hence power over them, and for the privileges granted to those who wielded such power. It was this new conception of photography as much more than a "handmaid" of the sciences that motivated Henry Snelling to portray photographic chemicals as therapeutic medications and others to draw parallels between the material practices of photographers and medical men. The following chapters explore these ideas about the *medicine of photography* by turning to the spaces in which commercial photography was practiced, from the operating room to the photographic laboratory. Analyzing the bodies within these environments, both those who operated and those who were operated upon, shows us how this metaphorical concept helped shape the kind of operation portrait photography was to become in the eyes of its practitioners, and the important contributions they could make to an ailing public in Civil War and postbellum America.

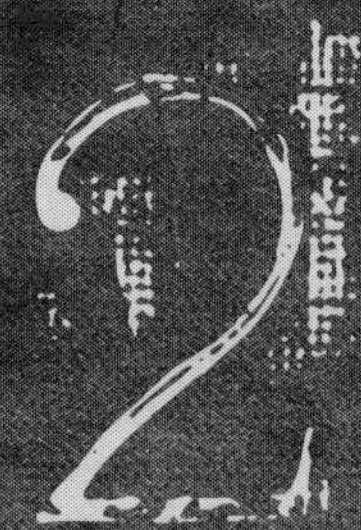

MAKING FACES AND TAKING OFF HEADS
The Operations of Photography and Medicine

In February 1854, the popular Philadelphia periodical *Arthur's Home Magazine* illustrated for its readers the experience of sitting for a daguerreotype (fig. 12).[1] According
to the description of the image published in the following issue, the portly, well-
dressed man seated for his portrait was a "well-conditioned" farmer from rural Pennsylvania who had been compelled by his wife and daughter to seek the services of a
daguerreotypist in Philadelphia. Upon arriving at the portrait studio of Marcus Aurelius Root, the farmer was invited to enter the "operation room." Taken aback, he asked
the daguerreotypist to repeat the invitation, as "it sounded to his ears very much as if
Mr. Root had said 'operating' room, and the only idea he had of 'operations' was the
cutting off of legs and arms." Although he was nervous about what might await him
upstairs, the man followed Root's instructions, allowing the well-dressed "operator"
to gaze coolly at his body beside the "muzzle of what seemed a small brass cannon"
(the camera), as an identically outfitted assistant gripped the farmer's head and "drew

it back into an iron clamp" (the headrest). The illustration in *Arthur's* depicts precisely that moment when the first-time sitter is thus confronted by the apparatus of the photographic studio, "the cold touch of which made the blood curdle in his veins."[2] Had the engraver shown the events that followed, we would have witnessed this sitter, suspecting foul play, bolt from his chair and abandon the operation altogether.

The farmer's fear, which caused him to experience the touch of the headrest as a physiological disturbance and to interpret portraiture as a violation of his body, stemmed from his confusion of the operations of portrait photography and surgery. The similarities that he imagined existed among the spaces, procedures, and performers associated with each technology, *Arthur's* suggests, were largely a product of his social class. Although his stout body and proper dress might have allowed the farmer to pass

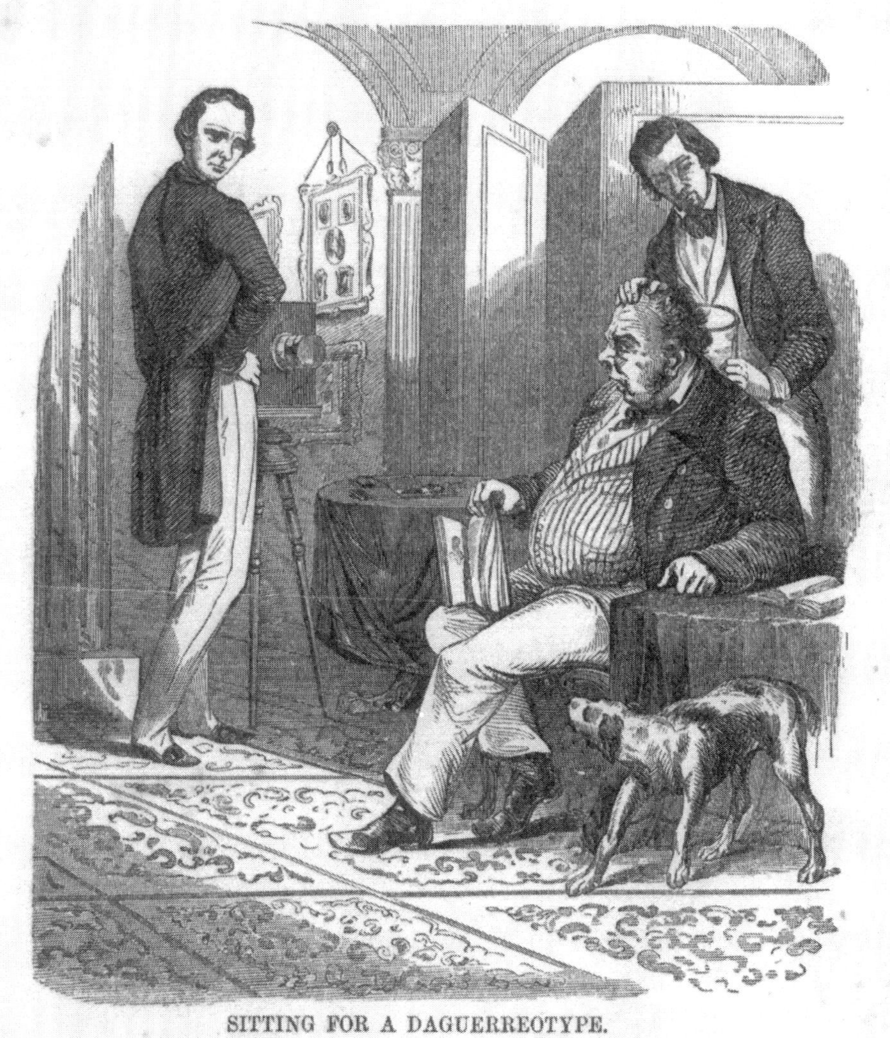

FIGURE 12 *Sitting for a Daguerreotype*, ca. 1849. Wood engraving. From *Arthur's Home Magazine* 3, no. 3 (February 1854).

as a typical middle-class studio patron, the mangy dog he brought into the operating room revealed his rural roots and ignorance of proper studio etiquette. Readers of the journal might have enjoyed what had become a common joke both within and outside photographic discourse. Made at the expense of unsophisticated rural Americans, such humor confirmed the unique ability of respectable city dwellers (the ideal consumers of *Arthur's*) to interpret social situations in modern life correctly; it also shows us that this group of readers imagined themselves to be the most appropriate clientele for Philadelphia's finest portrait studios. The city's photographic literature tells us, however, that studio patrons of *all* ages, origins, and social ranks persistently made connections between portrait photography and surgery throughout the nineteenth century, so much so that one photographer reportedly posted the following rule for visitors to his studio: "*Children should not be allowed to form an idea that to be photographed resembles a surgical operation.* The same remark is not inapplicable to adults."[3] For many sitters, the *Arthur's* farmer included, this resemblance was encouraged by portrait photographers themselves through their professional rhetoric; even Philadelphia's preeminent daguerreotypists spoke of "operating" on sitters in their studios.

The term "operation" had a number of uses in nineteenth-century Philadelphia that informed its cultural work in the practices and discussions of studio portraiture. It described, for instance, varieties of mechanical and scientific labor, at the same time that it figured prominently in the field of "operative medicine," which included surgery and branches of dentistry whose procedures were based on manual manipulations of the body. Also culturally prevalent was the idea that an "operation" signified a "performance," a "production of an effect" aided by instrumentation, and an expression of "agency" or "action."[4] Operations were defined, in other words, not only by the tools and methods they employed and the outcomes they produced but by the very fact that they constituted an assertion of power by an operator over the object of his manipulations. More recent uses of "operation" as a critical term suggest additional productive ways of interpreting its historical connotations. Michel Foucault, for example, sees "operations" as processes that are both subject to and expressions of disciplinary control; they embody forms of knowledge marked by order, discrete stages, internal conditions, and constituent elements that, taken together, make up a technology.[5] Lev Manovich has further defined "operations" as particular conceptual procedures embedded in a technology that are simultaneously "general ways of working, ways of thinking, and ways of existing" in a given culture.[6]

This chapter mobilizes these meanings to understand how, and to what effect, operative medicine became widely associated with posing and photographing sitters in urban portrait studios. While many sitters had objected to the material similarities between photographic and medical operations on the basis of their often painful physical experiences of them since the 1840s, photographers constructed positive epistemological connections between portrait photography and surgery beginning in the 1860s, imagining the ways in which these technologies embodied similar ways of knowing the body in the wake of the Civil War. What was at stake in this discourse of operations was the professional character of the photographer, the particular relationship that portrait photography was to have to the middle class, and the contributions that both operator and medium could make to the national project of (re)constructing physically and socially fit Americans.

CONSTRUCTING THE PAIN OF PORTRAITURE: PHOTOGRAPHY AS DENTISTRY

Of the countless complaints that Americans reportedly directed at the early practices of studio photography, comparisons to dentistry were among the most common; they were also the most troubling, yet often the most amusing, to commercial photographers.[7] A satirical want ad published in the *Philadelphia Photographer*, which sought a "party who can sit for their portrait without incidentally comparing the operation to one very often performed in a dentist's apartments," suggests that it was the exceptional sitter who did *not* associate photography with dentistry.[8] The perceived resemblance, as photographers understood it, represented in large part their patrons' reaction to "the 'thing' of all others that is looked upon with horror . . . [yet] one of the most necessary items of apparatus in the studio"—the posing stand and headrest.[9] Throughout much of the nineteenth century, American photographers consistently employed posing apparatuses like the one shown in figure 13, which gripped the back of a sitter's head and neck like a vice, supported his spine, and kept him still during the exposure of the plate. According to photographic literature, sitters regularly objected to the anxiety, physical discomfort, and even pain they experienced when posing in such devices; it was on this basis that they likened photographers' posing apparatuses to the instruments of tooth extraction, which were popularly associated in the nineteenth century with physical torture, decapitation, and even death. One year before the publication of "Sitting for a Daguerreotype," for instance, *Arthur's* shared with its readers a "parody" titled "The Dentist's Chair," which describes in verse with comic overtones the experience of a typical patient in that "fearful seat":

> 'Tis a fearful thing for the listening ear,
> Its ominous, rising squeak to hear—
> To see come forth from the little drawer,
> The weapons of torture, you've bargained for;
> [The dentist] scrapes and he cuts, and bores awhile,
> Then renews the attack with the horrid file.
> No one, though ever so vile, could dare
> To wish his worst foe in a dentist's chair.[10]

To imagine the experience of sitting before the camera in such terms was, of course, potentially damaging to the commercial success of portrait photography and its operators, since it suggested that both should be avoided at all costs. The very social group that photographers hoped to attract in large numbers to their studios—namely, the middle-class Americans who read "The Dentist's Chair"—would have been especially averse to a technology associated with bodily distress, given that anything from a minor ache to debilitating physical agony challenged notions of respectability. According to the historian Katherine C. Grier, the idea that respectable bodies should ideally be free of physical discomfort informed a wide range of social practices in modern America, such as the use of spring-seat upholstery in urban middle-class homes and the incorporation of lavish parlors into photographic studios and other commercial spaces.[11] This notion also dovetailed with what Karen Halttunen has identified as a "long-term transformation in the cultural significance of pain," through which physical suffering became "questionable, intolerable, disgusting, and obscene."[12] Citing the "uncivilizing" effects of pain on both the afflicted and those who observed them, Halttunen observes that Anglo-American humanitarian reformers and their white middle-class supporters opposed its "willful infliction" on a variety of "othered" subjects—particularly animals, criminals, the mentally insane, and black slaves—which implies that they could not even conceive of pain in relation to the bodies of ladies and gentleman. Photographic literature itself acknowledged the bourgeois distaste for bodily discomfort and pain when it described the social disfigurement that this class of sitters imagined posing would entail. As one

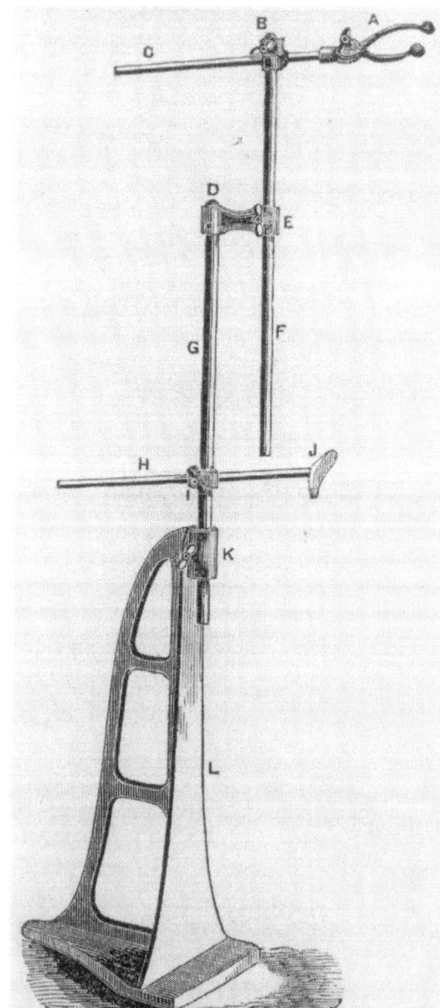

FIGURE 13 Harrison posing apparatus, ca. 1868. Wood engraving. From "Improved Photographic Rest," *Philadelphia Photographer* 5, no. 51 (March 1868): 74.

amateur photographer explained to the readers of the *Philadelphia Photographer* in 1864, the "photographer twists your head, and distorts your limbs, and sets you before the world an awkward and constrained creature"; gone are "an easy natural air, an intelligent countenance, [and] a respectable ladylike or gentlemanly carriage."[13] Because of the physical experiences they implied, popular comparisons of photography to dentistry seem to have similarly guaranteed that photographic operations were suitable only for socially "inferior" subjects.

Sitters' perceptions of photography as dentistry also challenged the social character of the photographer. The same middle-class Americans who looked upon bodily discomfort and pain with revulsion would have deemed an operator who inflicted them upon his subjects as unprofessional, if not lower class—either way, as someone socially unfit to manipulate their bodies. Such assumptions gained credence from the popular notion that both dental and photographic operators were essentially mechanical laborers; as such, they did not require the higher education or wield the cultural authority of professionals, whether fine artists or gentleman-scientists. For many regular physicians in Philadelphia, the fact that nineteenth-century dentists engaged in mere "tooth-plugging and tooth-pulling," rather than in performing "the most serious operations, involving life itself," excluded them from the category of "practitioners of medicine" altogether.[14] Similar perceptions of photography as "purely mechanical labor" were what studio portrait photographers sought to challenge through their professionalization, and what comparisons of photographic and dental operations threatened to reinforce; they also undermined the figure of the "doctor of photography" cultivated by Edward Wilson and other leaders of the Philadelphia photographic community.

In an effort to assert the high social character of their practice and increase their own social status, studio photographers launched a campaign in their trade literature against the insistence of middle-class Americans that they would "'rather go to the dentist than the photographer.'" Echoing the sentiment of many commercial operators, a regular columnist for the *Philadelphia Photographer* rejected any comparison between portrait photography and dentistry, explaining that the "operations are entirely dissimilar and there is no reason why the photographic chair should be associated with that of the dentist."[15] The arguments and evidence that photographers used to support such claims did, in fact, resemble those put forth by dentists in their own trade journals in defense of their place in the medical profession—a point of connection that arguably did more to reinforce than to sever the ties between them. Each group, for example, argued that the pain or injury patients experienced in their operations was due either to an operator's improper use of his instruments or to a patron's own insufficient care of her body.[16] This allowed dentists and studio photographers to claim that their operations could be made almost entirely painless through the use of an improved dental chair or posing apparatus; they could further assert that their work demanded professional expertise, even though such statements meant that they had simultaneously to question their professional legitimacy by admitting that there were indeed quacks among their ranks.[17]

In the case of studio photographers, mitigating the social effects of photography's apparent similarities to dental operations involved rhetorical assertions of power. "From the moment the sitter enters the studio," one photographic manual instructed commercial photographers, "bear well in mind that *you* are—or ought to be—master of the situation, not *he*." Such statements reminded photographers that verbal commands to "keep still!" and "look pleasant!" could silence sitters' claims that they "would prefer the dentist's chair."[18] Other photographers found that humor was the best means of disciplining sitters. As H. S. Keller joked bitterly in *Photographic Mosaics,* one way to mitigate the social effects of comparisons to dentistry was by killing the bodies that perpetuated them. "When a sitter mentions a toothless joke of breaking the camera, or preferring the dentist's chair," he quipped, "drown him in the developing tank."[19] To attribute serious work to Keller's joke—specifically the construction of photographic authority—is not to deny the fact that the scenario it describes belonged to the realm of fiction, or that it almost certainly made readers laugh; his instructions were clearly intended to entertain the Philadelphia photographic community rather than incite them to commit murder. Taking photographic humor seriously, rather, means acknowledging that it spoke to photographers' professional insecurities and their desires for social power in the second half of the nineteenth century, which informed the great lengths to which they were willing to go to keep sitters from interfering with their operations. It further involves reading photographers' jokes as metaphorically rich texts in which the cultural historian may interpret complex meanings.[20]

Such an approach reveals much about the following comparison between dental patients and soon-to-be-decapitated criminals that Edward Wilson published in the humor section of the *Philadelphia Photographer* in 1886: "An absent-minded dentist who, in addition to teeth pulling also took off heads, was called upon to pull a tooth for a young bride, who 'preferred to take the gas.' Upon presenting the nozzle [of] nitrous oxide to the nervous lady he said, 'Now just keep your eyes about there, and try and look pleasant, please.'"[21] In this scenario, a dentist who moonlights as an executioner confuses two procedures: the removal of teeth and the removal of heads. In his confusion, he preps his unsuspecting client for the "wrong" procedure, an operation that would tragicomically alter her body (it would take off her head), permanently freezing her facial features in what he hopes will be a pleasing expression. It would have been impossible for readers of the *Philadelphia Photographer* to interpret this instruction by the "dentist" that his patient "look pleasant" as anything but a thinly veiled reference to their own studio practices. Further encouraging such a reading was, of course, the studio public's fondness for comparing photographers and dentists as well as photographers and executioners, particularly hangmen and decapitators; the latter comparison informed the popular metaphorical conception of photographic operators as men who "make faces and take off heads for a living."[22]

Wilson's joke was all the funnier and more complex for coming from a photographer rather than someone posing for a portrait. Why would one of the most respected and outspoken leaders of the commercial photographic community deliberately invoke a set of comparisons so often used to disparage the social character of photographers and their studio practices? If we assume that the goal of the humor section in the *Philadelphia Photographer* was to entertain photographers while assuaging anxieties about their precarious authority, then we can read Wilson's joke as ironically *reinforcing* that authority. By articulating similarities among photographers, dentists, and executioners, Wilson effectively undermined sitters' complaints, presenting them as rhetoric that his readers could easily laugh away. Further, the act of "confusing" these different varieties of "operator" itself contributed to a fantasy of photographic authority in which sitters' bodies fell entirely under the control of the photographer, who might manipulate (or decapitate) them as he pleased. Aligning studio portraiture with the practices of medicine and the law, the joke can be said to function as a way of disciplining, "under the pain of portraiture," those sitters who challenged the photographic control over their bodies. Specifically, Wilson entertained studio photographers with the thought of subjecting their patrons to what Michel Foucault has defined as an "analogical punishment," or a form of discipline predicated on a relationship between the thought of committing a crime (conceiving of photography as an "operation") and the penalty (experiencing the removal of one's head).[23]

Outside the realm of humor, however, the fact that the *analogical* reasoning linking photography to dentistry and decapitation could function as *logical* reasoning supported by material effects presented a challenge to photographic authority. For even if photographers could silence their patrons' objections to the photographic apparatus, that rhetoric had the potential to alter bodies materially in portrait studios. Comparisons between the posing stand and the instruments of dentistry could quicken a sitter's breathing rate and pulse, which could blur the resulting image; they could also cause sitters to "assume a woe-begone expression or a nervous smile painfully suggestive of a sufferer in a dentist's chair as soon as they sit for a photograph," thereby hindering the photographer's primary aim of capturing pleasing expressions and likenesses.[24] Significantly, these reported changes to bodies seated before the camera were not confined to the pages of popular or photographic literature, given that the material outcome of any photographic "operation" in a commercial studio was the production of a portrait. In the *carte de visite* in figure 14, the boy's rigid body and petrified expression serve as visual reminders of the emotional and physical anguish sitters associated with the experience of posing, while the posing stand visible behind the boy's legs functions as their apparent object. In a matter of seconds, the Rhoads' New Photograph Gallery produced a seemingly permanent and circulatable image of an uneasy body subjected to the "pain of portraiture" that could have direct negative effects on the commercial success of the studio. Although Rhoads operated a profitable business in the 1860s, evidenced by the fact that this studio catered to a respectable class of sitters on Frankford Avenue for more than thirty years, portraits that conveyed the comfort and beauty of their sitters generally fetched higher prices and attracted more, and more affluent, customers than those that suggested the opposite.

Images further complicated photographers' insistence that there was no resemblance whatsoever between portrait photography, dentistry, and decapitation when one considers that vignette portraits were wildly popular in *cartes de visite* and later in cabinet cards (fig. 15). In this style of portraiture, the photographic medium produced a visual record of its fragmentation of the body in the form of a disembodied head, which would seem to confirm sitters' fears of photography's corporeal effects; a metaphorical

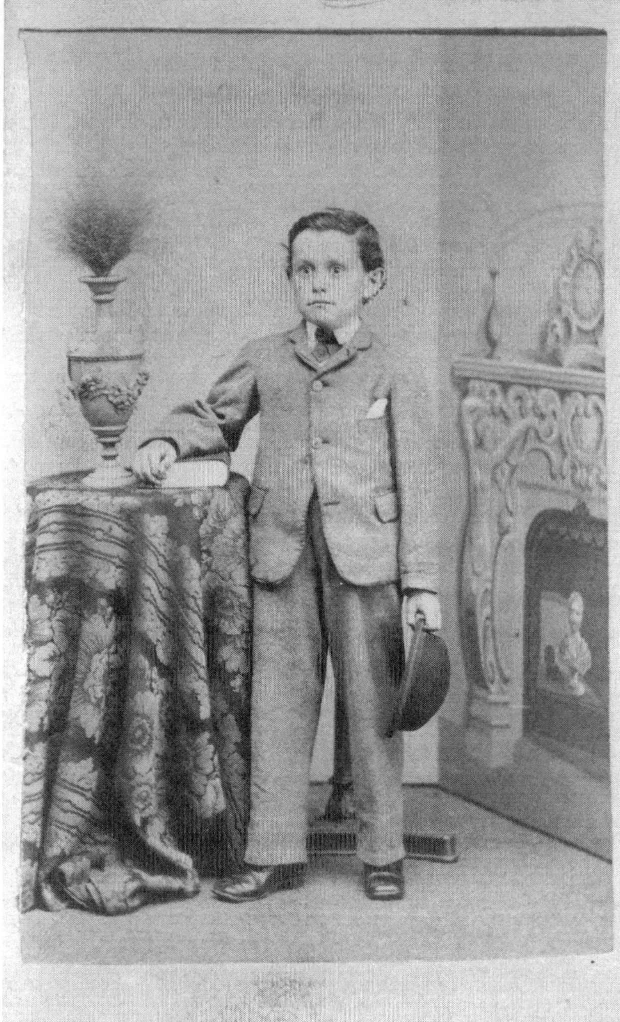

expression was thus materially confirmed by studio photography's aesthetic conventions. While photography was certainly not the first visual medium to produce images
of seeming decapitation, photographic literature suggests that sitters imagined the
technology's corporeal manipulations as operating uniquely on the level of representation *and* as materially affecting bodies themselves. In the lived experience of studio
photography, did a sitter ever expect the production of a vignette portrait to involve the
fatal fragmentation or dismemberment of her own body under the skylight? Probably
not, but as "Sitting for a Daguerreotype" tells us, the idea that photography could have
an unmediated relationship to sitters' bodies was not only conceivable but potentially
believable in ways that it rarely had been in the case of painting. The question that early
photographic discourse raises is whether this conception of the medium, underwritten
by the models and metaphors of operative medicine, did more to challenge or promote
its authority in nineteenth-century America.

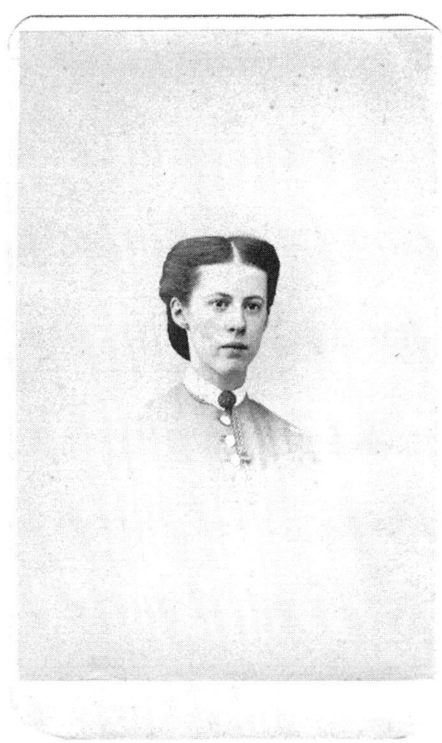

FIGURE 15 Henszey & Co., portrait of an unidentified woman, ca. 1860s. Albumen print on *carte de visite* mount. Private collection.

(RE)MAKING THE METAPHOR: PHOTOGRAPHY AS DIAGNOSIS AND CURE

Reflecting on a pair of *carte de visite* portraits in 1866, Walter C. North, a photographer well known in Philadelphia circles for his efforts to educate young operators, offered the following advice on how to prepare sitters for a photographic "operation":

> When your sitter enters, . . . allow him to sit down and make himself comfortable and feel at ease. Look pleasant, but do not talk too much as a general thing. . . . The only talking that is really needful, is to make your model forget he is sitting for a picture. We know of a very skilful physician who goes a little upon this plan. He visits his patient, says nothing, but listens. Looks at the tongue, feels the pulse, and writes his prescription. . . . It is to his interest to get his patients well as soon as he can. To do this, he must lead the mind away from the disease as much as he can, and so should the photographer do.[25]

North's characterization of studio photographers as physicians who systematically diagnose and cure rather than brutally dismember the body constructs a positive image of portrait photography as akin to a professional medical operation, one that was first introduced into commercial photographic discourse in the 1860s and attempted to discredit the comparisons of photography with dentistry. Educators like North proposed that photographic and medical operators shared a particular way of seeing and knowing the bodies of their subjects as well as a means of communicating that knowledge. Fighting metaphor with metaphor, these men fostered an association between studio portraiture and medicine in an effort to describe the power relations between operators and sitters and the ultimate aim of their operations: the eradication of physical and social disease. In this way they attempted to shift popular conceptions of photography away from the medium's perceived tendency to induce bodily dis-ease or pain, grounding it firmly in commercial photographers' ability to observe, diagnose, and restore bodies to health.

Marcus Aurelius Root, the same Philadelphia daguerreotypist whose reference to the "operation room" traumatized the Pennsylvanian farmer depicted in *Arthur's Home Magazine,* published one of the earliest efforts to relate photography to medicine in a way that emphasized the relationship's positive effects. Throughout *The Camera and the Pencil,* Root argued that the true character of a sitter was revealed through examination of the body itself, a belief he inherited from the sciences of physiognomy and phrenology.[26] He explained, for instance, that the photographer's first step in obtaining a good portrait was to "penetrate, by whatever means at his command, the fleshly mask, which envelopes the spiritual part of his model, and ascertain his real type and character." To accomplish this, Root instructed operators to follow the model of "an observant, acute physician [who] learns at once to detect, by the external appearances of his patient, what disease [a patient] is attacked with, and in what part of the organism this disease is seated."[27] Quoting a Philadelphia physician, he went on to list the various physical and mental ailments that write themselves on the body, along with the specific nature, location, and meaning of their inscription. "Morbid conditions of the chest write their signatures on the middle of the face—especially the nose," he explained, while the "mouth and the lips . . . show the presence of abdominal affections."[28]

Like North, Root invoked the photographer-physician metaphor to suggest that photographic operations subjected the sitter to a clinical gaze.[29] According to nineteenth-century descriptions of clinical observation published and widely read by the Philadelphia medical community, the rapid "glance" was the primary means of first acquiring knowledge of a patient's physical and mental characteristics—traits understood to be articulated directly on the surface of the body.[30] In *The Camera and the Pencil,* Root adapted this model of medical perception to a commercial photographic context, replacing the clinic with the portrait studio as the representation of that epistemological structure within physical space, and analogizing the procedures and bodies associated with those environments. Using language common to commercial photographic discourse of the period, Root concluded that "a sufficient amount of observation would detect distinctly marked signs indicative of *every* malady from which man suffers, so that a glance at the face and figure might determine the character and intensity of such malady. . . . The internal dispositions thus stamp themselves on the exterior."[31]

This seminal text in the historiography of American photography suggests a parallel between the birth of the clinic and the invention of photographic portraiture, one that speaks to a period preoccupation with new technologies equating an individual's body with his symptoms as well as with the visual representation thereof.[32] Like the medical doctors of his day, Root understood a sitter's "internal dispositions" and their external signs as his maladies—what North described as the patient's "disease"—or the collection of particular physical and mental traits that make up an individual's identity. It was precisely these markers of individuality, or the signs of pathology inscribed on the surface of the body that materially *constituted* the body itself, that were diagnosed and actively treated in the production of a portrait photograph. To put it another way, photographic and medical operations, as they were represented in nineteenth-century Philadelphia, embodied similar processes of identity formation, in that both physically altered the bodily appearance and identity of the subject in order to produce an ideal "normal" type.[33] As this chapter argues, one of the most readily available medical models for photographers' manipulations of sitters' bodies under the skylight was that of surgery, a technology of corporeal inscription that conceived of bodies as surfaces upon which sociocultural messages could be written and read, marking them with social identities.[34] In surgical operations, the patient's collection of visible deviations from a physical and social ideal was first identified through the doctor's case taking and subsequent diagnosis. These deviations, which collectively constituted a disease, could then be manually removed, and the body subsequently reconstructed into a sign of "normalcy."

In *The Normal and the Pathological* (1966), Georges Canguilhem dates this form of medical diagnosis and cure to the early nineteenth century. Fusing scientific and social authority, doctors in this period understood curing as "restoring a function or an organism to the norm from which they have deviated." According to Canguilhem, they took their conception of the "norm" chiefly from their "knowledge of physiology" and secondarily from "actual experience of organic functions, and from the common representation of the norm in a social milieu in a given moment."[35] Equipped with some knowledge of physiology from their professional literature, Philadelphia photographers relied heavily on the second authority in forming a "norm," while seeking to establish portrait photography—both the profession and its material objects—as the embodiment of that authority. To this end, they related the production of a medical diagnosis to their own visual cataloguing of bodily defects.[36] As one contributor to *Photographic Mosaics* put it, "I have learned to 'diagnose,' as the doctor would say, each case in hand, and adapt myself to the situation," translating sitters into pathological types set against a vision of health, respectability, and beauty.[37] Like the surgeons whose practices they modeled, studio photographers assumed that *all* of their patrons were inherently defective in body and manner, or "irregularly featured," as Root once put it; they also saw these bodies as inherently operable.[38]

THE BATTLEFIELD OF OPERATIONS

When considering the discussions of corporeal disorder and disease that began to dominate Philadelphia photographic literature in the 1860s, one must take into account not only the epistemological shift in medical operations that took place in the preceding decades but also the more immediate historical context of the U.S. Civil War. That its readership was preoccupied with the carnage that the war delivered to the city of Philadelphia, which was closely linked to the front by its extensive rail lines, is evident in the

very first issue of the *Philadelphia Photographer*, published in January 1864. In it, Edward
Wilson ran a poem titled "The Dead Soldier's Children," which opens with the following
verses:

> Upon a field which War's red hand
> Had strewn with dead and dying;
> When the foe, who late so boastfully
> Came on, in shame were flying;
> In a spot where thickest lay the dead,
> Most fierce had been the battle,
> Lay one who never more should hear
> The guns' death-dealing rattle.
>
> Three wounds, and all in front, told plain
> How bravely he had fought;
> One grazed his cheek, one broke an arm,
> The third his breast had sought.
> At night, when o'er the scene of strife
> The moon her pale rays shed,
> In hurrying groups, men moving round
> Are burying the dead.[39]

In an editorial comment, Wilson explained that these lines described the "terrible
slaughter at Gettysburg," where thousands of corpses, many horribly disfigured, were
strewn across the Pennsylvania landscape in July 1863. Referring to the remaining
verses of poem, he revealed their subject to be an unidentified Union soldier who had
been found dead on the battlefield grasping in his hand a photograph of his "three little
children." Just months before the *Philadelphia Photographer* began publication, both the
Philadelphia Inquirer and the *Philadelphia Press* had reported that the original ambrotype
found on the body of this soldier came into the possession of Dr. J. Francis Bourns, a
physician from the city, who arranged for it to be reproduced as *cartes de visite* by the
prominent studios of James E. McClees, H. C. Phillips & Brother, Wenderoth & Taylor,
and Frederick Gutekunst (fig. 16). The sale of these *cartes*, Bourns hoped, would help
reconnect the fatherless northern family with the fallen hero as well as offer them financial support.[40]

The debilitated body of the Union soldier continued to attract the attention of the
commercial photographic community as the war raged on. In April 1864, for example,
the *Philadelphia Photographer* published the first of a series of editorials urging readers
to support the work of the United States Sanitary Commission (USSC), which took "a
great and good national, as well as merciful object,—the alleviation of the sufferings
of our brave soldiers." Such support, the journal explained, should take the form of
photographs, especially "portraits of our Generals and distinguished persons, views
of battlefields and kindred subjects," that could be exhibited and sold during the first
week of June at the commission's Great Central Fair in Philadelphia.[41] That the city's
photographers participated in this event is not in itself remarkable, given that the USSC

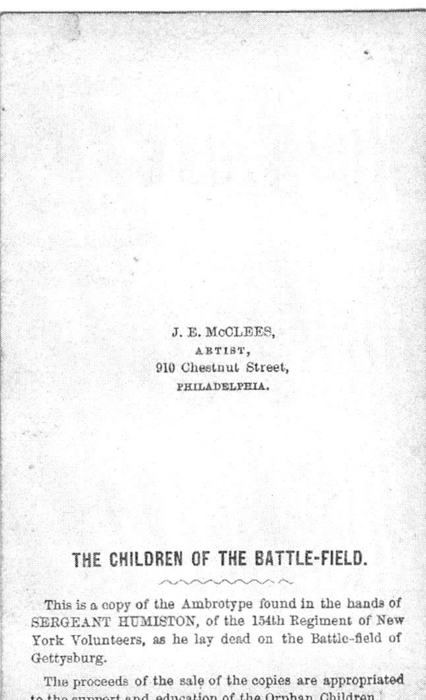

FIGURE 16a–b James McClees, *The Children of the Battle-Field,* ca. 1864. Albumen print on *carte de visite* mount (recto and verso). Collection of Mark H. Dunkelman.

called upon "all classes of citizens, of trades, and professions" to make contributions, although the fair's Philadelphia-based Committee on Photography represented its members as uniquely positioned to promote the health, and hence the military success, of the northern army. A flyer distributed to the local photographic community stated this position plainly, announcing that "none will respond more cheerfully to [the USSC's] call for aid than those interested in the beautiful and useful art of Photography."[42]

Contributors to Edward Wilson's journals also represented the value that the camera's records of bodies in pieces could have to the suffering nation by linking it to the achievements of surgery during the war. The majority of serious wounds that soldiers sustained in combat were the result of the soft lead bullet known as the minié ball, which did enormous physical damage to skin, bones, and muscles upon impact, often necessitating surgical intervention performed with minimal anesthesia in a military hospital, if not on the battlefield itself. Most of these operations targeted the body's extremities and led to gross disfigurement, bacterial infection, and considerable pain, like that suffered by the narrator in S. Weir Mitchell's "The Case of George Dedlow."[43] Although surgeons' propensity to amputate the limbs of the wounded revived old associations between surgery and butchery, the booming artificial limb industry in Philadelphia likened these operations to making "mutilated" bodies healthy and whole.[44] The significant number of face, head, and neck wounds incurred during the conflict also provided a valuable opportunity for surgeons to develop new reconstructive techniques that required specialized skills and produced remarkable visible results. Through their use of facial prosthetics and transplanted tissues to reconstruct eyelids, noses, cheeks, mouths, and chins, many men who had practiced dentistry before the war became pioneers in the burgeoning field of plastic surgery.[45] It was in this field that commercial photographers recognized surgeons' vital contributions to the advancement of the medical profession, the national project of reconstruction, and photography itself. In an article called "Photography as an Authority" in the December 1864 issue of the *Philadelphia Photographer,* for example, Reverend H. J. Morton reflected on his experiences as an associate member of the USSC, observing that "surgery has achieved some amazing triumphs of late years, particularly in providing new noses and lips and half faces for those who have been unfortunately injured by disease or accident." An active participant in the Philadelphia photographic community who lectured frequently at the Franklin Institute, Morton praised the authority of the medium when thus brought into the service of medicine, defining it in terms of its truth-telling capacity. "The operator desires to have a record of his skill," he explained to Wilson's readers, "and pictures of the former and latter state of the patients are produced. Is it in human nature not to exaggerate the original deformity, and increase the after loveliness? Photography will not do this. It gives the first and last state of the patient exactly, and refuses to flatter."[46]

In favoring the photographic study over the hand-drawn illustration, Morton may have had in mind the photographs taken for the Army Medical Museum in Washington, D.C., which had been established by the U.S. government in 1862 to document wartime injuries. The museum claimed to have set up a "full photographic outfit" within a year, but preparations for a designated studio, complete with props and equipment ordered from Philadelphia's Wilson & Hood and other major suppliers, continued through 1865, when chief photographer William H. Bell took over the museum's photographic department.[47] In 1866 Edward Wilson visited the museum's studio to view the work of this former Philadelphia daguerreotypist, which reportedly included depictions of "shattered bones, broken skulls, and living subjects, before and after surgical operations have been performed on them."[48] The experience of seeing Bell's photographs of wounded soldiers firsthand was a memorable one, Wilson told his readers. A particular pair of pictures stuck with him; one depicted a "poor fellow as he came from the field, with his face almost torn asunder by a shell," while the other was taken after "surgery had exercised its skill upon him." At this point the subject "was photographed again, and looked much better than any one could be expected to look with his lower jaw gone." Echoing Morton's celebration of the photograph's exactitude, Wilson concluded that "photography is the only medium by which surgery could so plainly make known its handiwork," confirming its status as a handmaid of the sciences. One detects in his editorial comments, however, a vision of photographic and surgical operators working together on the bodies of the grotesquely injured, ensuring that they could be restored to a state of physical and social fitness—as if the patient's reconstruction was not complete until "he was photographed again."

We can see how such a vision may have been applied to the photographs of Private Rowland Ward of Company E, 4th New York Heavy Artillery, which display the various stages of a "plastic" operation performed on the patient's mouth, chin, jaw, and neck after much of these were "destroyed" and "carried away" by a shell fragment (fig. 17). The "before" image of Ward, taken around August 1864 at Lincoln Hospital in

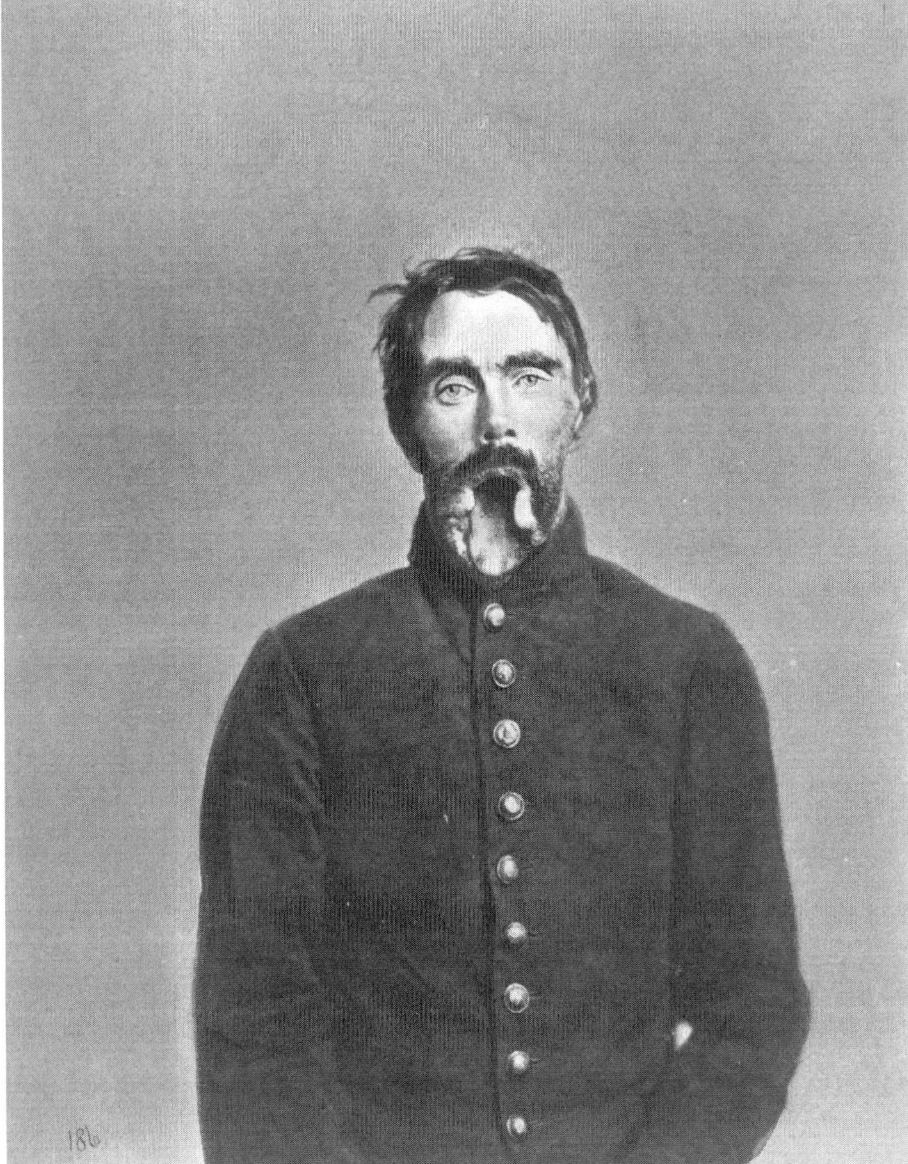

FIGURE 17a Unidentified photographer, *Case of Cheiloplasty (Private Rowland Ward, Co. E, 4th New York Heavy Artillery)*, ca. 1864. Albumen print. From Army Medical Museum, *Photographs of Surgical Cases and Specimens*, vol. 4, SP186.

Washington and contributed to the Army Medical Museum thereafter (fig. 17a), shows an impressively composed soldier in uniform facing the camera, his tongue hanging loosely where the bottom portion of his face had once been. The subsequent postoperative photographs, made under the direction of Surgeon J. C. McKee, record McKee's efforts to correct Ward's grotesque disfigurement by creating a series of skin flaps to close the gaping hole left by the shell (figs. 17b–c).[49] Although these "after" images suggest that the corporeal effects of the war could not be rendered entirely invisible—the

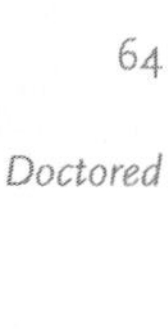

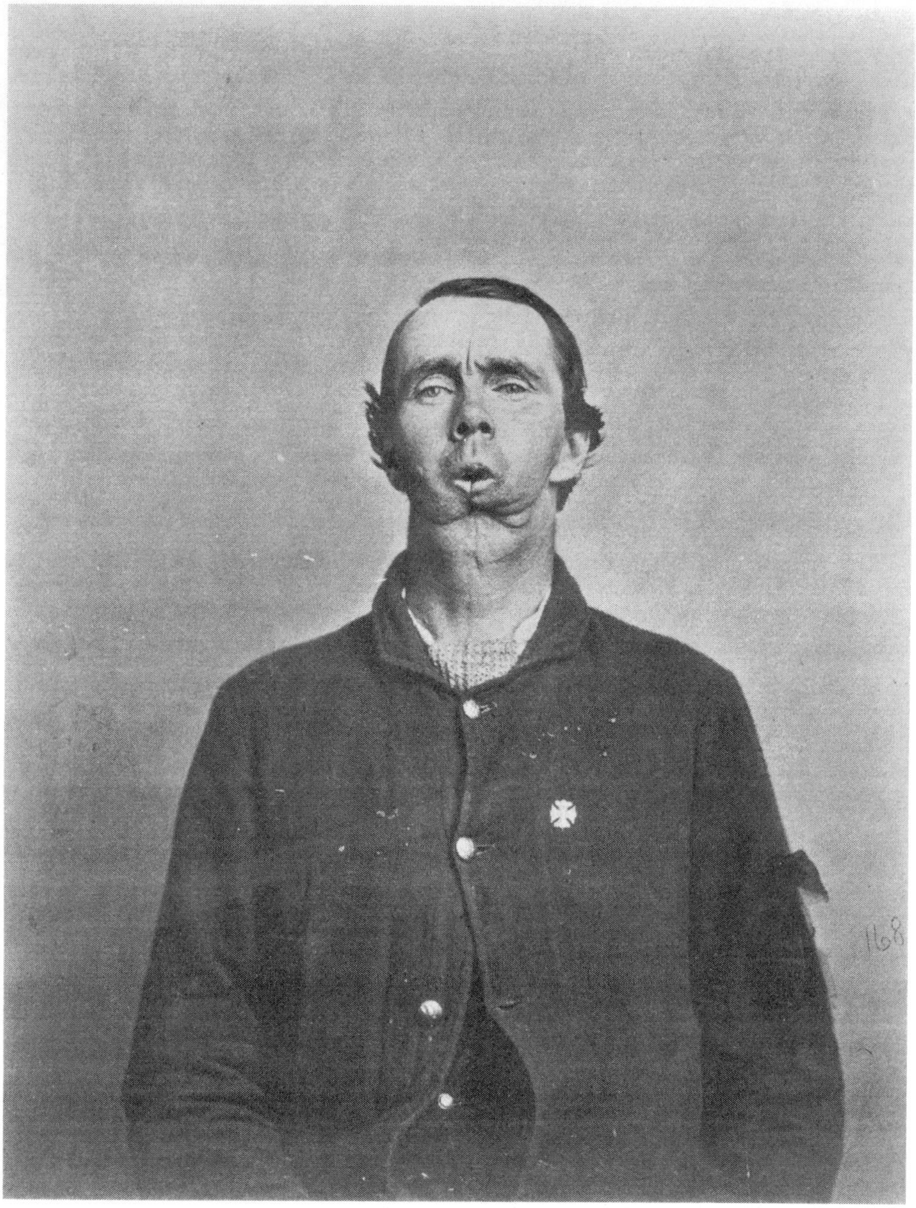

FIGURE 17b Unidentified photographer, *Case of Cheiloplasty (Private Rowland Ward, Co. E, 4th New York Heavy Artillery),* ca. 1865. Albumen print. From Army Medical Museum, *Photographs of Surgical Cases and Specimens,* vol. 4, SP168.

viewer may find himself dwelling on Ward's recessed chin—the reconstruction of Ward's lower face undoubtedly had significant consequences for the patient. Ward appears to us human and whole, the surgeon's case notes tell us, having regained the ability to speak and to consume food normally, thus rebuilding his physical strength and reintegrating him into social life. It is this social makeover of the wounded soldier that the medical photographer aided most directly by employing the aesthetic conventions of studio portraiture, however subtly. Indeed, the most favorable postoperative images of Ward, in which his body most closely adheres to ideal physical norms, are those in

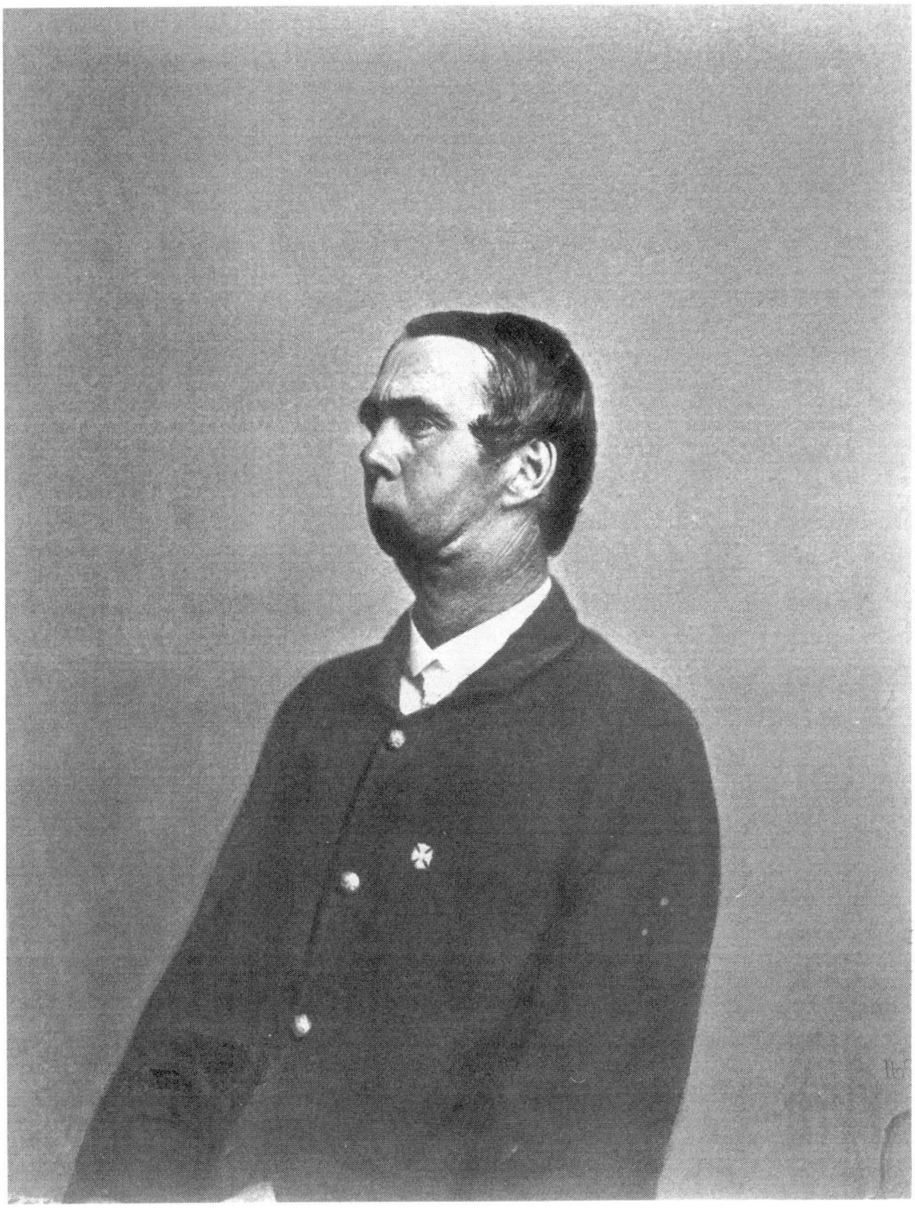

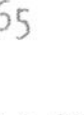

FIGURE 17C Unidentified photographer, *Case of Cheiloplasty (Private Rowland Ward, Co. E, 4th New York Heavy Artillery)*, ca. 1865. Albumen print. From Army Medical Museum, *Photographs of Surgical Cases and Specimens*, vol. 4, SP169.

which he is posed, dressed, and lit in the manner associated at the time with proper gentlemen; with his hair neatly trimmed and his mouth closed for the first time in the series, he appears to us in three-quarter profile, gazing coolly out of the frame of the shot, his thoughts apparently far from the military hospital in which he still sits. That figure 17c could, formally speaking, be a portrait of any respectable studio patron in the 1860s contributed to Ward's social reconstruction and the larger project of piecing together the nation, symbolized by the military medal conspicuously pinned on his jacket. Like so many other photographic studies overseen and collected by the Army

Medical Museum, the representation of Ward's body across this series of images thus relies on and reinforces the slippage between medical and vernacular studio portraiture, one that works to "increase the after loveliness," if not also "exaggerate the original deformity."

This slippage belongs to what Sander Gilman has described as the "constant bleed between the world of the medical photograph and the general world of visual culture," and it accounts for the influence of studio portraiture on clinical photography so often noted in recent scholarship on the latter.[50] Historians have largely ignored, however, the innumerable ways in which the visual culture of the military hospital and the bodily horrors it represented shaped ideas about "everyday" photographic practices. Such horrors, after all, were literally present during the war in Philadelphia portrait studios, as some of the city's most reputable operators had, like Frederick Gutekunst, themselves witnessed the war and had photographed rehabilitated Union soldiers and respectable

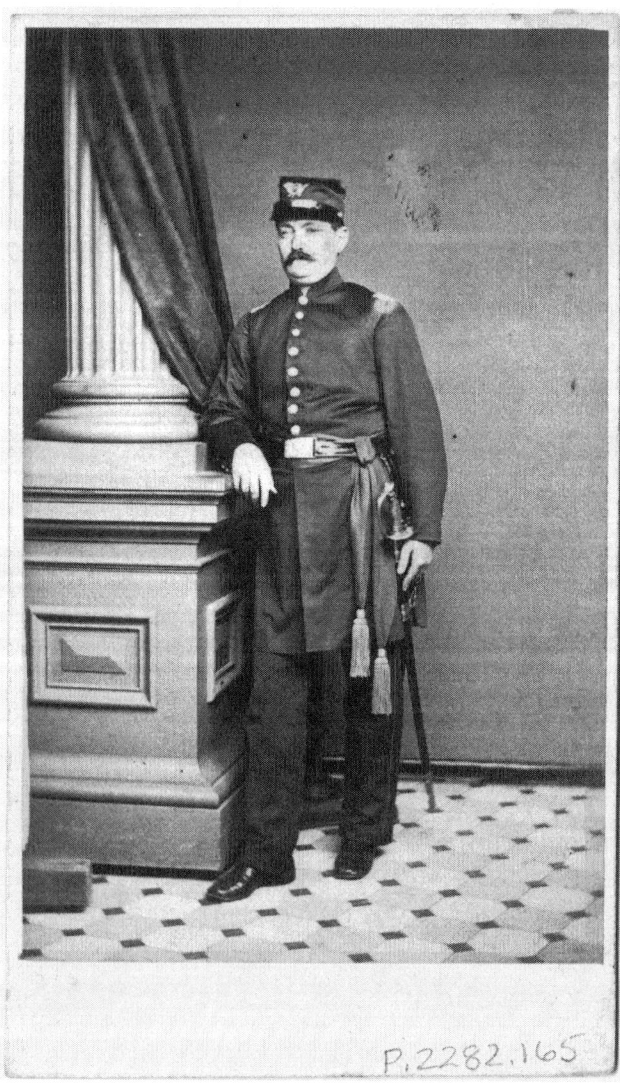

FIGURE 18 Frederick Gutekunst, *Portrait of an Unidentified Soldier*, ca. 1860s. Albumen print on *carte de visite* mount. The Library Company of Philadelphia.

Philadelphians in precisely the same space, often with the same props and poses (figs. 18 and 19).[51] Others, including James Cremer, actively encouraged the co-presence of these bodies under their skylights by advertising their portrait practices in army publications like the *West Philadelphia Hospital Register*, where they offered a "discount of $1.00 to wounded soldiers."[52] The work of the medical and commercial portrait photographer would continue to overlap after the war ended, when men like Bell resumed their studio work in Philadelphia, all the while sending photographs of clinical cases in the city's hospitals back to the Army Medical Museum.[53]

In the form of references to bloody battles, northern heroes, and military burial grounds, the war and its carnage remained present in photographers' trade literature throughout the postbellum period. On multiple occasions Wilson selected one of these subjects for the original photographic print that appeared at the front of each issue of the *Philadelphia Photographer*, including a view of Richmond, Virginia, in ruins shortly

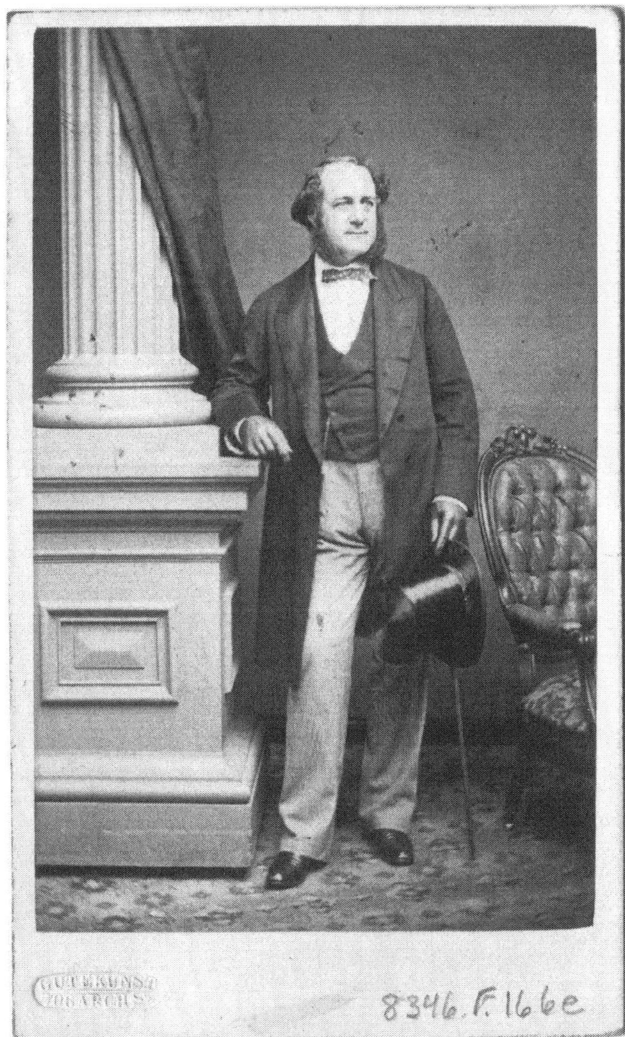

FIGURE 19 Frederick Gutekunst, *Portrait of an Unidentified Man*, ca. 1860s. Albumen print on *carte de visite* mount. The Library Company of Philadelphia.

after a battle devastated the city in April 1865, and a portrait of Civil War hero Lieutenant-General Philip Henry Sheridan taken in 1877.[54] As long as two decades after the last shot was fired, photographer William H. Rau (son-in-law and former apprentice of William Bell) shared with Wilson's readers his experience of leading a photographic party from Philadelphia back to Antietam, "where our army led by McClellan defeated the Confederates." Led on a tour of the battlefield by Colonel Boteler, the group learned that "he saw men carry out legs, arms, and parts of bodies . . . and load them on carts to haul them away for burial. The fighting at this place was terrific," Rau explained; "the troops were so badly mutilated that scarcely a man escaped without a wound."[55]

That Wilson, Rau, and others found themselves returning to such memories should come as no surprise, for, as art historian Sarah Burns has observed, "it is difficult to imagine that living in the midst of a wartime hospital city with its thousands of wounded, broken bodies—bodies on stumps and crutches, truncated bodies—would leave no trace."[56] What is remarkable are the ways in which Philadelphia photographers re-created the experience of the war every time they manipulated bodies under the skylight by imagining that all studio sitters were in need of "surgical" rehabilitation. Through their discourse of operations, these men represented vernacular studio portraiture as an invaluable contribution to the national project of remaking bodies, while promoting themselves as its agents.

PHOTOGRAPHIC RETOUCHING AND SOCIAL REMAKING

As Civil War surgeons were being praised for their construction of "new noses and lips and half faces" on the pages of the *Philadelphia Photographer,* contributors to the journal focused their daily operations on a similar set of bodily features. When photographing patrons who entered one's studio, Roland Vanweike explained in his column, the "peculiarities of faces are what we want to consider. . . . Thin face with high cheekbones; retreating forehead and prominent nose; crooked nose—generally two noses; pug nose; turn-up nose; large mouth; large ears; staring eyes; weak and squinting eyes; cross eyes; sunken eyes; very light eyes with sunburnt face; retreating chin; [and] long neck"—these were "the more prominent peculiarities we meet with, that require special treatment."[57] In order to remedy these visible defects, or at the very least to offset their deviations from an ideal norm, portrait photographers had many techniques at their disposal. These included using certain lighting effects, applying makeup to sitters' faces, or rubbing their skin with a flannel cloth to produce an artificial blush. They could also strategically position bodies away from or near the camera to highlight certain features and conceal others. Beginning in the 1870s, the most common yet controversial photographic remedy was retouching, known then and now as "doctoring" photographs.[58]

The retouching techniques developed in the 1870s were of a very different character from the over-painting practices of earlier decades, which involved applying loose broad strokes of color onto the surface of an albumen print to produce a portrait that closely resembled a miniature painting. Securing the photographic negative in an adjustable frame or stand, like the one illustrated in figure 20, the retoucher would first apply a varnish to create an abraded surface, and then work with a pencil or brush on the collodion film, as if applying a scalpel to human skin. Because most retouching was performed directly on the negative, the printed portrait typically bore little evidence—few discernable pencil marks or brushstrokes—of the retoucher's hand.

Whether the retoucher doctored photographs manually or with the aid of newly marketed retouching machines, this "operator" aimed to remove two kinds of defects from the negative: blemishes produced by the photographic process, and those apparent on and peculiar to the sitter himself. The first class of defects included areas of the negative that were under- or overexposed, scratches on the film, and dark spots caused by dirt or dust on the photographer's equipment. The second class comprised a range of anatomical and dermatological abnormalities that compromised a sitter's apparent physical beauty and social status. In a pair of portraits printed before and after retouching, which appeared in Hermann Vogel's widely read photographic manual from 1875, we find that both kinds of defects—the photographic and the corporeal—are visible in the portrait on the left and have been touched out on the right (fig. 21). Several spots on the negative have been removed, one of which produced a prominent white mark on the young lady's cheek in the untouched print. The retoucher also softened the heavy contrast of light and shade, probably caused by an improper diffusion of light at the time of exposure and exacerbated by the deep contours of the sitter's face. The result is the appearance of smoother, blemish-free skin with even pigmentation, fuller cheeks, a straighter mouth, and well-rested eyes, which contribute to our reading of the subject as youthful, racially white, feminine, and middle class. In her retouched portrait Mlle. Artot becomes, quite simply, the picture of health, as it was defined in medical and popular discourses of the period.

In treating the second class of defects, the work of the nineteenth-century retoucher bore a striking resemblance to that of the reconstructive surgeon, who, as we have seen, relied heavily on pre- and postoperative photographs to illustrate his transformation of the pathological into the normal. While the surgeon's use of photography was meant to prove the operation's success to medical professionals and the patient, the studio photographer's job was to conceal the reconstructive process from the public eye.

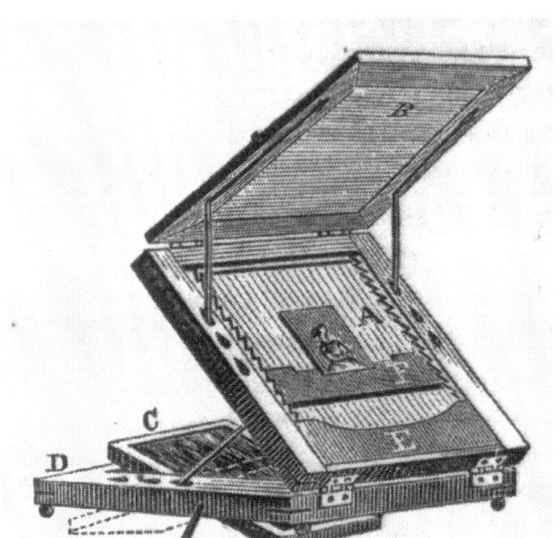

FIGURE 20 Retouching frame, ca. 1870. Wood engraving. From "Our Picture," *Philadelphia Photographer* 7, no. 75 (March 1870): 92.

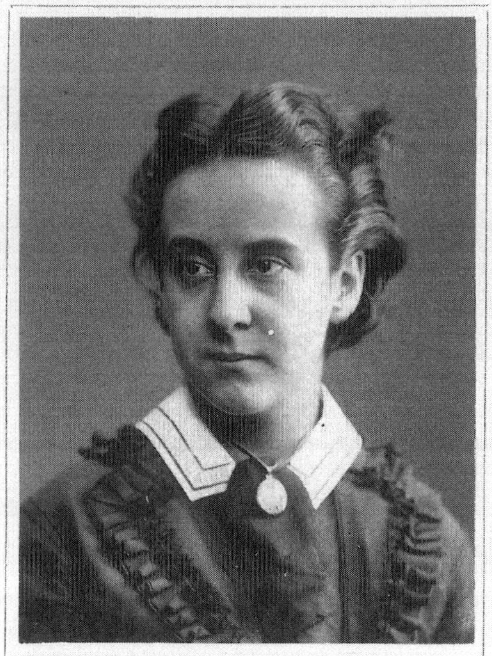

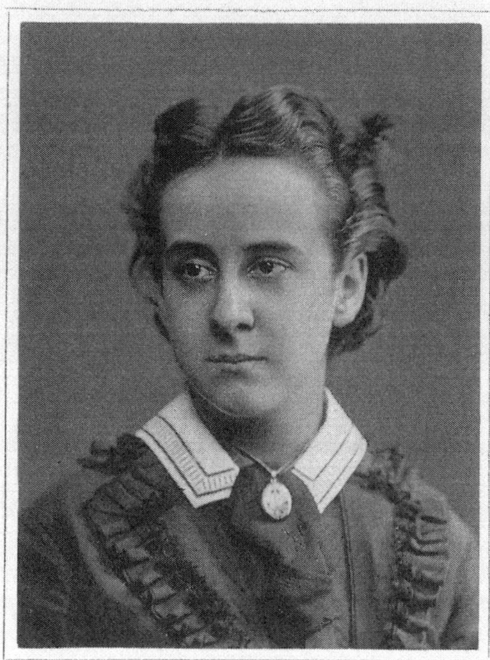

FIGURE 21 Portrait of Mlle. Artot, untouched and retouched, ca. 1875. Albumen print. From Hermann Vogel, *The Chemistry of Light and Photography* (New York: D. Appleton and Co., 1875), 245.

The public display of before-and-after photographs was, in fact, rare in the nineteenth century; intended to be seen only by commercial photographers, the pair in figure 21 is one of a few examples that appear in American photographic literature of the period.[59] The invisibility of these photographic transformations does not mean that a medicalized process of physical and social rehabilitation has failed to take place. Rather, early photographic discourse sought to embed that process within the material practices, and indeed in the very idea, of photography such that the "conventional" studio portrait would be understood as essentially *post*operative. When we look at *any* portrait from the 1870s and 1880s, then, what we see is always-already an "after," or the result of a series of manipulations intended to rid the sitter's face of its (pathological) signs of individuality and produce a "pleasing" (idealized) likeness; it is this reconstructed image that the photographer, if not also the sitter, hoped would be read by viewers as her "true" self.

The dialogue between studio portraiture and reconstructive surgery became a powerful means of making over the studio public *and* the body of commercial operators entrusted to its care. As discussed in chapter 1, one of the most important things that the idea of a "doctor of photography" could do in the 1870s was to support portrait photographers' professional legitimacy. When it came to the practice of "doctoring" photographs, the figure of the "doctor" indeed embodied the specialized knowledge and skills of a gentleman-scientist, whose practices promoted the physical and social fitness of the nation's growing middle class. While acknowledging that a retoucher required the skills of a fine artist, members of the Philadelphia photographic community also increasingly advocated acquiring knowledge of anatomy and a "more or less perfect understanding of the principles of physiognomy and phrenology."[60] This would allow the good "doctor" to diagnose a sitter's abnormalities "at a glance," to correct them in such a way that they "harmonized" with the rest of the sitter's face, and to determine which traits to retain in the negative to ensure that the portrait would be deemed both flattering and "truthful."[61] It was therefore common for popular manuals on retouching to include anatomical illustrations of the head and face, while insisting that the retoucher's work was still an artistic endeavor (fig. 22).

Ensuring that the "doctoring" of portraits would contribute positively to photographers' professionalization, however, required considerable work. First, something had to be done about the fact that amateur female artists performed nearly all of the retouching in portrait studios not only in Philadelphia but in cities across the country. While women continued to play a primary role in remaking the faces of studio patrons throughout the nineteenth century, photographers' trade literature consistently masculinized the figure and qualifications of the retoucher so as to promote photography's links to the male-dominated scientific profession.[62] It was not only women's hand in retouching that had to be negotiated; ironically, the popular belief that retouchers should produce

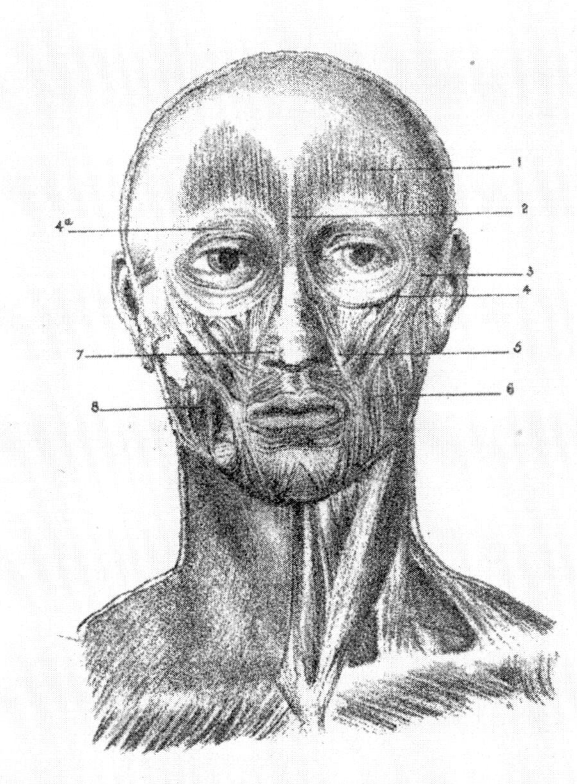

FIGURE 22 Anatomical diagram of the face, ca. 1876. Lithograph. From J. P. Ourdan, *The Art of Retouching* (New York: E. & H. T. Anthony, 1880), plate 2.

remarkable results on the order of those ideally achieved by the newest forms of reconstructive surgery had the potential to threaten studio photographers' reputation as professionals. Whereas surgeons who performed "plastic operations" during and immediately after the Civil War were careful to define them as "the reparation or restoration of some lost, defective, mutilated, or deformed part of the body" in order to establish the legitimacy and necessity of their practices, portrait photographers were increasingly expected to operate with few limitations, and often without reference to a lost original.[63]

Disagreements about the precise limits photographers should place on their retouching makeovers sparked heated arguments in the pages of Wilson's journals beginning in the 1870s. One of the most vociferous opponents of liberal retouching was the author of "Doctor Photo," Henry Snelling, who summarized the terms of these debates in 1872 by posing a series of questions to the readers of the *Philadelphia Photographer*. "If a person has an habitual freckled face, and you touch out the freckles in the picture, is the original rendered correctly? If one has high cheek-bones, do you give a correct representation of the individual by 'judiciously touching out the shadows in the negative that reproduce them in the photograph'? If one has a 'snub' nose, or a broken nose, do you make a correct likeness by 'touching out' the defect?" Snelling's response: "Certainly not."[64] Within the debate he fueled, Snelling did not deny photography's power to alter appearances; rather, he and his supporters questioned the ethics of exercising it, often citing the higher authority of "truth," which they believed was essential to photography's cultural identity and authority as a *science*.[65] Insofar as the so-called truthfulness of early photography was tied to a cultural belief in the camera's ability to record a sitter's *every* facial feature, this aspect of photographic authority was greatly challenged by the practice of "doctoring" portraits, which reminded the public that the medium was, after all, precisely that—an artful medium of *representation*. Opponents of radical retouching associated this practice with a host of other undesirable results. A doctored portrait, they predicted, could conflict with an individual's perception of her own identity, causing a sitter to point to her portrait and say, "that's not me," thereby rendering the operation a failure. This group of photographers also feared that their patrons would consistently define the "right" operation as that which made visible signs of difference virtually disappear from *any* body; if catering to vanity in this way fostered sitters' upward social mobility, they imagined, it was likely to do so at the expense of their own professional character.

That fear underlies the following list of instructions for a retoucher, which Edward Wilson published in the humor section of the *Philadelphia Photographer* in 1887. Supposedly constructed by a group of schoolgirls, the list of one hundred operations included:

No. 90.	Pug nose; pull it down.
No. 91.	Put dimple in her chin.
No. 92.	She wants a new ear.
No. 93.	Too much foot; pare it.
No. 94.	Insert teeth in her smile.
No. 95.	Cross eyed; change 'em.
No. 96.	Big nose; change to retroussé [upturned nose].

No. 97.   Too much mouth.

No. 98.   Improve bust.

No. 99.   Wants to be made pretty; doubt if it's possible; extra pay.

No. 100.   Arch eyebrows; pout her lips and fatten her arms.[66]

The indignant and clearly overworked retoucher went on to explain, "I am . . . used to being asked to put new eyebrows on a woman. But the expectations of people who get 'took' are growing to such a size that it wouldn't surprise me to have a darkey come in and ask to have his complexion made white." As fictional and obviously satirical as Wilson's joke about the photographer-dentist-executioner, this list articulates the social implications of retouching as a cosmetic operation and the anxieties they produced for studio operators. It was one thing to correct the blemishes that photography created or exaggerated on a sitter's face, they argued; it was quite another to touch out those features that were essential to the sitter's personal character, as both she and others perceived it—a character that was closely linked to perceptions of her class, race, and gender. If retouching was to authorize portrait photographers' healing powers, then the bodies in their care had to fall within broadly defined limits of normalcy; if they exceeded those limits, photography would connote artifice instead of truth and its operations would become associated with the "wrong" kind of medicine—an outcome with serious implications for what Snelling called the "photographic body politic."[67]

DEALING WITH THE PAIN: PHOTOGRAPHY AS ANESTHESIA

By imagining the studio environment as populated by diseased bodies and introducing elements of the surgical into the act of having one's portrait taken, professionalizing photographers represented their seemingly prosaic practices under the skylight as vital to the health of the studio public. Through this effort to connect photographic operations with reconstructing the "face" of the social body, however, the pain of portraiture continually resurfaced in early photographic discourse, leading both operators and sitters to ask whether photography could ever be a painless procedure. The persistence of this question throughout the second half of the nineteenth century brings us back to the posing apparatus, which we can now understand as a device designed to promote social rehabilitation—that is, to mold the body into an ideal form associated with the middle class.[68] Complicating that reading, however, are the perceived similarities between photography and dentistry with which this chapter began, as they suggest that the posing apparatus simultaneously *disrupted* the inscription of respectability on the bodies of sitters by contorting their faces and frames while disfiguring the gentlemanly and professional character of operators. As a result, studio photographers faced an unavoidable conflict in their use of this device, a difficult choice between making a pleasing portrait and maintaining the comfort and gentility of their sitters.[69]

Studio photographers' acknowledgment of this conflict accounts for another important feature of their discourse of operations, as it was constructed in nineteenth-century Philadelphia—namely, the conception of portrait photography as relying upon power relations and procedures similar to those associated with surgical anesthesia. This idea depended on the following logic: if photographers were to persuade a respectable class of patrons to trust in the healing powers of their operations, then something had to be done about their sitters' perception of pain in portraiture; like the surgeons to whom they were so often compared, photographers needed to equip themselves with the rhetorical and material means, as well as the social justification, for rendering sitters' bodies insensible to pain. Out of this logic emerged fantasies of sitters' bodies as anesthetized, docile objects, and of operators as agents of their control. These fantasies came to be seen as prerequisites for photographically remedying disease and alleviating any physical and social suffering it implied.

The impact of the introduction of anesthetics on the professional identity of American surgeons in the mid-nineteenth century is well known and shares many similarities with photographers' efforts to elevate their own social standing through analogies to anesthesia.[70] Measures taken by studio photographers and surgeons to mitigate the pain associated with their operations, for example, were both effects of and contributions to a distinctly modern obsession with physical pain as a visible marker of social dis-ease. The technology of anesthesia was, moreover, born out of a professional debate over heroic versus conservative uses of an apparatus that was considered necessary but nonetheless had the potential to disfigure the body; in the case of portraiture, that apparatus was the posing stand, while in the field of operative medicine it typically took the form of amputation instruments or a tooth-extraction kit. Debates over operating practices stood alongside a question that both photographic and medical operators faced with respect to their definitions of professional duty: does curing physical or social disease, as it was written on the body, take precedence over relieving suffering? The development of ether anesthesia (by an American dentist) and the proliferation of improved posing apparatuses in portrait studios allowed operators to accomplish both purposes, thereby increasing the likelihood that respectable patrons would willingly subject themselves to their operations and that those operations would be deemed successful. Uninterrupted by cries of agony from the bodies in their care, photographers and surgeons could then focus on the manipulations at hand and, ultimately, increase their social power.

In both surgical anesthesia and efforts to relieve the pain of portraiture, operators imagined that control over a subject was directly tied to their possession of knowledge concerning bodily pain and even of the operation itself. We can see this connection when we compare the first description of the use of ether in surgery, reported in 1846, to an advertisement for a new photographic posing apparatus published twenty years later. In "Insensibility During Surgical Operations Produced by Inhalation," Henry Jacob Bigelow, a young surgeon from Boston, recounted his experience as a witness of the first public demonstration of the use of ether. Bigelow observed that patients under the influence of the drug were "rendered completely insensible" during certain operations, including painful procedures like amputations and tooth extractions, while others were "performed without the knowledge of the patients." He went on to describe the peculiar "character of the lethargic state" resulting from inhalation: "The patient loses his individuality and awakes after a certain period, either entirely unconscious of what has taken place, or retaining only a faint recollection of it. Severe pain is sometimes remembered as being of a dull character; sometimes the operation is supposed by the patient to be performed upon somebody else."[71] The administration of ether, as described in this passage, is tied to the transfer of knowledge away from the patient, along with the translation of his subjectivity (he "loses his individuality") into objectivity (the misrecognition of his body for that of "somebody else"). This translation is accompanied by a shift in power relations and perception; as a result, the agency of the operators, their technology, and the operating theater itself replaces the loss of control observed on the patient's body.[72] Early advocates of anesthetics thus represented the loss of one's individuality as a means of protecting individuals from the "severe pain" that knowledge of the radical disruption to one's body and self would inflict upon them; in this way, anesthetics in the nineteenth century authorized operators' claims to epistemological control.

In advertisements for his new and improved posing apparatus published in Wilson's photographic journals, the renowned New York City studio owner Napoleon Sarony invoked comparisons between photographic and surgical operations in the era of anesthesia to similarly justify the control over minds and bodies that his device would make possible. Reflecting on the state of relaxation and comfort provided by his posing machine, he appealed to the public value of technological progress: "Those of you who have taken laughing gas to ease the pangs of tooth-pulling, know what an improvement it is upon the old plan." The advertisement concludes with language remarkably similar to that of Bigelow, praising the Sarony machine for its capacity to make you "forget you are having a picture taken."[73]

There were certainly different stakes associated with photographic and surgical anesthesia in the mid-nineteenth century, which point to the important differences between the two practices. According to medical reports, doctors in Bigelow's circle were merely puzzled by the fact that some anesthetized patients occasionally scowled or frowned, uttered a cry, or tried to get up from their chairs; the operation, and even the effort to relieve pain, was still a success. However, if a studio patron were to resist a photographer's efforts to anesthetize her body—that is, his efforts to make her unaware of the physically and socially transformative process she was undergoing—then that resistance would necessarily be visible in the resulting portrait. Returning to the *carte de visite* in figure 14, one might argue that the portrait functioned as the only permanent visual record of the sitter's transformation from diseased subject to object of respectability, such that a visible disruption of the photographic operation would have signified a failure of the operation itself. It was only on the relatively rare occasions when photographers were invited to enter the surgical operation room that the medical patient's transformative *process* under anesthesia was visually recorded; even then, the consistently docile surgical bodies in these photographs were represented exclusively for the eyes of medical operators, to document the success of their efforts to discipline and rehabilitate the public.[74] Early clinical photographs of anesthetized patients, most of which date from the invention of anesthesia (1846–47) and the Civil War period, also speak to the fact that the visible inscription of bodily insensibility had become a precondition of photographic portraiture by the 1860s, within both surgical and photographic operating theaters.

In their trade literature, studio photographers identified two primary methods of securing the social benefits associated with rendering sitters insensible. The first, as we have seen in the case of Sarony's advertising campaign, involved reconfiguring the material apparatus of photography and its relation to time. The technical requirements of the camera, a machine without which photographic portraiture would not be possible, determined the manner and speed with which the operation was performed, and necessitated the use of all other equipment in the studio, including the posing stand. Just as radical surgeons sought to reduce the duration of pain by working quickly, photographic operators as early as the daguerreotype period began to construct a fantasy of "instantaneous photography." In this fantasy, the speed of exposure could be increased to such a point that the camera's presence, along with the often morbid effects of its presence on the sitter's body, could be entirely erased; in Foucauldian terms, one could say that, through instantaneity, the disciplinary apparatus of portrait photography could be made to seem invisible to the bodies upon which it acted.[75]

Expressing this desire for instantaneity, one studio photographer observed in the *Philadelphia Photographer* in 1866 that the "constrained position of the sitter, as he waits with his head pressing against the iron rest, and eye fixed painfully on some designated object, interferes materially with the success of the operation." The possibility of capturing a sitter "in a natural and easy attitude, with no watchful and strained expression of face, is a great desideratum, and rarely to be secured, we think, without the instantaneous process, which would make it always attainable."[76] Another contributor to the journal, recalling his experience managing sitters in a prominent New York City studio, declared that "the present time [1871] is the most auspicious for agitating the subject," because the "long wished for time when instantaneous sittings could be made, or sittings so nearly instantaneous as to be practically so," had yet to arrive. It was only when that time did come that one could finally say "good-bye" to the "much-abused head-rest," the dreaded experience of being conscious of one's transformation into a "living mummy," and the "unnatural expressions" that these conditions produced—all of which constituted significant threats to photographic authority.[77] The idea of portraiture as social cure was therefore seen as impossible without insensibility, which implied studio photographers' complete control over and knowledge of the body; and many of them considered insensibility impossible without instantaneity, a fantasy that the material conditions of knowledge production could be made entirely imperceptible to the general public. What we find in these early discussions of photographic instantaneity, then, is the social basis of the seemingly self-evident desire for a technical development, a desire that persisted throughout the nineteenth and twentieth centuries as the speed of photography continued to increase and photographic operations came to take virtually no time at all.

The second method studio photographers used to relieve their sitters' pain and simultaneously manufacture respectable bodies for both themselves and their patrons involved cultivating an image of the operator as "a gentleman possessing great and varied conversational powers."[78] When such discourse was attached to medical models, as in the case of North's and Root's portrayals of the portrait photographer as medical case taker, its social value was twofold: while transforming the operator into a respected authority who controlled the manner in which his operations were conducted, certain modes of conversation during a sitting had the effect of removing the patron's mind from his "disease." In photographic terms, this often amounted to the eradication of dis-ease itself, together with its fatal effects on expression and posture.[79] As operators regularly noted when advising colleagues on the proper management of sitters, taking the time to listen to patrons' stories and allowing them to engage in a lively conversation with the operator on topics unrelated to the manipulations at hand was, as the British photographer H. P. Robinson bluntly put it, "the best method of having your own way at last."[80] Such conversation, in other words, created the illusion for sitters that they were full participants in the event, rather than virtual participants under anesthesia. This allowed the studio patron to imagine himself in control of his body yet forget about the operation, his peculiar abnormalities, and his resulting "pain," thereby transforming him into an affable and obliging subject willing to "believe wholly and heartily in photography."[81] Like an etherized patient on an operating table, he would ideally be compelled, in the words of Roland Vanweike, to "unconditional[ly] surrender to the photographer's superior knowledge of what he is doing."[82] Through gentlemanly discourse, the operator thus constructed the conditions under which to make his observations and diagnosis, all the while unimpeded by the sitter's attempts to influence one or the other.

The particular social benefits that early studio photographers derived from the metaphorical concept of photographic anesthesia were largely tied to their adoption of a "calculus of suffering," which, according to the medical historian Martin Pernick, was constructed by surgeons of the same period to determine which patients would receive the most (or any) anesthesia in an operation. Studio photographers, in other words, based their anesthetic treatment of individual sitters on the notion that different social types experience different sensitivities to the pain of portraiture, suggesting once again that photographic portraiture was intimately connected to social politics. White women and children of the educated, respectable classes were considered especially prone to agitation in the portrait studio, which, as figure 14 reminds us, tended to promote their disfigurement before the camera. Photographers therefore shared with the medical profession a belief that this class of patrons was the most susceptible to bodily pain.[83] While surgeons often claimed that nonwhite races, particularly the American "negro," "bear operation the best" in order to justify their practice of selective anesthesia, photographic operators and their public similarly maintained that, of all the visitors to the portrait studio, "beautiful" white bodies had the most to lose in an operation.[84] "It is difficult to lay down rules of general application," explained one contributor to the domestic magazine *Godey's Lady's Book,* "but it may be safely said that the people who come out of the photographic struggle the best, and who are least injured in the engagement, are people of ordinary appearance, from whom we do not expect much." People who were generally acknowledged as "pretty," the author reasoned, had a greater likelihood of being disappointed by their looks in a portrait.[85] Most likely to equate portraiture with pain and inspire all of the attending challenges to photographic authority, the dominant social group "required" operators to administer their most powerful anesthetics—that is, to maximize technological efficiency and comfort, as well as promote a general atmosphere of gentility through their professional discourse, bodily comportment, and manipulations. It appears, then, that in operating on the most respectable classes of patrons, studio photographers also had the most to lose with respect to social status, as well as the most to gain.

HISTORY IN THEORY, THEORY IN HISTORY

Unlike previous discussions of photography's surgical character that appear in twentieth-century theories of the photographic image, this chapter has attempted to reconstruct the complex history of the medium's resemblance to operative medicine as it emerged in the photographic literature and practices of a specific time and place: Philadelphia of the 1860s and '70s.[86] Walter Benjamin's well-known analogy between a cameraman and a surgeon, like later highly suggestive comparisons of early portraiture to surgical operations, leaves out several important features of that history.[87] Among those features is the agency that studio patrons and photographers exercised in representing portrait photography as similar to operative medicine. A critical reading of early photographic discourse shows us, in other words, that relating photography to dentistry or surgery does not measure the medium's inherent properties, as most theoretical writing on the subject suggests; rather, it constructs photography's epistemological and social character, which served the particular desires and anxieties of social actors in a given historical moment.

Second, Philadelphia photographic literature offers an alternative to theoretical conceptions of photographic authority in relation to the medium's corporeal effects. From the early writings of André Bazin to the later reflections of Roland Barthes and Susan Sontag, photographic theory consistently tells us that, since the first decades of photography's popularity, the knowledge that the camera produces indexical traces of objects themselves has accounted for a perceived equivalence between portrait and self, as well as a conception of the medium as unnaturally fixing, marring, touching, and even penetrating the body. Considered the primary marker of its ontological identity and authority, photography's indexicality thus allows the medium to produce very real effects on the bodies of its subjects. The heavy breathing, palpitations, anxious expressions, and bodily discomfort that nineteenth-century studio patrons reportedly manifested before the camera suggest, however, that it was the physical experience of sitting for one's portrait that guaranteed photography's authority on and over the body. If sitters could feel pain or even *conceive* of portrait photography as a painful surgical operation, then photography, through a further series of metaphorical relations that tie subject to likeness, could be seen as a particular kind of technology of representation—one that penetrated deeply and directly into the body, seemingly without mediation. As a result, the medium's much-discussed indexicality becomes a matter of cultural belief as well as a side effect of the pain of portraiture.

Although theory would seem to have placed the cart before the horse in seeing indexicality as a precondition of photography's authority, it complicates my historical interpretation of pain in the portrait studio by raising the possibility that such pain operated as a marker of the real. Whether as a physical sensation or a mental fantasy, sitters' perceptions of pain can be said to register an unmediated relationship between the photographic apparatus and the body and, ultimately, between the body and its photographed image.[88] According to this logic, we can read the rigid torso and pained facial expression of the boy in figure 14 *not* as signs of an unsuccessful (in the sense of unpleasing) portrait, but as testaments to the culturally constructed authority of portrait photography and its operators—a pleasing result, indeed. The same logic may explain why posing stands were used at all, once exposure times had been reduced to mere seconds after the 1850s; it would seem that the pain of portraiture had become not only a cultural expectation that sitters grudgingly endured but one with potentially positive implications for the construction of photographic authority.

The many complexities suggested by the metaphors of operative medicine generally remain uninterrogated in theories of photography, however, even though a series of contradictions can be read across this body of literature. Lev Manovich, for instance, has suggested that the introduction of the headrest into the photographic studio marks the moment at which portrait photography became surgical, thus revising Roland Barthes's earlier claim that the photography-surgery metaphor was forged in the years well *before* the apparatus was employed. For Barthes, the pain of portraiture is inherent in the process of surrendering oneself to objectification before the camera, while the headrest merely "supports" the suffering sitter in his experience of this process; the posing apparatus is not, as Manovich would argue, the instrument of torture and pain itself.[89] These authors also propose different conceptions of portrait photography as anesthetizing the body, ideas further complicated by Susan Sontag's discussion of the subject. While Barthes and Manovich attribute photography's anesthetic effects to its incapacitation and objectification of the sitter, Sontag proposes that it is the *viewer* of a photograph who becomes anesthetized. Photographs of suffering, she claims, corrupt the viewer's ability to be passionate, impairing the viewer's sensitivity; through the concept of the *punctum,* by contrast, Barthes accounts for the viewer's experience of pain and trauma in the contemplation of a photographic image.[90]

As this chapter demonstrates, the instability of the relationship between photography and operative medicine suggested by twentieth-century theory is in fact an important feature of photography's early history. I have aimed to account for this instability by acknowledging the intimate connection and tension among the identities of nineteenth-century studio photographers, patrons, and portrait photography itself, and observing that these identities were inseparable from a generally unstable social context. We have seen, for instance, how the object of comparisons to dentistry and surgery depended on who was articulating them, or whose social identity they were called upon to support. Sitters, I have argued, were drawn to the models and metaphors of operative medicine as a means of expressing their apprehension about the new technology of portrait photography and the corporeal effects of its apparatus, whereas studio photographers were largely motivated by their professional insecurities. The public's acknowledgment of photography's resemblance to medical operations therefore challenged photographers' status as respectable professionals, while photographers' discussions of that resemblance aimed to confirm their ability to produce desired radical cures. In this way it was possible for the posing stand both to function (as Manovich suggests) as an instrument of torture in the eyes of studio patrons and to "support" sitters' bodies in photographers' (and Barthes's) estimation.

The discourse of the pain of portraiture that developed in Philadelphia further demonstrates that, when it came to the social body in the Civil War and Reconstruction periods, there was a fine line between rehabilitation and debilitation, figuration and disfigurement. As a result, the perception of studio photographers as making faces and taking off heads for a living, which was underwritten by medical metaphor, placed the photographic profession in a simultaneously powerful and weak position with respect to treating the American public. On one hand, the notion that portrait photographers could "make faces" was arguably the key to their commercial success; the possibility that a trip to the photographic studio would result in the visible inscription of a desirable social identity inspired hordes of subjects to place their faces in the hands of photographic operators. The proliferation of portrait studios in major cities like Philadelphia occurred at a historical moment when the social body was believed to be in need of rehabilitation and when many Americans, particularly the middle class, promoted technologies of the body as the best means of getting the job done.

Accompanying the public's desire to have their faces and social identities remade, on the other hand, was a widespread anxiety about the physical and social trauma associated with such rehabilitation, and particularly the possibility of representing trauma in photographic portraits. This remaking could not be made visible—certainly not to others, but perhaps even not to studio patrons themselves—if newly constructed selves were to pass for "real" selves. If reconstructions under the skylight were too radical, moreover, then the markers of social difference upon which Americans relied to structure their notions of the "real" would come under threat. In this way, comparisons of photographic operations to those of medicine generated a continuous negotiation of competing analogies and desires, resulting in a paradox that framed the very idea of photographic authority in the nineteenth century. In attempting to relieve the pain of portraiture, that is, early studio photographers violently induced it; in making faces for a living, they also took off heads.

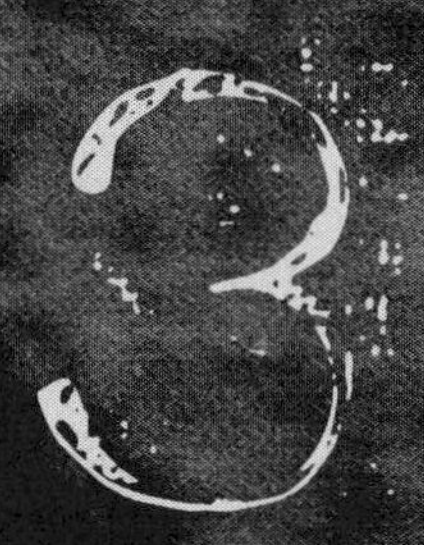

"PANES CURING PAINS"
Light as Medicine in the Photographic Studio

In 1871, the former brigadier general and Philadelphia native Augustus J. Pleasonton first shared his findings on the chemical properties of colored light with the American scientific community. Addressing his remarks to the Philadelphia Society for Promoting Agriculture, Pleasonton described a series of experiments he had been conducting since 1860 in which he tested the effects of blue light on the development of grapes and pigs. Having observed their growth in a greenhouse structure fitted with a combination of clear and blue glass, he reported that the organisms within that environment grew significantly faster and more robustly than those he placed under clear glass only (fig. 23). This dramatic difference, Pleasonton argued, was due to the fact that the blue and violet rays alone contain the "magnetic, electric, and thermic powers of the Sun"—or the "actinic" powers of sunlight that produce physical and chemical changes.[1] In his application to the U.S. Patent Office later that year, Pleasonton extended his claims about blue light's health benefits to humans, who suffered from

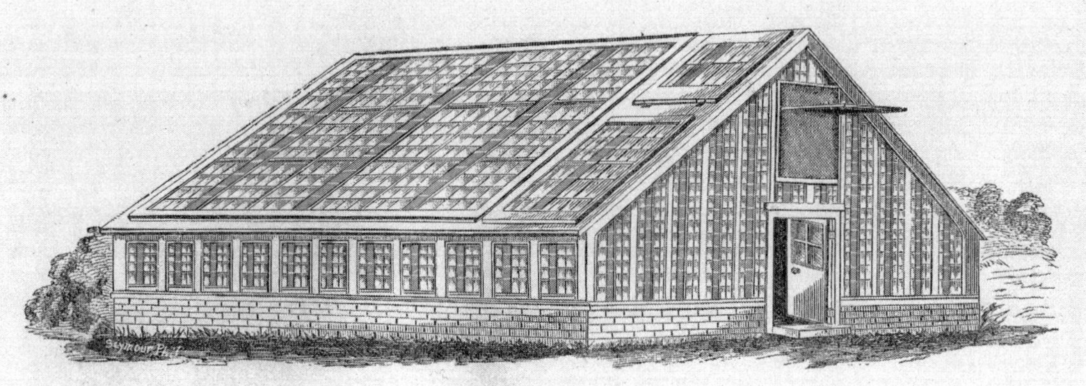

FIGURE 23 *Sketch of Gen. A. J. Pleasonton's Grapery, in the 24th Ward of the City of Philadelphia, Displaying the Arrangement of Blue and Transparent Glasses*, ca. 1876. Color lithograph. From Augustus J. Pleasonton, *The Influence of the Blue Ray of the Sunlight and of the Blue Color of the Sky* . . . (Philadelphia: Claxton, Remsen and Haffelfinger, 1876), frontispiece.

a host of ailments that the American medical profession had failed to cure. Prescribing approximately four hours a day of sunbathing under panes of blue glass, he reported that "spinal meningitis, hemorrhages from the lungs, nervous debility, partial paralysis, [and] rheumatic affections of all kinds . . . yielded to this treatment."[2] Prematurely born children grew rapidly in strength and size, the bedridden rose upon rejuvenated legs, sleep and appetite were restored after years of deprivation, and hair even grew on bald heads!

With the mass publication of these findings in 1876, news spread quickly of Pleasonton's alleged cure-all from Philadelphia to other U.S. cities, generating a blue-glass "craze" that took hold of America's urban middle class. Purchasing panes of cobalt and mazarine blue from door-to-door salesmen or commercial glass warehouses, many members of this social group transformed their drawing rooms into blue-glass conservatories (fig. 24), where they would ideally spend several hours a day luxuriating in blue light; others wore blue-glass spectacles in the hope of healing weak eyes.[3] Those with access to Philadelphia's commercial district had the unique opportunity to purchase blue-light treatments at Markoe House, a popular hotel for ladies and gentleman located at the corner of Ninth and Chestnut streets, which functioned for a short time as a phototherapeutic clinic (fig. 25). There, in Parlor B, the Philadelphia physician H. M. Beidler "scientifically administered" blue-light baths to invalids between the hours of 10:00 A.M. and 3:00 P.M.; he also sold a "portable bath" for regular use in the home, which consisted simply of a framed piece of blue glass.[4]

The support Pleasonton's phototherapy enjoyed among many outspoken and wildly popular practitioners of alternative medicine like Beidler fueled the frenzied consumption of blue glass. Some distinguished Philadelphia doctors were reportedly so impressed by its therapeutic effects (so Pleasonton claimed) that they, too, adopted

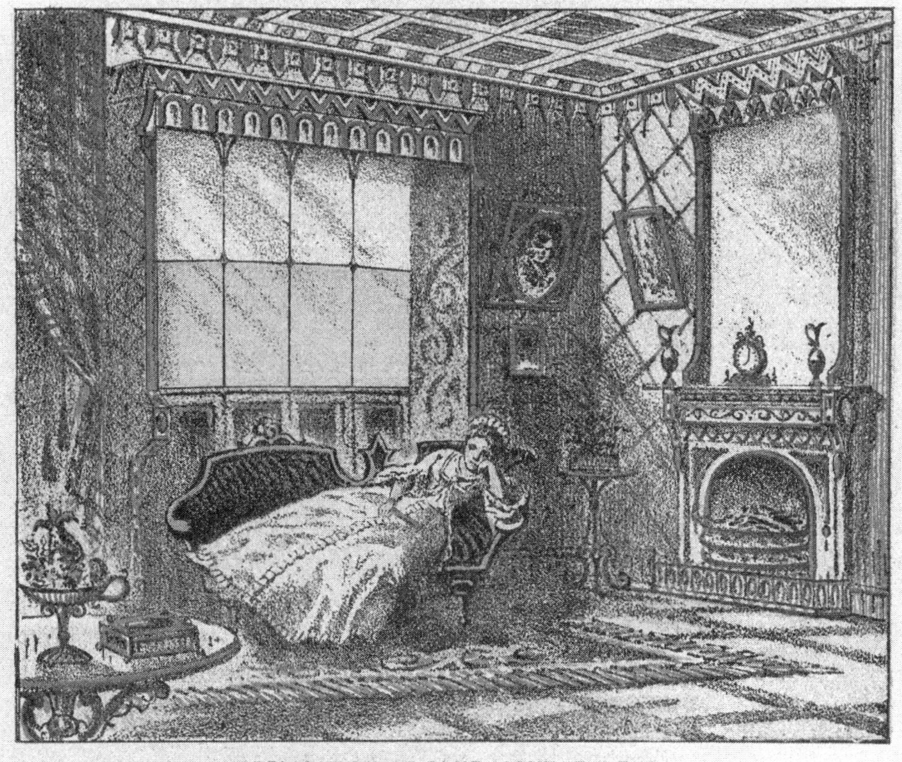

FIGURE 24 *Application of Blue Light, Full Bath*, ca. 1877. Color lithograph. From Seth Pancoast, *Blue and Red Light, or Light and Its Rays as Medicine* . . . (Philadelphia: J. M. Stoddard and Co., 1877).

the treatment as an alternative to pharmaceutical and surgical remedies in the city's hospitals.[5] Whether it ever featured in orthodox medicine, blue glass undoubtedly preoccupied professional scientific and medical authorities in the 1870s, who often described the treatment itself as an "epidemic" that plagued the American public. At the same time, it captivated the cultural imagination of middle-class city dwellers, as it became the subject of musical scores, satires, and even theatrical productions.[6]

Despite its immense popularity and controversy at the time, Pleasonton's supposed panacea has remained a rather unpopular topic among modern scholars.[7] This chapter argues for the importance of restoring it and other early phototherapies to our cultural memory by establishing their relevance to ongoing discussions of the cultural authority and social value of technologies of the body consumed by the American middle class.[8] What follows, then, is not a history of the blue-glass craze as an isolated phenomenon but the story of two technologies of light: phototherapy and studio portrait photography. This story centers on the complex relationship that first developed between these practices in the literature and visual culture of nineteenth-century Philadelphia. Unlike the surgical models and metaphors that featured in early photographic discourse, however, the idea that portrait photography and blue-light therapy constituted similar

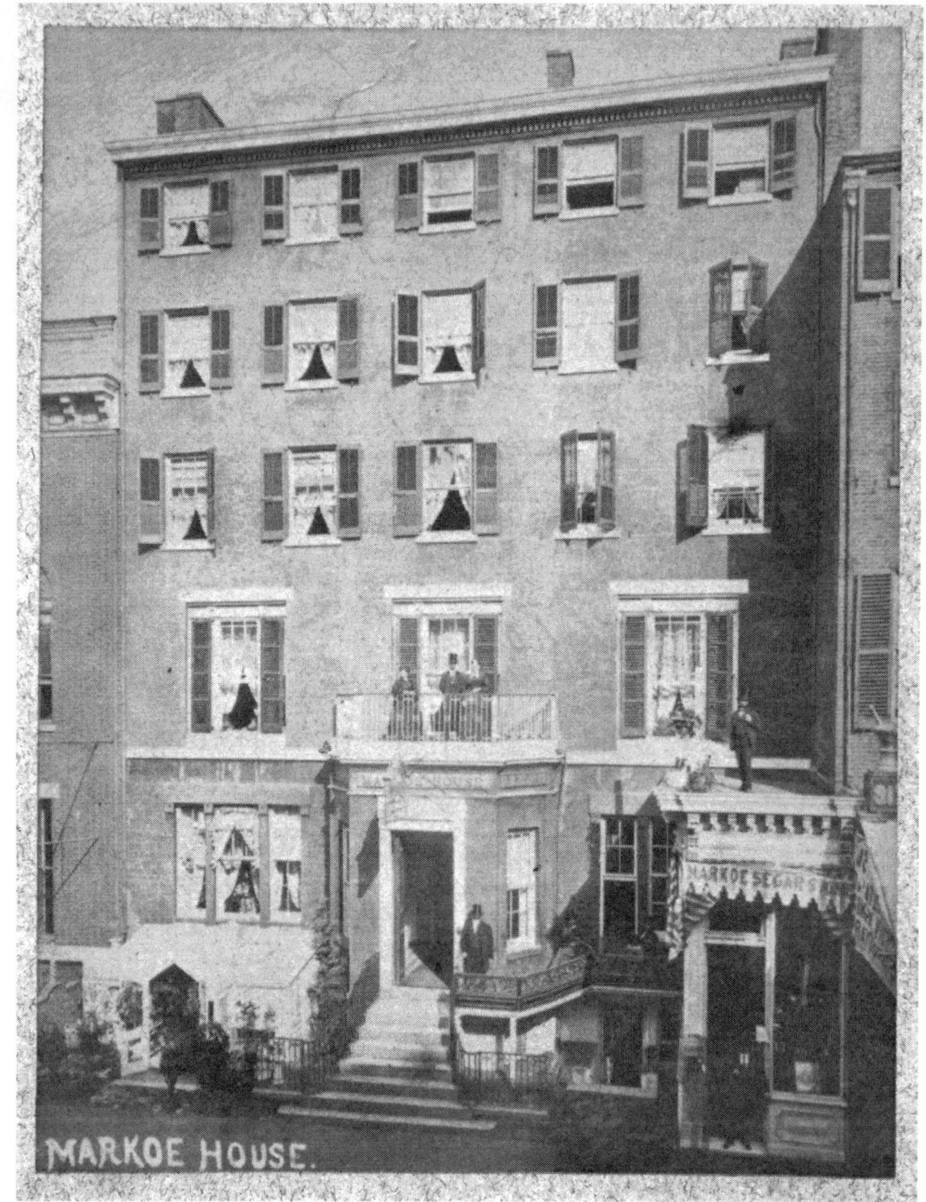

FIGURE 25 Unidentified photographer, *Markoe House, 919 Chestnut Street, Philadelphia*, ca. 1875. Albumen print mounted on cardboard. The Historical Society of Pennsylvania, Philadelphia.

methods of treating diseased bodies was never explicitly articulated by photographers or their public. The largely unspoken analogies between the two practices nevertheless structured what could be said about the light-filled urban studio, at the same time that they defined what Americans could see (or, more precisely, wanted to see) in commercial photographic portraits.

In the second half of the nineteenth century, when photographic studios were both numerous and profitable in American cities like Philadelphia, the connections between phototherapy and portrait photography were based in part on a material resemblance, one that made the physical experience of sitting under a studio skylight similar to that of sitting in a medicinal blue-light bath. Additional similarities resulted from the particular social effects that phototherapists, photographers, and their shared public desired from corporeal applications of light. These points of connection supported perceptions of photographic lighting as ridding sitters' bodies of social ills, particularly deviations from the ideal of whiteness. In the popular imagination as well as in the rhetoric and material practices of commercial photographers, portrait photography thus emerged as a powerful phototherapy that, like Pleasonton's blue glass, was called upon to rehabilitate an ailing social body in the aftermath of the Civil War.

BLUE LIGHT AND THE PHOTOGRAPHIC STUDIO

For evidence of the material similarities between photographic and phototherapeutic environments, we need look no further than General Pleasonton's 1876 treatise, *The Influence of the Blue Ray of the Sunlight and of the Blue Colour of the Sky, in Developing Animal and Vegetable Life; in Arresting Disease, and in Restoring Health in Acute and Chronic Disorders to Human and Domestic Animals.* In the only footnote in this text, Pleasonton recalls a letter to the *Boston Evening Transcript* from George Shove, a fellow advocate of phototherapy. A longtime sufferer from lung disease, Shove explains in his letter that he discovered the healing properties of blue light by accident in 1863 while on sick leave from the army and in the habit of visiting a photographic studio. According to Pleasonton, Shove observed that "the operating room of the gallery was lighted by a skylight of light blue glass, and the walls were tinted of the same colour. [Shove] soon noticed, that he invariably felt better after an hour or two passed in the gallery, and he was firmly convinced that the beneficial effect was largely due to blue light."[9]

The commercial photographic studio that Shove visited in the 1860s employed a lighting arrangement in its operating room that was typical of urban American studios at that time. Although their design and position with respect to the sun varied, all studios contained overhead and/or side skylights made of glass; in Philadelphia, they were usually situated on the top floor of multistory row houses. Such was the case at Henszey & Co., a major photographic firm whose operation room was hailed as "one of the very best arrangements and a safe model to go by" (fig. 26).[10] Henszey's primary goals in manipulating the light in his studio, like those of any early portrait photographer, were to reduce the time required to expose a photographic plate and in turn to produce a pleasing likeness of his sitter. A single principle governed these aims: the higher the light's actinism, or its potential power to effect chemical changes on light-sensitive silver nitrate, the shorter the exposure time. Studios like Henszey & Co. found that they could admit the greatest amount of the sun's actinic rays into their operating rooms, without overexposing the plate, by installing into their skylights "what is almost universally used, namely, a good article of window glass, frosted blue."[11] The presence of blue glazing and thin blue shades also reportedly filtered and softened the light that fell on sitters' bodies. According to the *Philadelphia Photographer,* these blue materials produced "a variety of soft, artistic, and satisfactory effects" in the resulting portraits.[12]

Philadelphia's photographic literature thus encouraged its readers to use blue glass in their studios well before the height of the blue-glass craze in the late 1870s. It did, however, respond to the popularity of General Pleasonton's therapy by observing the material resemblance between portrait studios with blue skylights and therapeutic blue-glass parlors, and expanding upon Shove's observations concerning the healthful properties of studio lighting. Robert Chute, a regular contributor to the *Philadelphia Photographer,* went so far as to emphasize the interest in the body that members of his profession shared with phototherapists by noting the therapeutic physiological applications of photographic blue light. "Some rather singular revelations have recently been made in this city," Chute announced in 1877, "which seem to indicate that the same property of light by which the photographic plate is impressioned, is also a very potent remedial agent for disease." Referring, of course, to Pleasonton's experiments, Chute explained that blue glass transmitted "that peculiar quality known as actinism, which possesses such chemical and medicinal properties . . . and, combining with the clear sunlight, produces the wonderful effects referred to" in Pleasonton's treatise. Chute's reference to Pleasonton and his phototherapy will probably strike the modern reader as irrelevant to the technical operations of the studio, which were the primary focus of the Philadelphia photographic press at the time. Indeed, Chute must have anticipated a similar reaction from his nineteenth-century readers, for he concluded his discussion of "health and actinism" by justifying its place in the *Philadelphia Photographer.* "We refer to this," he wrote, so that photographers "may have a more thorough understanding of

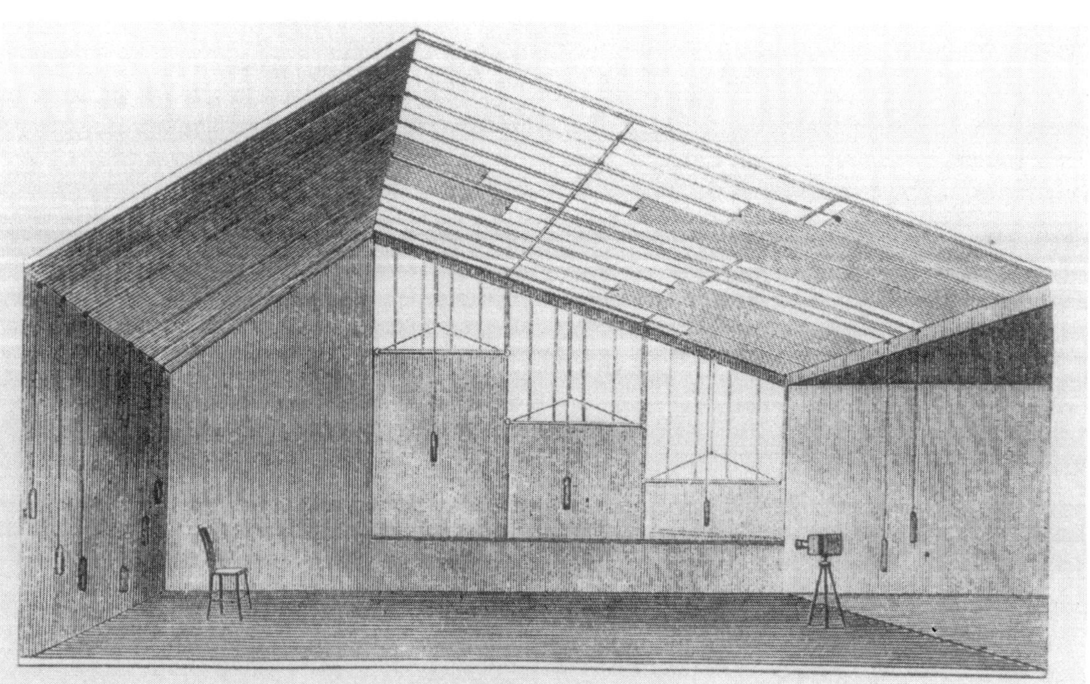

FIGURE 26 The glass-house of Henszey & Co., 812 Arch Street, Philadelphia, ca. 1865. Wood engraving. From "The Glass-House," *Philadelphia Photographer* 3, no. 30 (June 1866): 162.

the beautiful agent with which they all have so much to do and have any advantages that may be derived from it in relieving 'the ills that flesh is heir to.'"[13]

The physical "ills" associated with the early photographic studio were, in fact, many—and perhaps Chute had these in mind when describing the therapeutic benefits of blue glass. Urban Americans in the 1870s were repeatedly told that the adverse health consequences of living in an environment like the darkroom, where photographers worked under a small amount of hazy yellow or red light, were numerous and severe. The idea of living in a light-deprived room carried further connotations of mental disease; this was particularly the case in Philadelphia, where it was public knowledge that the Insane Department of Blockley Almshouse employed a "dark-room" to isolate, confine, and calm their most maniacal patients.[14] Outside the darkroom, studio patrons commonly complained that the intense concentration of rays under the skylight impaired their eyesight and, in rare cases documented by the medical profession, even rendered them permanently blind.[15] Although the studio environment often contributed to these afflictions, it also offered patrons a means of potentially remedying them, if only temporarily. According to *Scientific American,* the ability of blue glass to transmit an "exceedingly mild light" made the material particularly beneficial to the eyes, both within and outside the photographic studio.[16]

According to the so-called scientific literature on blue glass, the medium was also capable of alleviating the nervousness that people experienced in anticipation of being photographed, especially in response to the posing stand. The collection of disorders that sitters reportedly developed in the presence of this apparatus—the pained facial expressions, rigid torsos, paled or flushed complexions, and accelerated heart rate, pulse, and breathing—were not, of course, associated exclusively with portrait photography in the late nineteenth century. Rather, they were among the pathological corporeal effects associated with urban life in modern America, effects to which white middle-class women and children were seen as most susceptible.[17] Popularly diagnosed as neuralgia and neurasthenia, these "nervous and excitable conditions" were also among the "ills" that the practitioners of blue-light therapy claimed to remedy most successfully.[18]

For our purposes, what matters is not whether the Philadelphia photographic community ever marketed the therapeutic applications of blue glass but that its members widely employed a material that was part of a popular discourse on health and the body, which meant that it carried a particular set of cultural connotations into the portrait studio in the 1870s. These would have been available for a specific class of sitters to read during their experiences under the skylight, marking that space as one in which their desires for rehabilitation could take shape, even if only in the realm of fantasy. That this social group was the urban middle class, photographers' most desirable clientele, also meant that the use of blue glass endowed photographers with a considerable social "advantage," as Robert Chute had put it, helping to promote the respectability of photography as a practice and burgeoning profession.

The near ubiquity of blue panes in the city's portrait studios before the 1880s did not always support photographers' professional aspirations, however. Pleasonton's therapy, after all, figured prominently in popular discussions and visual representations of quack medicine in the years during and after the height of the blue-glass craze, among them

Joseph Keppler's *Death's-Head Doctors* (fig. 2). At the same time, Pleasonton's theories had come under harsh attack in respectable journals that were widely circulated among men of science; and it was as artists and men of science, rather than as artisans and mechanics, that photographers most often represented themselves in their professional literature.[19] Several outspoken critics of blue glass who published in the scientific, medical, and photographic press appealed directly to photographers' desires for cultural authority in the hope that they would condemn blue light as quackery.[20] The outcome of using blue light, these critics argued, would be the same for a portrait photographer or a physician—it would call into question his professional status as well as the scientific legitimacy of his theories and operations. If studio photographers were to accept the pseudoscientific theories underlying blue-light medicine, in other words, portrait photography would be placed, alongside Pleasonton's cure, "among the many burlesques of science and inductive investigation."[21] Such arguments managed to persuade a small but growing number of urban portrait photographers to rebel against the "orthodox blue." These photographers expressed a desire to align photography with institutions and knowledge that could stand the test of time, rather than with passing fads.[22]

For the middle-class Philadelphians who flocked to their city's many photographic studios and who also put stock in Pleasonton's cure, however, the authority of portrait photographers and phototherapists alike was not tied exclusively to the experimental verifiability of their theories or their endorsement by the scientific profession. Instead, these patrons expressed faith in the possibilities of portrait photography and blue-light therapy in part because of their novelty, which was tied to their *appearance* of scientism; at the same time, they demonstrated their seemingly insatiable desire for modern technologies that promised radical, rapid, uninvasive, and relatively cheap rehabilitations of their bodies.[23] Of the many media upon which the American middle class relied for this rehabilitation, technologies of light were among the most popular; they were also generally believed to be among the most powerful in relieving the physical and social ills associated with modern life in American cities. It was thus precisely their combination of the quasi-scientific, the fashionable, and the conveniently curative that contributed to the immense popularity of both photography and phototherapy in the 1870s. The authority that the urban middle class granted these technologies and their operators in matters of the body, moreover, was constructed within a wide-ranging, conflicted discourse on light, health, and social identity. It is to this discourse that we must turn in order to understand how light in the photographic studio came to function as socially therapeutic.

PHOTOTHERAPY AS SOCIAL MEDICINE

As they evolved between the 1840s and the 1880s, the idea and practices of phototherapy were tied to the development of the public health movement, which saw poor lighting, inadequate ventilation, and improper sanitation as the greatest threats to the lives of Americans, particularly those living in crowded cities. According to an 1848 survey of the sanitary condition of Philadelphia commissioned by the American Medical Association, the material changes that Philadelphians made to the city to accommodate the rapid growth of industrialization, trade, and immigration had given rise to these unhealthy living conditions. Of particular concern to the AMA was the construction of massive buildings and tenement houses along the Schuylkill River and in small courts and alleys throughout the city, which prevented light and fresh air from reaching inhabitants.[24] In the decades that followed the publication of this report, advocates of alternative and home remedies, including men and women of letters who had a stake in the health of the nation, would continue to portray the light-deprived urban dwelling as detrimental to physical and mental fitness. In his influential book *Light: Its Influence on Life and Health* (1868), the phototherapy advocate Forbes Winslow offered a common conclusion concerning the fate of American families in this period. Without the life-giving properties of light, he explained, there could "be no persistent vitality nor healthfully developed bodily structure." Under such conditions, racially white subjects became the victims of a pathological blanching known as "etiolation," which was associated with deathlike pallor, nervous disorders, emaciation, and severe physical deformity.[25]

Around the time of the Civil War, American treatises on light and health consistently interpreted these pathological symptoms as having significant social effects, on both individuals and entire populations. For Winslow, the material effects of confining middle-class whites in unhealthy urban homes were always accompanied by *"moral* and *mental"* etiolation, which took the form of "intellectual deterioration," criminality, and other threats to respectability.[26] Popular medical manuals further linked any "tax upon daylight" to "a direct tax on Public Health and National Prosperity," assuming a direct connection between the light-starved individual and an ailing social body.[27] Unsurprisingly, this assumption runs through state discourse on sanitation and public hygiene. As the *Philadelphia Medical Times* reminded readers in 1873, the surgeon general of the U.S. Army had warned Americans a decade earlier that barring light from their houses would make it "impossible to rear well-formed, strong, and robust children." Without light, William Hammond proposed in his *Treatise on Hygiene* (1863), the country could not ensure the reproduction of physically, mentally, and morally fit citizens.[28]

Although public health advocates promoted the transformation of the urban middle-class home into a light-filled environment, they also acknowledged, and often with concern, the powerful effects that changes in light could have on social identities. In his popular treatise *Human Health,* published in 1844, the prominent Philadelphia physician Robley Dunglison promoted the idea that one's environment of origin and the qualities of light associated with it are primarily responsible for determining one's physical health *and* one's "race."[29] As Dunglison put it, the "great diversity of colour in the different races of mankind" is "ascribable to the difference in the intensity of the solar rays across regional climates. . . . The difference between one, who has been for some time exposed to a tropical sun, and his brethren of the more temperate climes, is a matter of universal observation."[30] Observing that tropical climates generally yielded "darker" races, including "the Arab race" and the "negro race," Dunglison also expressed the much-debated idea that "artificial" transplantations of "dark" individuals to cold or light-deprived environments could make them appear "as white as the fairest Europeans." In the mid-nineteenth century, the most commonly cited transplantation was, unsurprisingly, that of Africans to the North American continent.

The fundamental question that drove Dunglison's observations—what was the nature of the relationship between environment and race?—would preoccupy American authorities on public health for decades. The new line of questioning that they pursued in the 1860s and '70s, and that stimulated a variety of anxious responses, asked whether changes in light conditions would alter an affected individual's "original character," which William Hammond had defined in racial terms. According to the army's surgeon general, a sun-induced blackening or bleaching of the hair and skin could *not* "cause a race of men to lose their identity," since race is dependent on certain "fixed" corporeal features such as "the form of the cranium, the shape and size of the features, and the mental organization."[31] By treating skin color as an "accessory" that could be taken on and off without changing one's "essential character," Hammond was able to mitigate the transformative effects of climate-induced changes, effects that would have destabilized contemporary perceptions of whiteness.

Other writings on light and health treated acclimatization's threat to social difference differently, ironically by emphasizing that threat in an effort to control it. "That the influence of the solar heat materially modifies the national character cannot for a moment be doubted," Forbes Winslow declared in 1868, noting that the climate, which was tied to the light conditions, of a given environment determined an individual's "physiognomy, dialect, and habits of life, as well as his mode of subsistence."[32] That certain races could develop different pigments in response to a modification in their "natural" light conditions blurred the lines between the "savage" darker races and the "intelligent" lighter races by allowing one race to take on the essential characteristics of another. Predictably, Winslow's text, published in the immediate wake of the Civil War, focused its attention and anxieties on the mutability of "the black color of the negro race." "The black pigment has been known during attacks of severe illness to be entirely absorbed," Winslow wrote, "and a white pigment cell developed in its place, thus affording a remarkable illustration of a *black person being suddenly bleached into a white man!*" Revising Hammond's conclusions, this statement suggested that a black man could actually *become* white through light-induced bleaching, albeit pathologically so.[33] The possibility of such racial reconstruction was so radically disruptive to Winslow's conception of the natural order of things that it warranted italics and an exclamation point.

Although there was disagreement about whether light could change character superficially or essentially, these writers on light and health consistently promoted phototherapy as a means of rescuing white bodies from their decrepit states, while safeguarding, and rehabilitating, the social value of whiteness. Confronted with the effects of widespread etiolation, they expressed growing concern that popular notions of whiteness as an unfailing index of physical fitness and respectability were becoming mere fantasies, without acknowledging that connections between health and social identity had always been social constructions. As Winslow's text in particular reminds us, however, the racial anxieties that fueled interest in the social effects of climate were as much about whiteness as they were about blackness. The idea of placing middle-class whites in light conditions unlike those of the relatively sun-deprived cities of North America, in other words, sought to ensure that white skin pigmentation would never replace black as a sign of physical and social disease.[34]

In his popular treatise *Life Under Glass* (1874), George Shove, who reportedly discovered the healing properties of blue glass while visiting a photographic studio, proposed what was arguably the most elaborate materialization of those fantasies: the construction of enormous structures made of steel and glass to accommodate each state's population of invalids. Shove explained to his American readers that the most destructive diseases ravaging England and the northern states of America in the nineteenth century were products of their cold, harsh climates and dramatic variations in temperature. Rather than migrate south for the winter, residents of these regions could live within isolated artificial environments that would "bottle up sunshine" and its heat, as if one were "in one's grapery or conservatory."[35] In Shove's estimation, the thousands of residents in one of these massive urban greenhouses would benefit not only from the uniform temperature and light provided by the clear glass but from an entire program aimed to promote physical and social fitness. He expected that the features of his "Winter Garden," including proper ventilation, gardens, gymnasia, libraries, easy chairs, and soothing music, would particularly appeal to white middle-class Americans. Shove's dream of providing this group with a segregated "life under glass" offered a corrective to what he and his contemporaries described as an unjust concentration of sunlight in the "less civilized" areas of the globe. While "exotic plants" and "brutes" received the health benefits of intensive exposure to the solar rays, Shove observed, the white population of northern America was needlessly lost to disease, as if it were of lesser social importance. Further, in the face of a growing influx of "Old World" immigrants to America's "hospitable shores," Shove's proposed phototherapeutic facility would ensure that the country did not waste sunlight on such "human raw material" but instead promoted the productivity, prosperity, and general happiness of its citizens.[36] Shove thus expressed the popular notion that America's natural resources and their health benefits, along with citizenship itself, should be reserved exclusively for its "native-born population."

The blue panes marketed by Philadelphia's glass manufacturers and phototherapists offered these "natives" a relatively cheap and simple means of reversing the many ills to which their bodies were prone, one that did not require mass withdrawal into an artificial environment like the Winter Garden—or even removal from one's drawing room. Following Shove's example, advocates of blue glass created a need for technologies of light by appealing to the growing anxiety that white middle-class Philadelphians were at risk of physical debilitation as well as social contamination. Not only was this group particularly susceptible to etiolation, they argued, but the city they called home attracted masses of working-class immigrants from Ireland, Germany, and other parts of Europe throughout the nineteenth century who, according to the popular and scientific thought of the period, were at best problematically "white."[37] Significantly, Philadelphia also supported the largest African American community in the north around the time of the Civil War; in 1860, the U.S. Census counted roughly twenty thousand free blacks in the city, or 3.7 percent of its total population. While there was a significant concentration of blacks in southern Philadelphia as well as in the Seventh Ward throughout the second half of the nineteenth century, their growing numbers remained largely dispersed and thus in close proximity to businesses and residences belonging to whites of all classes. As historians Michael Katz and Thomas Sugre have observed, "On the bustling streets of Philadelphia, it was nearly impossible for the well-to-do to avoid the less fortunate, for whites to avoid blacks."[38]

Before the war, the coexistence of different classes and ethnic groups in the heart of the city had led to vociferous public debates and frequent race riots. While many of these concerned Irish Catholics and Protestants, most involved African Americans, white abolitionists, and "native" Philadelphians whose support of slavery stemmed from their significant investments in the southern economy. Augustus Pleasanton himself recalled in his diary the racial violence that erupted in the city in the 1830s and '40s, which resulted in the destruction of black churches and abolitionist meeting places as well as numerous injuries and deaths.[39] The riots against blacks in this period were sparked by occupational competition between blacks and whites, public celebrations in the African American community, and even a mixed-race marriage; once the war began, and the mayor appointed Pleasonton commander of the Home Guard, such events became increasingly focused on the civil rights of free blacks. After their offer to enlist in the Union army was reluctantly accepted in July 1863, black Philadelphians fought to desegregate the city's streetcars and to exercise the freedom to vote granted to them by the Fifteenth Amendment in 1870.[40] Although they were ultimately successful on these fronts, largely owing to the efforts of the African American leader Octavius V. Catto, anti-black sentiments continued to disrupt social order in the city. Racial tensions reached a particularly violent climax during the October 1871 election. With no federal troops on hand, the local police were unable to control the fighting that broke out between white and black voters, which led to the fatal shooting of Catto.[41]

Promising remarkable physical cures and social reform in the wake of these events, those who fueled the blue-glass craze attempted to inspire hope in the idea that a change in light conditions could, as Forbes Winslow predicted, radically and essentially alter—that is, "whiten"—Philadelphia's economic and racial character. In this way, they offered an alternative to physical violence yet reinforced the belief in the superiority of "pure" whiteness that had stimulated the city's race riots and previously thwarted its abolitionist activities. The literature on the blue-glass craze articulates this aim through its emphasis on the many social indications of Pleasonton's remedy. The general had suggested these in his 1871 patent letter, in which he specified the primary reasons why one would apply to him for a license: first, for "treating diseases in hospitals, lunatic asylums, or medical practice by physicians and surgeons as a profession," and second, for "purifying the vitiated atmosphere in public schools, halls of legislation, court rooms, and other places where crowds of persons are commonly assembled in badly ventilated apartments."[42] By situating blue glass within the spaces of "professional" medicine and civic authority, Pleasonton defined the object of his patented therapy as the revitalization and discipline of an ailing social body. Others who claimed to use blue glass to cure everything from mental disease to skin abnormalities similarly linked the specific actinic properties of blue light to the rehabilitation of what Pleasonton called the "disordered or deranged." Understanding physical disease as profoundly and adversely affecting the social lives of the afflicted, these phototherapists aimed to reinsert their subjects into the larger social group, which, they argued, would ultimately contribute to the health of the nation.[43]

The racial anxieties that fueled midcentury scientific discourse on light and health certainly informed phototherapists' conception of social disorder and derangement, but it is in the many popular satires of blue glass published in 1877, which highlight the absurdity of the therapy's seemingly universal applications and limitless social potential, that we find their most colorful illustration. Modeling itself on a contemporary blue-glass treatise, one satirical book by John Carboy, entitled *Blue Glass, a Sure Cure for the Blues* (1877), transformed Pleasonton into "Brigadier-General Bottleton," an idiot-savant who claims that blue glass will remedy consumption, cure a house of its mortgage payments, and grow a tail on a horse (or its owner).[44] Although his remedy deforms or kills nearly every white subject he treats, Carboy's General Bottleton achieves remarkable results with an emancipated black slave, or a "fifteenth amendment" who "had been suffering terrible pain from softening of the brain."[45] This "awfully black individual" agrees to try bathing in the general's blue-glass facility for four hours a day, free of charge. To his benefactor's surprise and delight, the man's skin color changes visibly each day, "becoming lighter and whiter in hue. To Mulatto—or dark chocolate. Then to quadroon, like a well-browned peanut. Then to the hue of an octoroon. And then, most wonderful of all, he became white—as Caucasian as the snow of the Caucasus. . . . Blue Glass could, by its powerful influence and reflective qualities, when acted upon by the sun's rays, make an Ethiopian change his skin. . . . That 'nigger' went out of that room after his fifth sitting a white man, with a soft head and a reorganized brain."[46]

In this satire, the patient's skin decreases in its quantity of blackness by half at each stage of the treatment, as if the black pigment were bred out of him. By inducing a virtual breeding of this sort, the blue glass appears to produce Forbes Winslow's feared scenario: a black man is bleached to *become* white, dramatically cured of his racial "disease." At the same time, the satire's visual illustration supports competing claims that the essential traits of the "negro" remain unchanged, despite his transplantation to the blue-light-filled environment (fig. 27). Although the man appears "white," his body retains legible traces of stereotypically "black" features, including a broad nose, short woolly hair, and full lips. As the surgeon general predicted, the black man's skin color may be merely an "accessory"; only through an actual and infinite regression of miscegenation, as opposed to one that is photochemically induced, can the man and his progeny be cured of their blackness.[47]

Carboy and other popular critics of the blue-glass craze thus amused white urban Americans by proposing that the black body would always be recognized as pathological, despite the work of supposed panaceas like Pleasonton's phototherapy. But by entertaining the idea that blue light could cure bodies of their social difference, these writers expressed serious sentiments concerning the instability of social, and particularly racial, categories at the close of Reconstruction. As Saidiya Hartman explains in her analysis of period legislation, which aimed to define a place for the four million emancipated blacks in the American social body, these sentiments included "outrage that the bottom rail seemed to be on top, anger at the assault on white ownership of property in black persons, [and] fear that whiteness as it had once existed was endangered or doomed." Laws promoting racial segregation in cities like Philadelphia, in other words, at once expressed and assuaged anxieties about the social effects of literally "mixing" the races, or allowing blacks to become the social equals of native-born whites.[48] The freed slave in Carboy's satire articulates this prospect when he announces that as a result of his "bleachin' under de Blue Glass. . . . Dar ain't ter gwine to be no mo' niggers!" The general corroborates his claim by sending a letter to Congress offering "for two dollars a head, to bleach out the entire Negro population of the country."[49] While these statements clearly derived their entertainment value from their apparent absurdity, they ultimately delivered stern warnings to Carboy's readers. *Any* technology that promised social reform through its manipulation of light, the satire suggests, is a technology whose operators would have to manage with extreme care, lest it bring about unwanted alterations in the complexion of the nation—namely, an irreversible "whitening" of blacks and "darkening" of whites. As the Philadelphia photographic community regularly observed, studio portrait photography was no exception.

THE CURATIVE POWERS OF PHOTOGRAPHIC LIGHT

In order to explore the analogous social implications of phototherapy and photography in postbellum Philadelphia, we must remember the technical premises that these

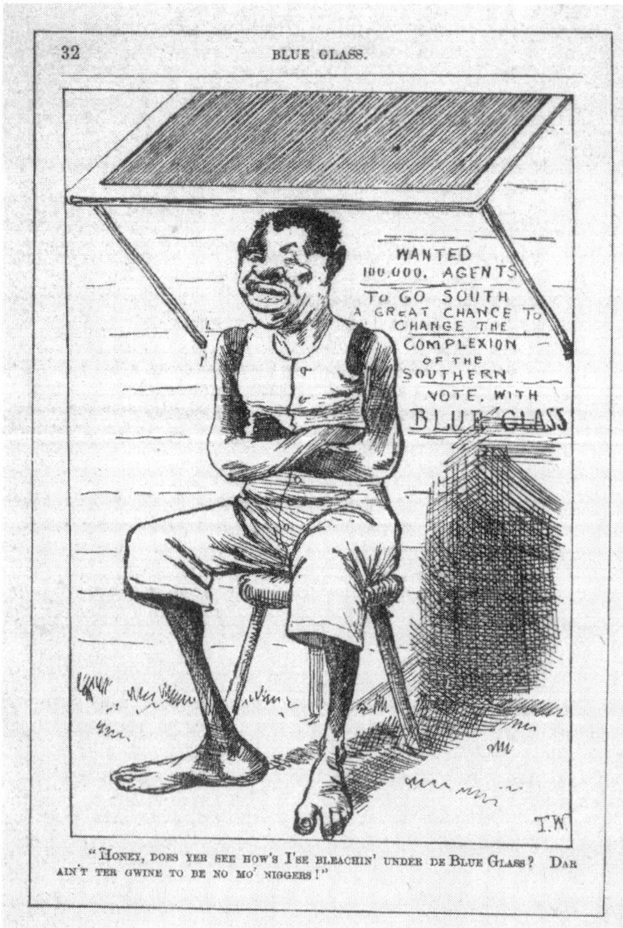

FIGURE 27 Thomas Worth, *Honey, Does Yer See How's I'se Bleachin' Under de Blue Glass?* 1877. Lithograph. From John Carboy [John A. Harrington], *Blue Glass, a Sure Cure for the Blues* (New York: J. B. Collin, 1877), 32.

practices shared. The first premise can be stated thus: when light operates chemically on a photosensitive surface, the surface retains an indexical trace of the exposure. In phototherapy, the photosensitive surface was the patient's skin, while in the case of portrait photography light operates on two surfaces: the body of the sitter and the photographic plate. Building upon this shared principle of indexicality, the second premise concerns the degree to which a body darkens in the presence of light. Both early photographers and phototherapists assumed that the degree of darkening depended on the photochemical properties of the solar rays as well as on the body's unique ability to absorb light. By exposing a body to light under blue glass, they aimed to alter its absorptive properties, thereby changing its relative lightness or darkness. A phototherapist would typically apply blue light to an etiolated patient to increase her body's absorption of light and subtly darken her deathly pale skin. A studio photographer could likewise darken, but most often whiten, the appearance of his sitter's skin by manipulating the lighting conditions of his operating room and then controlling the development of the resulting portrait. Such alterations performed in a blue-light clinic or portrait studio promised a remarkable rehabilitation of an individual's physical and social health, since the visible effects of light on the human body, or the degree to which it appeared "white," functioned as an index of a person's physiological condition *and* social identity.

In developing a vocabulary with which to describe the effects of photographic lighting on bodies, Philadelphia's photographic literature suggested a similar resemblance between portrait photography and photomedicine based on the social effects of their physical transformations. Consider the particular qualities and properties of photographic lighting that Hermann Vogel proposed in *The Chemistry of Light and Photography* (1875). Light, Vogel explained, can produce either "chemical" changes, whereby bodies become essentially different materials, or "physical" changes, which alter the appearance of a body while its substance or matter remains the same.[50] According to commercial portrait photographers, much of their work in the operation room was aimed at preventing the "physical" effects of sunlight on sitters' bodies from developing into "chemical" effects. By using light to reduce the shadows or tan on a gentleman's face, in other words, they aimed to represent his "original" (or racial) whiteness in the resulting portrait, thereby preventing a change of pigment from becoming a change of race. This is not to say that operations under the skylight never led to "chemical" changes that fundamentally transformed sitters' self-presentation. In fact, radical changes in social class were reportedly what patrons most desired from their sittings in the portrait studio, transformations that could be achieved by making their dress, pose, and even skin color conform to ideal norms. As Vogel put it, "The rascal wishes to appear an honourable man in his picture . . . the maid-servant plays the fine lady in the atelier; the tradesman's daughter would be a court lady, [and] the street-sweeper a gentleman."[51]

The social rehabilitations that Vogel describes in this passage bear a striking resemblance to those promised by blue-light therapies, in both satirical and scientific literature. There is, however, an important distinction between portrait photography and the phototherapies marketed in the 1870s, which stems from the unique characteristics of photography as a medium of representation. Since light in the portrait studio operated on two photosensitive surfaces (the body of the sitter and the photographic plate or print), photographers could offer patrons "physical" (or nonessential) changes to their bodies under the skylight, while also providing them with visual evidence of the remarkable "chemical" (or essential) changes they supposedly desired. The photographic print could therefore signify a change in race and class, recording a light-induced rehabilitation analogous to that of a phototherapeutic treatment, but the sitter could leave the studio with his body intact and unaltered. Even though photographers' whitening or darkening of bodies occurred within the space of representation, their operations nevertheless had to be carefully negotiated so that a visit to the portrait studio would be seen as socially therapeutic rather than socially threatening. This is largely because we are encouraged to read a photograph as an indexical trace of a sitter's body—a reading that contributes to the realist fantasy that the subject *himself* has been permanently rehabilitated, or debilitated, by his exposure under the skylight. Cultural belief in a direct relationship between photograph and skin thus allows for an individual's appearance in a portrait to be seen as an imprint of his physical and social condition.

Within their trade literature, Philadelphia photographers obsessively discussed the challenges they faced in lighting studio sitters, which stemmed from this perceived relationship between image and body, on the one hand, and health and social identity, on the other. On the whole, their observations about light speak to the pathological status of nonwhite bodies upon which photographic practices have been predicated since the 1840s.[52] Throughout the nineteenth century, the classification system they used to determine the "difficulties" individuals presented with respect to studio lighting relied primarily upon perceptions of racial difference. In 1868, *Photographic Mosaics* summarized this taxonomy of race under the skylight with the following "hints on lighting": in order to preserve a sitter's "roundness" and "fairness," one must employ a "full exposure" on the body, but the light must not be intensified "to any great extent"; when photographing "darker individuals" with "prominent features," however, "a much greater body of light, with more diffusion, will soften down the strongly-lined features, and so produce a more pleasing likeness."[53] The specific arrangement of top and side lights that a studio photographer would employ on a given subject therefore depended upon the degree to which the sitter conformed to the characteristics stereotypical of a robust white gentleman, a man with a "rather fair complexion," "regular features," and "standard nerves."[54] In this way portrait photographers, like phototherapists, allowed the degree of exposure a sitter "required" to function as an index of his social identity and its particular deviations from a standard picture of health—but with one important difference. Since the bodies of light-complexioned sitters would imprint themselves on a photographic plate more rapidly and were more likely to yield a "healthy" print than those of dark-complexioned sitters, white skin was understood as an unequivocal technical advantage in the early portrait studio. It was almost impossible for a sitter's body to be *too* white, or for whiteness itself to operate in early photographic discourse as anything other than a sign of physical and social wellness.

Two highly conventional portraits of African American sitters allow us to illustrate visually the long history of photography's pathologizing of dark skin: the first is an albumen print from the mid-1860s of a Philadelphia waiter named William Lancaster (fig. 28); the second, a cabinet card of an unidentified sitter taken by William Withers's studio, which operated on Chestnut Street in the 1890s (fig. 29). In the details of both photographs we can see the effects of the photographers' labors as they attempted to produce "pleasing" portraits of their racially black patrons. In addition to dressing the men in proper clothing to portray their respectability, each photographer exposed his sitter's body to the chemical effects of studio lighting to the degree that his dark eyes and skin would have "required"—that is, at a much greater intensity than with white patrons. The effect of this treatment is a visible whitening of each man's skin, so much so that there is little distinction between the background, which we are to read as naturally white, and the sitters' faces. The two photographers took different measures, however, when it came to making visible their efforts to cure these African American men of their social "disease." Like many albumen prints of black sitters taken in the 1860s, Lancaster's portrait has been heavily retouched on the surface of the print, with dark areas added to define the outlines of his hair and suit, compensating for the overwhitening of his body; his moustache and eyebrows, which would have received the same exposure as Lancaster's face, have been almost entirely redrawn. The Withers cabinet card, by contrast, visually documents the side effects of the sitter's photo treatments through the bleached appearance of his tie and collar. One could say that these bleached details represent the cost, as it were, of the black sitter's prolonged exposure in the studio; they are the largely unavoidable results of his social rehabilitation.

The modern viewer is left to wonder whether the light-induced rehabilitation of racially nonwhite subjects was deemed necessary by photographers alone, regardless of their own racial identities, or whether it was desired by the subjects themselves. This question of who controlled the photographic representation of black sitters has been at the center of scholarship on early commercial portraits of African Americans, much of which has celebrated the opportunities for positive self-making that the medium of photography uniquely provided them. Most consistently, Deborah Willis has pointed to the "counterimages of African-American life," or the "images of dignity, pride, success, and beauty," which contradict dominant racist stereotypes, produced by both black and white commercial photographers in the second half of the nineteenth century. It was through studio portraiture, Willis argues, that black sitters were able to control how they were portrayed, often improving perceptions of their social class and idealizing images of their race as a whole.[55] The pathologizing of black bodies in discussions of early photographic lighting complicates faith in the positive impact of photography on the black community after emancipation. While it would be a mistake to assume that all African American sitters entered commercial photographic studios with the intention of making themselves "white," they always ran up against the fact that the technical success of photographic operations was predicated on the presence of a light-complexioned body before the camera. For this reason, historians of photography should be wary of reading even the most seemingly honorific portraits of African American sitters as unproblematic instruments of agency.

My reading of the Lancaster and Withers portraits suggests that commercial group portraiture was a particularly rich, yet generally untapped, source of racial anxiety in early photographic discourse, given that the complexion of each sitter who entered the studio necessitated a different diagnosis and light treatment. The "difficulty," as photographers described it, was producing a healthy print without overexposing "the light-complexioned subject" or "underexposing the darker subject."[56] James Cremer avoided this difficulty in his portrait of the Arms family, taken in his Philadelphia studio (fig. 30), since their fair complexions required roughly the same exposure time to portray the whiteness of each family member. The photographer H. J. Rodgers recounted in his popular memoir a very different case, however, one in which a studio operator was asked to photograph a "gentleman of dark brown complexion and black hair" with "two ladies of blonde complexion and hair." When the operator presented the picture to the group, the dark-skinned sitter declared the portrait

> "horrid! altogether too dark and the ladies too light" and at the same time with an air of dignity taking a faint, indistinct vignette card picture of himself from his pocket, "There! that's white. I want mine in the group white as that." . . . The artist politely informs him that all things are *not* possible with a photographer; that by sitting him *alone,* with a view of producing a "white picture," he would be required to sit longer. The clear white and rosy complexion of the ladies did not require *one half* as much time in the light, as his dark hued features, black hair and coat absorbing the rays of light.[57]

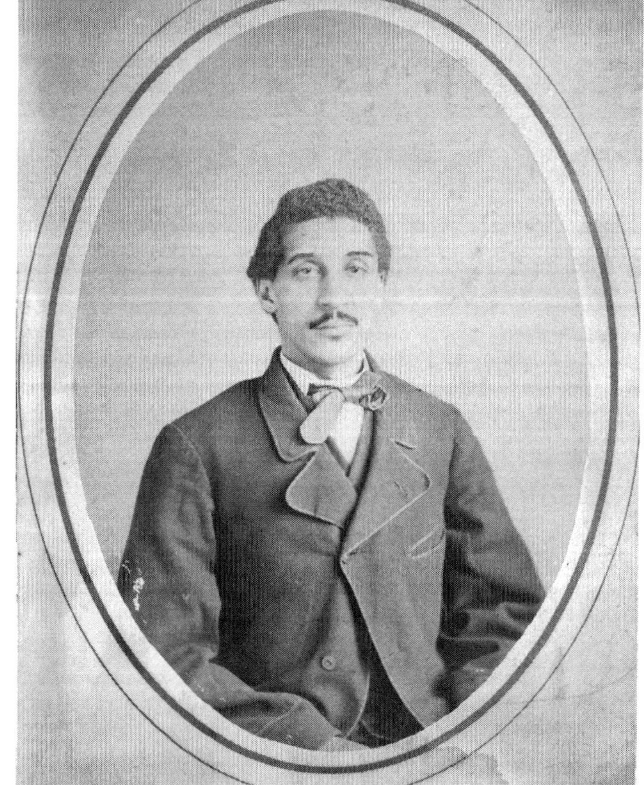

FIGURE 28 Unidentified photographer, *Portrait of William I. Lancaster,* ca. 1865. Albumen print mounted on cardboard. From *Portrait Album of Well Known Nineteenth Century African American Men of Philadelphia, 1865–1885.*

As we see in this exchange, the fact that studio patrons expected photographers to "whiten" their bodies became a professional problem when the public failed to recognize the limits of photographers' ability to foster social transformations. Although most urban photographers in postbellum America offered their services to sitters of all complexions, there was a point at which the reconstructive powers of studio lighting no longer contributed to the popularity of photography but opened it to charges of quackery. As satires on the blue-glass craze warned the middle class, the social outcome of bleaching the black population was a deeply undesirable darkening of whiteness itself, which threatened the stability of social categories and the visibility of difference. Similarly, the photo treatment that would cure the dark-complexioned sitter could compromise the racial identity, and hence the social health, of his white companions, not to mention threaten the professional reputation of the photographer. Many photographers felt that the best way to avoid such an outcome *and* ensure that each sitter received the treatment that he or she "required" was to subject the group to a lighting scheme "proper" for the white bodies, remove those bodies from the picture, and then complete the exposure.[58] They might also avoid such groupings altogether, and the extant

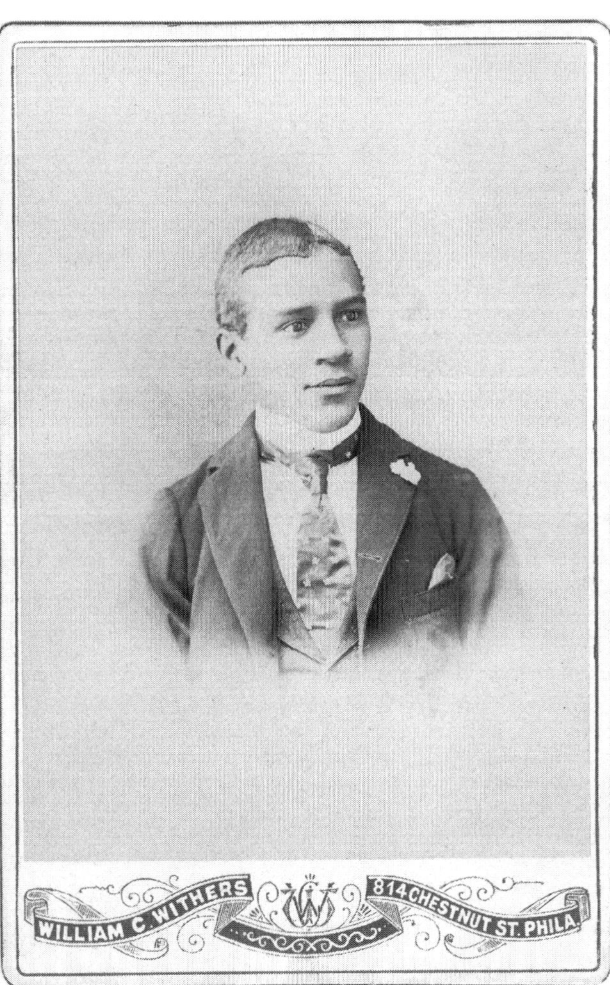

FIGURE 29 William C. Withers, portrait of an African American man, ca. 1890s. Albumen print on cabinet card mount. Private collection.

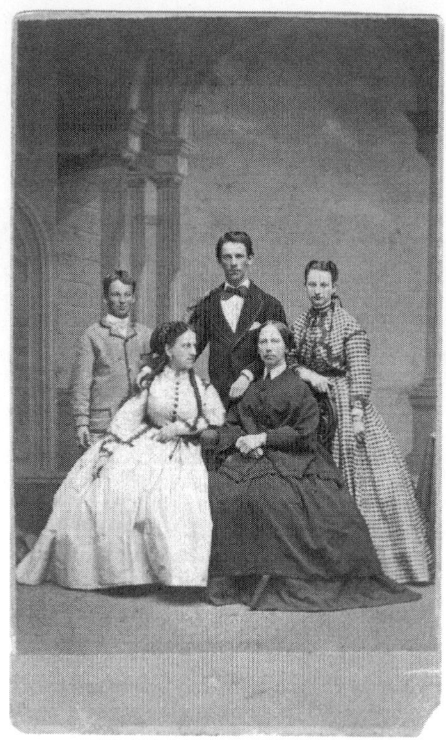

FIGURE 30 James Cremer, portrait of the Arms family, ca. 1865. Albumen print on *carte de visite* mount. Private collection.

photographic record shows that they generally did. In this way, the technical require-ments of the portrait studio supported dominant anxieties associated with mixing differ-ent races within the American social body that found popular expression in the Civil War and Reconstruction periods.

A significant exception to the photographic segregation of blacks and whites was the practice of depicting white children with their black caretakers. Rather than express a utopian vision of racial equality, the black skin of the servants literally frames the bodies of these children, allowing them to perform their whiteness. In figure 31, the Philadelphia firm of W. L. Germon made an exposure "proper" to the African American subject, one that ensured that her blackness made visible the social superiority of the white family who commissioned the portrait.[59] Beyond this peculiar practice, however, the Philadelphia photographic community ascribed a particular urgency to photographic segregation, and indeed to the very practice of portrait photography, when it came to posing white babies. Since the whiteness of the child's skin ideally functioned as a stable sign of social dominance, its exposure to light both in and outside the portrait studio was an operation that had to be handled with considerable care. Typically posed alone (or with their crudely concealed parents) and dressed in a sea of white clothing, white children were exposed to such a degree that their skin appeared unnaturally light, if not translucent, in the resulting picture. In a conventional *carte de visite* portrait such as figure 32, the child's left arm is almost indistinguishable from her white dress, both of which function as alibis for the whiteness of her mother, who crouches behind the chair; for (albeit rare) material evidence that this photographer was especially concerned to

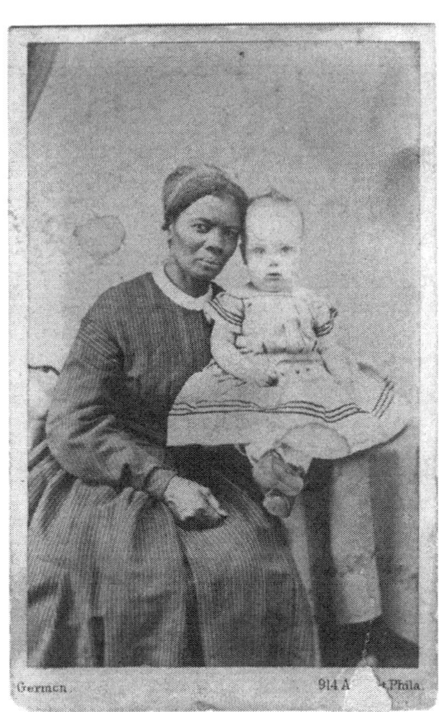

FIGURE 31 W. L. Germon, portrait of a servant with baby, ca. 1865. Albumen print on *carte de visite* mount. Private collection.

portray the child as "white," we need only refer to the note he inscribed to her parents on the verso, which explains that the barely decipherable "spot on her face is in the paper"—that is, not inherent in the subject—and "the picture can be made without it." In other cases where patrons insisted on a family portrait, as in figure 33, photographers could selectively expose areas of the print to light so as to avoid what one Philadelphia operator described as the "evil arising from difference in exposure."[60] Despite such efforts to preserve—one might even say promote—the whiteness of each family member, however, studio photographers generally represented babies as glowing white objects that lacked the corporeal delineation of their darker parents.

With respect to the representation of white children, portrait studio practices in the second half of the nineteenth century thus seem to contradict writing on light and health from the same period, which typically warned parents that their children's bodies were becoming *too* white, even cadaverous, as a result of insufficient light and air in American cities. Such warnings were common in Philadelphia in the 1870s, when public health officials pointed increasingly to the environmental factors that contributed to the city's significant infant mortality rate.[61] The few instances in which photography is explicitly mentioned within the literature of phototherapy, however, suggest otherwise. Their authors, in fact, envisioned a scenario in which the portrait studio could be seen as a therapeutic environment for white children by creating a distinction between studio lighting and its visible effects in photographic portraits; that is, they implicitly acknowledged that portraits of glowing white babies resulted *not* from depriving little ones of light but from exposing them to a considerable, and indeed a healthy, dose of the sun's rays. In an article that was reprinted in several American treatises on phototherapy

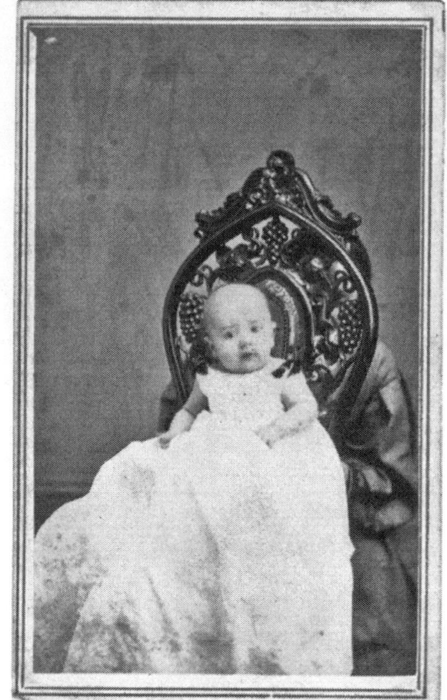

FIGURE 32a–b Draper & Husted, portrait of a baby, ca. 1865. Albumen print on *carte de visite* mount (recto and verso). Private collection.

from the 1860s, one British physician went as far as to propose a remedy for the urban epidemic of etiolation that involved modeling urban nurseries on photographic studios: "When we see the glass-rooms of the photographers in every street high up on the topmost story, we grudge them their application to a mere personal vanity. Why should not our nurseries be constructed in the same manner? If mothers knew the value of light to the skin in childhood, especially to children of the scrofulous tendency, we should have plenty of these glass-house nurseries, where children may run about in a proper temperature, free of much of [their] clothing."[62]

This transformation of the early portrait studio into a pediatric health facility attributes a newfound social purpose, as well as a medical justification, to the seemingly superficial craze for photographing children. Rather than serve "mere personal vanity," the light-filled environment of the studio, according to the distinguished physician, could offer countless little ones phototherapeutic treatment, if only for several minutes. The technical requirements of photography that would make this possible could also help offset what was seen as an unfair advantage conferred by nature onto "savage" races, whose children were believed to enjoy good health thanks to their frequent exposure to the sun.[63] These texts thus suggest that lighting a child's body had profoundly racial implications—implications, I would add, that have contributed to the popularity and social importance of American portrait photography, both then and now.[64] Although it is unlikely that nineteenth-century Americans ever mistook photographic studios for phototherapeutic clinics, photographers offered white middle-class patrons a means

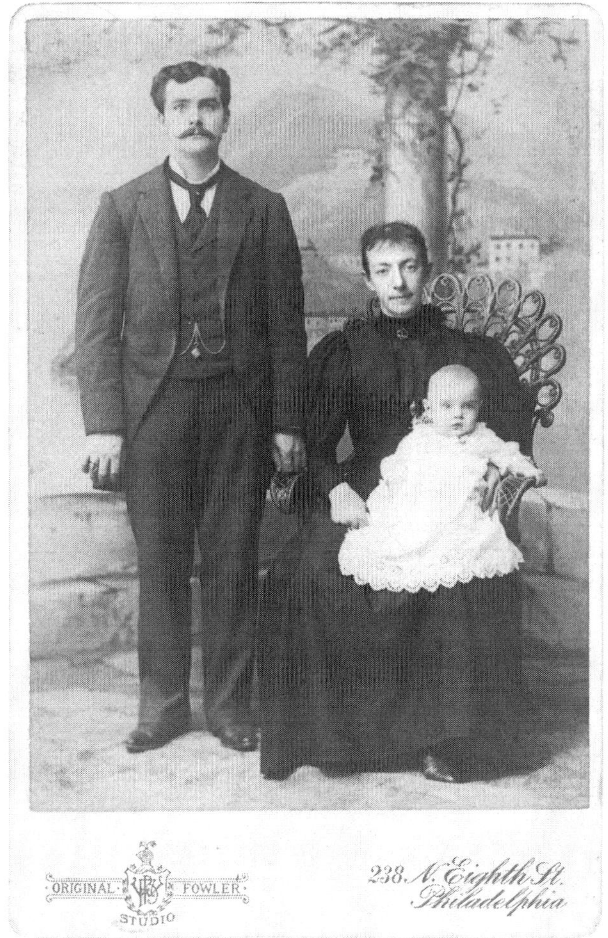

FIGURE 33 Fowler Studio, portrait of a family with baby, ca. 1892. Albumen print on cabinet card mount. Private collection.

of stabilizing their social identities by representing a robust and fully developed race of urban children. The social goals of photographing young Americans therefore resembled those of subjecting them to blue-light baths.

CURTAILING QUACKERY

Despite its potential contributions to public health reform and its efforts to rehabilitate racially marked bodies, photographic lighting routinely failed to produce socially desirable results. As photographers often observed in the 1860s and '70s, an excess of top light could make "prominent in the face all the most unlovely features" in addition to casting deep black shadows that disfigured the head and body of a sitter and in some cases called into question his racial identity.[65] Even in the absence of such effects, a growing expectation of photography to represent bodies "as they were" and to embody subjects themselves inspired feelings of revolt in some sitters who examined their exposures. Like practitioners of blue-light medicine in this period, studio photographers always ran the risk that the public would condemn their work as quackery if their photo reconstructions contradicted a sitter's perception of his own (always idealized) physical and social health.

According to the Philadelphia photographic community, such responses might be avoided if photographers, rather than studio patrons, possessed intimate knowledge of the social transformations inherent in photographic processes. Using the photographic negative as a metaphor for those processes, Hermann Vogel suggested that the racial changes sitters involuntarily underwent under the skylight should *never* be made visible to a given subject or to the general public. "However interesting . . . a negative could be, it could not satisfy the purchaser of a portrait, because it showed everything reversed," Vogel explained. "No one would hang up on his wall a picture representing him as a Moor."[66] If such undesirable racial reversals became commonly associated with portrait photography, then the professional character of the popular technology that American photographers cultivated would probably be tossed out with the offending picture, along with public faith in photography's truth effects, its cultural authority over the body, and its growing importance to affirmations of white middle-class identity. The light-induced social changes that helped define the medium of photography in the nineteenth century were therefore precisely what threatened to undermine it—if, that is, they did not remain sufficiently contained by the photographic medium *and* its practitioners.

Reading nineteenth-century discussions of phototherapy alongside contemporary writings on photographic lighting thus shows us how ideas about sunlight, race, and health shaped studio photographers' power to remake bodies and social identities. It further demonstrates that such power was not constructed without significant effort and contradiction, given that light and its social effects were the objects of much optimism and much anxiety in the scientific and popular discourse of the period. Studio photographers and phototherapists in Philadelphia responded similarly to the collective desire of the middle class for rehabilitation during Reconstruction. Those who frequented portrait studios in the city or luxuriated in their own blue-paned drawing rooms, in turn, put their faith in the idea that filtered sunlight could restore health to white bodies. At the same time, the quick cures that technologies of light promised patrons posed a serious threat to "native" whiteness. The rays of the sun, after all, had dramatically different effects on bodies of different races and classes, which made their universal application potentially hazardous in a social sense. While light could rescue etiolated bodies from their pathological state, moreover, it also had the potential to close the perceived gap between the races, thus threatening to break down the crucial boundaries that defined social difference. As a result, phototherapeutic and photographic light had the power to darken and lighten, compose and decompose, as well as physically and chemically alter the complexion of a nation.

What was particular to commercial portrait photography, then, was its promise to conceal, if not entirely erase, the perceived social drawbacks associated with "exposing" the American public on a mass scale; this promise shaped the cultural authority of portrait photographers and their medium, rescuing them from the fate of Pleasonton and his blue glass, which twenty-first-century Americans have almost entirely forgotten. In their professional rhetoric and material practices, the Philadelphia photographic community attempted to represent the corporeal application of photographic light as having only socially therapeutic effects for the bodies in its care. Whether studio photographers communicated this successfully to their public, they sought to ensure that analogies between studio lighting and phototherapy would legitimize their professional identities and endow photographic representation with enormous social potential—namely, the potential to replace the darkness and disease plaguing urban Americans with lightness, whiteness, and health.

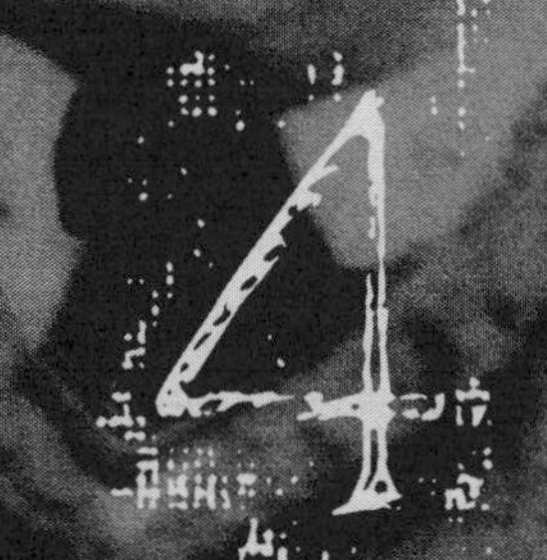

A MATTER OF PUBLIC HEALTH
Photographic Chemistry and the (Re)production of Healthy Bodies

The relationships between commercial portrait photography and the practices of operative medicine and phototherapy in nineteenth-century Philadelphia share an important focus in shaping perceptions of operations under the skylight. There, photographers posed and lit bodies in a setting modeled on the ideal domestic parlor, which encouraged studio patrons to perform their respectability and whiteness before the camera. Henry Snelling's "Doctor Photo" takes us out of the genteel, light-filled environment of the glass house, however, and into an area immediately adjacent to it that was constructed exclusively for the operator: the photographic laboratory. Typically measuring no larger than eight by ten feet, the principal space in that laboratory was the darkroom, where the photographer performed chemical operations on light-sensitive materials. Given the nature of this work, the only light that could enter the room was that provided by a window with yellow or red glass, or by a lamp that offered similar illumination. In place of the finely upholstered furniture, framed portraits, and velvet curtains of the studio, it contained a dizzying array of chemical apparatuses, including sinks, tanks, funnels, beakers, and dishes. Bottles were arranged on shelves or in a cupboard or adjacent chemical storeroom; these were designed to hold sensitizing, developing, and fixing solutions, which emitted their vapors into the air.

Among the visual representations of the photographic laboratory published in the second half of the nineteenth century, the wood engraving in figure 34 was among the most widely known. It first appeared in Gaston Tissandier's *History and Handbook of Photography* (1876), which quickly became a standard reference book in both American and international photographic circles, and was reprinted several years later in Edward Wilson's practical manual, *Wilson's Photographics* (1881).[1] While presented as an "admirable model" that showed readers what a darkroom looked like, the illustration is remarkable for what it does not, and arguably could not, represent. The rigorous linear perspective and the positioning of the viewer at the center of an invisible fourth wall encourage him to see the room not as a confined space but as one that extends well

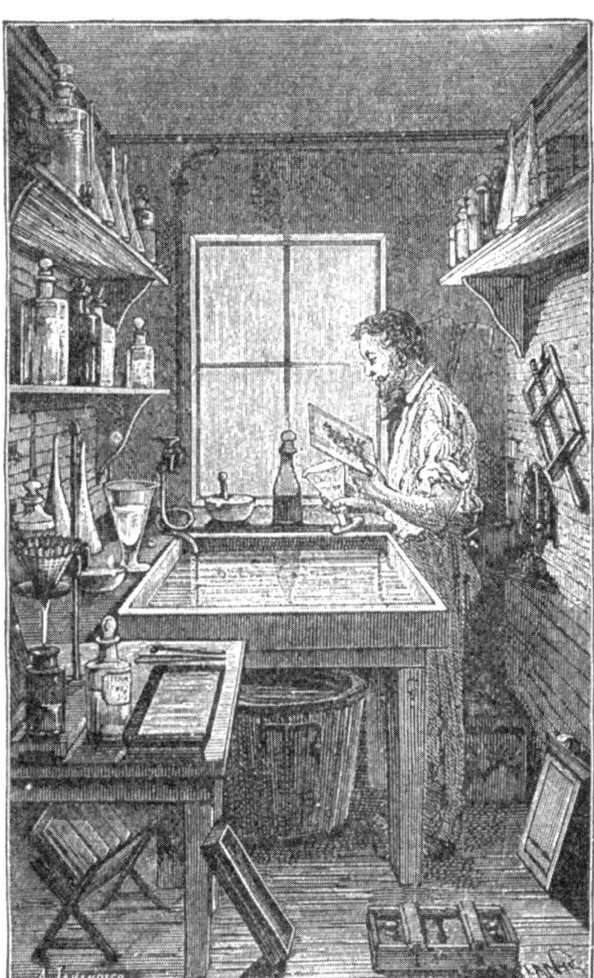

FIGURE 34 Interior of darkroom, ca. 1874. Wood engraving. From Edward L. Wilson, *Wilson's Photographics; A Series of Lessons, Accompanied by Notes, on All the Processes Which Are Needful in the Art of Photography* (Philadelphia: Edward L. Wilson, 1881), 91, fig. 34.

beyond the limits of the picture frame. The central window, moreover, ensures that this "darkroom" is anything but dark, precipitating Wilson's observation that it is "supplied with rather more [light] than properly belongs to the work" performed therein.[2] Illuminated for the viewer is an impossibly well-ordered space in which neatly stopped bottles contain the fumes of highly flammable and poisonous chemicals. Shown washing a newly developed print, the operator displays no evidence of having spent hours a day absorbing these substances; the skin exposed by his rolled-up shirtsleeves is free of dark stains or ulcerations, while his body appears physically erect and able. Taken together, these details contribute to a highly idealized vision of a modern laboratory embraced by the American middle class, one that imagined a man of science working patiently and carefully to maintain control over his delicate manipulations.[3]

Missing from this illustration is everything that threatened to invade the darkroom, and precisely what the Philadelphia photographic community worked hard to control at the time of its circulation. In the 1870 issue of *Photographic Mosaics,* Edward Wilson gave this threat a name: *dirt.* Invoking its once common definition as "matter out of place," he used the term to describe everything from impure air, water, or chemical baths, toxic chemical fumes, dampness, and dust anywhere, to aspects of the operator himself, such as a lack of patience or attention.[4] As Mary Douglas famously argued in *Purity and Danger* (1966), this traditional definition of "dirt" more generally implied the existence of "a set of ordered relations and a contravention of that order." It constituted, in other words, the "inappropriate elements" that must be excluded from a system of ordering and classifying matter so that matter would have integrity and meaning in a given social context.[5] Portraying the darkroom and chemical storeroom as spaces of potential danger and pollution, Wilson's discussion of "matter out of place" expresses such a desire for organization and system in laboratory operations aimed at carefully controlling two movements: first, that of matter in and out of the body, as in the absorption of chemicals through the operator's skin and lungs; and second, that of bodies and matter in and out of the space itself, as in the wafting fumes of ammonia and ether. Allowing the chemical contents of the photographic laboratory to escape their strictly defined boundaries had profound consequences for bodies in the portrait studio as well as for the social order that space ideally embodied. At best, such transgression interrupted the parlorlike atmosphere and fantasies of bourgeois respectability that operators and sitters cultivated under the skylight; at worst, it caused physical debilitation or even death.

While Douglas's analysis focuses on pollution rituals in primitive religions, Wilson's reflections on "dirt" support her observation that defining and maintaining the boundaries between order and disorder continue to have an important and highly symbolic place in modern Western culture. They further support Douglas's claim that "dirt avoidance" for modern subjects has been bound up with the discourse of public health, and more specifically with ideas about "pathogenicity and hygiene."[6] On the pages of *Photographic Mosaics,* Wilson referred to such concepts as metaphors and models for laboratory work; "dirt," he explained, is "a chronic *disease* with which [photographers] are afflicted—a *sickness* which they seem to enjoy, judging from their work. . . . Nothing but the utmost care and cleanliness and watchfulness will rid us of it."[7] Others in the Philadelphia photographic community made similar references in their discussions of darkroom operations, connecting the "dirty" appearance and habits of the operator to not only his poor bodily condition and social status but also the deplorable state of his materials. The principles of public health reform, particularly those associated with sanitary science, simultaneously informed commercial portrait photographers' collective effort to represent the photographic laboratory and the "matter" within it as conducive to physical and social fitness. These efforts resulted in visions of sanitized darkrooms (e.g., fig. 34), as well as representations of photographic chemicals as therapeutic medicines that cured a host of epidemic diseases. Such connections between photographers' laboratory work and public health reform had important practical implications for the Philadelphia photographic community, which came to see itself as capable of diagnosing accidental poisonings, administering antidotes, and ultimately preventing untimely deaths in portrait studios. At a historical moment when sanitary science and hygiene were linked to ideas about social fitness, this group further portrayed itself, and its chemical operations, as promoting the health of an ailing nation.

While photographers had acknowledged photographic chemistry's various threats and benefits to health since the invention of the medium, this chapter shows why they gained new meaning and social significance in postbellum Philadelphia. More specifically, it asks, how did discussions of "matter out of place," which photographers expressed through the language of public health in this period, respond not only to the state of the photographic profession but also to the urban context in which it operated? More specifically, how did ideas about dirt and disease in the photographic laboratory intersect with anxieties about the recent effects of civil war on the bodies of American soldiers, the newly emancipated black population, and poverty and mass immigration in major cities like Philadelphia? What emerges from these questions is an understanding of the laboratory as a symbolic boundary in early photographic discourse, or what sociologist David Armstrong has described as an "unruly region [that] separates and defines the fundamental spaces of social life."[8] As such, it distinguished the comfortable environment of the ideal middle-class parlor, as it was re-created in the reception room and glass house of the portrait studio, from the bustling, filthy space of labor and production that had become the modern American city. The setting of photographers' chemical operations was thus precariously situated between a fantasy of health and a fantasy of disease.

SANITIZING THE CITY

In the mid-nineteenth century, as Philadelphians were developing creative approaches to promoting the connection between light and health across the city, they were also confronting the fact that many of its dwellings were overcrowded, filthy, excessively hot in both summer and winter, and plagued by foul smells from domestic and human waste. In his 1849 report to the American Medical Association on the sanitary conditions of Philadelphia, Isaac Parrish also observed that relatively few private homes had access to clean water, despite the "abundant supply of excellent water" available from the Schuylkill at the time. Likewise, the city had established a good system of drainage in the form of an open sewer system, but its cesspools regularly backed up with "putrid filth" that had to be collected and deposited onto the streets, which were difficult to clean properly; this caused "the surrounding atmosphere to be charged with a sickening effluvium" in hot weather.[9] In Parrish's estimation, unsanitary conditions were responsible for Philadelphia's high rates of infant mortality as well as outbreaks of influenza and cholera in the 1840s.

These sobering observations about public health in Philadelphia were largely confirmed in the following decade, when the city was struck several times by yellow fever and experienced one of the severest influenza epidemics to date. The Board of Health responded in 1857 by organizing the first national convention devoted to improving sanitation and controlling epidemic disease in American cities.[10] To further these goals, the seventy-five delegates who attended the meeting set about revising the system of quarantine that controlled the entry of contaminated foreign ships into U.S. harbors. These "foul vessels," they observed, regularly contained "stagnant and putrid bilge water," poorly ventilated air, and filthy cargo, and were marked by overcrowded conditions that encouraged diseases like smallpox, cholera, and yellow fever to proliferate on board.[11] In the case of the port of Philadelphia, preventing an epidemic from reaching America's shores involved close examination of all ships several miles from the city, especially those coming from foreign ports. People with symptoms of contagious infection were treated at a quarantine hospital on Little Tinicum Island known as the Lazaretto, which was built in the late eighteenth century in response to devastating epidemics of yellow fever. But the city's Board of Health acknowledged in the 1850s that quarantine was simply not enough to prevent "foreign" diseases from infecting the city as long as certain unsanitary conditions persisted within it. Like the "foul vessels" that delivered laborers and other passengers from Europe and the West Indies, America's "filthy," overcrowded cities required a thorough cleansing and purification.[12]

Running through these official reports on public health in Philadelphia at midcentury was a tendency to associate a lack of sanitation and its detrimental health effects with poor immigrant communities. This association was supported by staggering differences in the rate of disease and death across the city, due in part to the uneven geographic distribution of its population. As Sam Alewitz notes in his history of sanitation in Philadelphia, one out of sixty-one inhabitants in the "densely populated Fourth Ward" died in 1860, compared to one out of 163 in the "more affluent and uncrowded Thirteenth Ward."[13] These statistics correlate with the rates of epidemic diseases in the two districts. While officials had sympathy for the plight of those in the poorest neighborhoods and pledged to improve their living conditions, they were generally critical of their hygienic practices. Parrish had observed in 1849, for instance, that the tenement houses along Water Street, where "the accumulation of filth and offal . . . must inevitably take place," boasted "a population peculiarly liable, from their habits, to disease."[14] Authorities on public health in antebellum Philadelphia therefore imagined that curing the city of its many ills required rigorous sanitary *and* social reform.

Although the national conventions on quarantines and sanitation held between 1857 and 1860 expressed a collective commitment to such reform and yielded numerous specific proposals, they did not find widespread application until the onset of civil war in 1861. Throughout the conflict, the number of deaths from infectious disease among Union soldiers was staggering, exceeding deaths from gunshot wounds and serious injuries alone. The army's medical personnel often performed operations on the battlefield, where clean instruments, proper dressings, and drugs to treat infections were rarely available. The confinement of soldiers in camps meant that even the uninjured routinely contracted measles, malaria, spotted fever, and typhoid fever, while the passage of regiments through Philadelphia enabled these afflictions to spread quickly to the city's general population.[15] It became the mission of the United States Sanitary Commission (USSC) to convince the army's Medical Bureau, the War Department, and the civilians who supported their efforts that "camp disease is by far the most dangerous enemy [military officers] have to fear." In the war to preserve "our national unity and national territory," the USSC adopted as its weapons of choice the "fullest and ripest teachings of Sanitary Science" and applied them to the care of the sick and wounded. Among the subjects they oversaw were "Diet, Cooking, Cooks, Clothing, Tents, Camping Grounds, Transports, Transitory Depots. . . . Everything appertaining to outfit, cleanliness, precautions against damp, cold, heat, malaria, infection; crude, unvaried, or ill-cooked food, and an irregular or careless regimental commissariat, would fall under this head."[16]

The successful efforts of the USSC and other charitable organizations in Philadelphia that offered material support to ailing soldiers contributed to the wider dissemination of hygienic principles. After the war, for instance, practitioners of regular medicine in Philadelphia introduced hygiene as an elective subject in medical schools, adopted antiseptic practices in their operations, and gradually accepted the germ theory of disease. Prominent physicians like Henry Bowditch, who served as president of the Massachusetts State Board of Health, were particularly strong advocates of public health reform; Bowditch declared in 1876 that it was "the most important matter any community can discuss, for upon it, in its perfection, depend all the powers, moral, intellectual, and physical, of a State." Speaking before his peers at the International Medical Congress in Philadelphia, Bowditch acknowledged that studying and preventing disease could not be accomplished by medical professionals alone but should be the concern of "experts, professional and scientific, chosen . . . from any class of life in which the requisite scientific or other appropriate knowledge can be found."[17] Indeed, some of the most outspoken proponents of public health reform after the war were military officers, engineers, and city officials, who often criticized regular physicians for failing to teach the suffering public how to protect themselves from illness. These men aimed to correct this perceived failure and worked hard to bring important lessons from the battlefield into the daily lives of urban Americans.[18] As Lewis W. Leeds told audiences at the Franklin Institute in the late 1860s, the "greatest enemy" of the city was no longer the camp disease he had often observed as a health consultant in the army hospitals; rather, it was "our own breath," or the exhalations of city dwellers confined in unventilated homes and crowded public spaces, that accounted for 40 percent of Philadelphia's total deaths in 1865 alone. While the "regular old school Philadelphia physician" certainly knew about recent developments in sanitary science, Leeds explained, he preferred to rely on his chemical prescriptions, "no matter of how much public utility" new hygienic practices might be. Leeds thus took it upon himself to bring public health reform to "the people, the laboring man, the bone and sinew of the nation," so that he might "lecture every day" to his suffering friends on "the value of health and how to preserve it."[19] Reinforcing Leeds's efforts in the following decades were countless articles in domestic magazines as well as popular treatises on the "unhealthy home" published in Philadelphia. Taking up such subjects as maintaining the temperature of one's home throughout the year, designing a model sick room, setting up proper drainage and filtration systems, and generally keeping clean, this vast body of literature aimed to teach urban Americans that exposure to clean air and water saved lives.[20]

In the decades after the war, then, popular discourse on sanitation and hygiene increasingly represented public health as a matter of national concern that required both individual and collective action. The idea that every citizen should be armed with knowledge of what made people sick acquired particular social value in Philadelphia, which was experiencing an alarming environmental and health crisis as a result of massive increases in industrial production and population. As the art historian Alan Braddock has observed, Philadelphia's image makers were among the many groups who responded directly to these changing conditions by reimagining the physical and social space of the city. While millions of gallons of sewage and industrial waste were being pumped daily into the Delaware and Schuylkill rivers, contributing to the proliferation of typhoid and other epidemics, the celebrated painter Thomas Eakins included subtle references to these realities in paintings like *William Rush Carving His Allegorical Figure of the Schuylkill River* (1877); at the same time, Eakins performed what Braddock describes as an "aesthetic filtration" of the marshes and fisheries in the southern part of the city, "which were increasingly marked by pollution, disease, and [social] difference."[21] In so doing, the painter spoke to the civic values of his wealthy patrons, who were concerned to forge discrete spaces for whiteness and health in the city and its suburbs. As I argue in this chapter, similar environmental conditions and social values set the stage for the Philadelphia photographic community's frequent references to sanitary science in its trade literature. Endowing themselves with the power to shape, disseminate, and put the ideas associated with the movement into practice, the leaders of this community embraced Lewis Leeds's vision of delivering medicalized knowledge into the hands of every American. Desiring to become more than educated laborers who tended to the ill within their own trade, they also sought to join the "large corpus of able and earnest agents" that Henry Bowditch called upon to study and prevent the many illnesses afflicting the nation.[22] Medical models and metaphors facilitated these goals insofar as they enabled commercial photographers to imagine themselves as continuously fighting epidemic disease in their laboratories.

MAKING SPACE FOR PUBLIC HEALTH IN THE PHOTOGRAPHIC LABORATORY

In April 1886, Edward Wilson published an announcement of the Pennsylvania Board of Health's National Sanitary Convention, which was to be held in the city the following month. That it appeared on the pages of the *Philadelphia Photographer* suggests that— in the opinion of Wilson and Dr. Joseph F. Edwards, the convention's chairman, who submitted the announcement—the readers of the journal were invested in the event's goal, which was "to afford an opportunity for an expression of opinion on matters relating to the public health and the discussion of methods looking toward an advancement in the sanitary condition of the Commonwealth, the prevention of sickness and avoidable death, and the improvement of the conditions of the living." Among the topics to be discussed, and of apparent interest to photographers, were the "water supply of towns and cities; ventilation; sanitary plumbing and drainage; tests for impurities in water, the use of filters; city *versus* country life, from a hygienic point of view."[23] Although remarkable for the ease with which it assumed and outlined a close connection between public health and the Philadelphia photographic community, this brief announcement was not the first instance in which its leaders had conceived of unclean air, water, and bodies as urban-*cum*-photographic problems in the second half of the nineteenth century. Significantly, it was in the immediate wake of the Civil War that commercial photographers began discussing the practical and social implications of sanitation and hygiene for everyone associated with the burgeoning profession.

The renowned Philadelphia chemist Mathew Carey Lea was one of the first and most prolific writers on the subject, to which he devoted an entire chapter in his widely read *Manual of Photography* (1868) as well as numerous articles in Edward Wilson's journals. As Lea explained to studio operators, the primary cause of their debilitation and death was prolonged exposure to noisome and highly toxic chemicals in a confined environment. "All physicians know that the proper ventilation of the blood through the lungs is one of the most indispensible conditions of health," he reported in the *Philadelphia Photographer*, but when the air was "vitiated" by chemical fumes, any number of "evil" effects on the body could result.[24] Lea's *Manual* offered readers a concise, sobering summary of those effects: "Vapors of ammonia disorganize and paralyze the blood corpuscles. Vapor of ether is very injurious to the nervous system, and depresses the whole tone of the body. Nitric acid is highly poisonous; its fumes, when inhaled, in even a moderately strong form, may cause death in a few hours."[25] By the time the second edition of the manual was published in 1871, countless contributors to Wilson's journals were echoing its observations about the detrimental health consequences of working with photographic chemicals. The Boston photographer Robert Chute, who had also alerted commercial photographers to the health benefits of blue glass, sympathized with the "poor operator" who "has been for months buried, as it were, in that chemical den, till almost crazed with headaches, and emaciated from loss of sleep and appetite . . . and all this time drinking in the fumes from the collodion till his clothes and even his breath seem saturated with it." As a result of this experience, Chute imagined that photographers' knowledge of disease mechanism exceeded that of a "disciple of Galen," who, upon hearing of the chemicals to which he was exposed daily, "strokes his beard and says he 'don't think those would have any injurious effect.'"[26]

Such observations prompted proposals from across the Philadelphia photographic community, all of which emphasized the importance of letting fresh air into, and foul air out of, the darkroom. The ventilation schemes that operators developed to transform their "dens of science" into healthful or at least livable environments ranged from simple to elaborate. Very often they resembled those that public health officials proposed for use within the urban domestic interior. Like the ideal bourgeois subject in his sitting room, a photographer could open a window or a door in his darkroom, or maintain a continuous open fire to warm and remove the contaminated air. He could also install a ventilating apparatus along the walls or near the floor and ceiling of the room that consisted of a series of pipes, valves, and other means of mechanically controlling air circulation.[27] Photographers turned to additional models associated with sanitary reform to prevent light and dust from entering the laboratory and spoiling their work. According to Edward Wilson, these included the "plan in common use for ventilating the holds of vessels *i.e.*, a canvas tube, reaching from the dark-room floor to the air, so bent as to prevent the admission of the light."[28] Another was proposed by Norman Bridge, the well-known physician who was invited to speak at the annual meeting of the Photographers' Association of America in 1880. Introducing a discussion of "the hygiene of the business of the photographer" and the "sanitary improvements that might be made in the way in which business is conducted," Bridge explained, "there is one thing you can always do with the vapors and gases" in the photographic laboratory, "and that is the thing that well-ordered cities do with their sewage. They cannot get rid of it; it is forever accumulating; it is always noxious; but . . . we can dilute it."[29]

By comparing the noxious fumes of photographic chemicals to those of an unhealthy home, a quarantine ship, and sewerage, the Philadelphia photographic community connected laboratory work in commercial portrait studios to the larger social project of cleaning up the filthy city in postbellum America. In each space (urban and photographic), self-appointed authorities on the body defined sanitation in more than physical terms; together they participated in an anxious discourse about public health at a time when sanitary reform had become a matter of urgent social and moral concern to middle-class city dwellers. In alerting readers to the contaminating presence and unsavory bodily practices of urban immigrant populations, popular literature was deeply concerned to equate health with racial whiteness, respectability, and masculinity. At the same time, photographers urged one another to police the boundaries between their bodies and their chemical work in order to save lives in the darkroom and promote their own professional identity. In this way, both public health and photographic discourse advocated sanitation after the Civil War as part of an effort to safeguard an ideal physical and social body perceived to be constantly under threat.

According to Mathew Carey Lea, Edward Wilson, and other authorities on photography and health, an operator could not promote this ideal through ventilation alone; he must always practice bodily hygiene as well. According to popular treatises on the subject, this involved washing and clothing the skin properly, exercising the muscles, regulating diet and alcohol intake, and engaging in other bodily practices associated with moral, gentlemanly behavior.[30] Photographic literature observed, however, that operators too often failed to meet these ideal standards of hygiene by bathing infrequently and by smoking in their laboratories, and even using them as lavatories. Like the improper ventilation of chemical fumes, each of these practices contributed to the "nauseating atmosphere clinging to self and studio" that jeopardized photographers' physical health and the success of their operations.[31] What made them especially unacceptable were their social implications for a class of aspiring professionals who sought to attract a respectable clientele; to put it plainly, the unclean habit of polluting the darkroom with one's own excrement corrupted the "air" of gentility that photographers cultivated for themselves and their patrons in urban portrait studios.

In the 1880 issue of *Photographic Mosaics,* Samuel V. Allen articulated the social implications of practicing such poor hygiene when he admonished his fellow operators for allowing their laboratories to smell like an "emigrant car," a second-class railroad carriage with minimal comforts that carried passengers of various races and low economic status between New York, Philadelphia, and points west.[32] In his lectures at the Franklin Institute, Lewis Leeds had already alerted Philadelphians to the grave dangers that the city's overcrowded, unventilated "cars" posed to the health of educated, respectable urbanites like himself. "I am obliged to sit in the foul offensive atmosphere, and breathe the poisonous exhalations of my own lungs, and that from dozens of others, some of them, it may be, badly diseased," he wrote. "Thus in one half hour, I have inhaled six hundred times of this foul and poisonous air, and the blood has carried it to every portion of my body, so that my entire system is completely saturated, poisoned."[33] The unsanitary conditions and resulting dangers to the body of which Leeds warned were even more strongly associated with the emigrant car in the late nineteenth century, in both public health discourse and the popular imagination. Working to mitigate their threat to respectability on the rails through visual humor, the satiric illustration in figure 35 catalogues these dangers by filling "the American emigrant car" with caricatured blacks, Irish, Jews, and a variety of peasant folk. The men fight, drink, sleep with their feet propped on the seats or other passengers, and fill what little space remains with smoke; while the women make some effort to maintain order, most of the children are left to fend for themselves, unsure where to turn for food or comfort. Comparing the photographic laboratory to such a public space, as Samuel Allen did in 1880, evoked anxieties about filth and contagion in the multiethnic American city, at the same time that it suggested a parallel between the "unclean" inhabitants in each environment. Like authorities on public health who often blamed the poor health of immigrant communities on their dirty and immoral habits, Allen urged photographers to take responsibility for what he saw as a public health crisis in their laboratories. "Cleanse at once the room that has been defiled," he counseled his readers, "and then go your way, and break stones upon the public street until want and a sense of shame shall teach you never again to use that room for other than the purpose to which it was first dedicated."[34]

The same literature that instructed city dwellers to be wary of foul air called upon them to attend to their visual appearance, arguing that how one looked was just as important as how one smelled when it came to cultivating a particular social identity. For this reason, the Philadelphia photographic community worried about the dark stains that their chemicals produced on bodies in the portrait studio. Among the most troubling of these chemical marks were those associated with silver nitrate, a light-sensitive substance essential to photography's chemical operations. Unsurprisingly, frequent discussions of this material's ability to darken white skin, particularly around the time of the Civil War, articulated widespread anxiety about public health and racial identity. In 1866, for example, Edward Wilson published two reports in the *Philadelphia Photographer* that present a change of race as the unfortunate side effect of the white

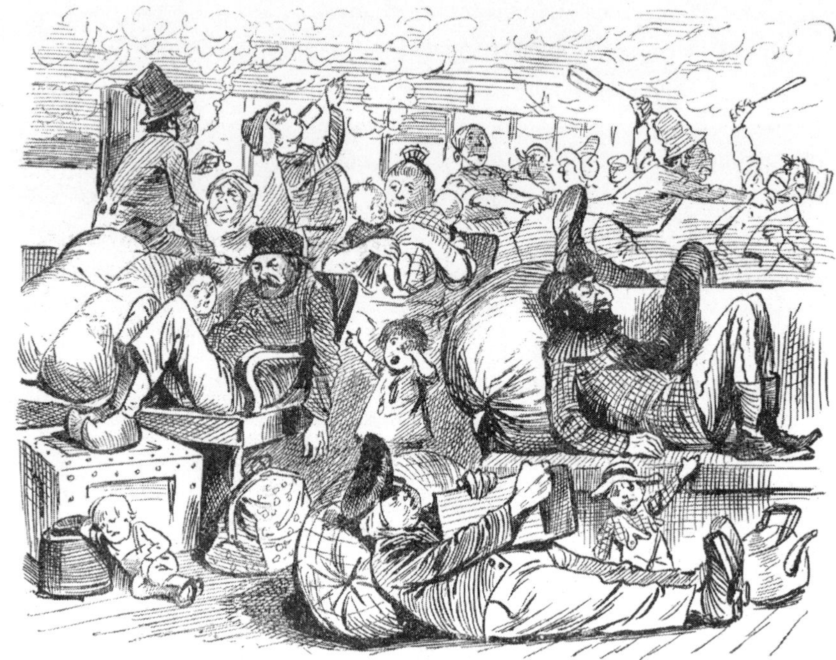

FIGURE 35 *The American Emigrant Car,* ca. 1882. Wood engraving. From *Puck* 11, no. 277 (June 28, 1882): 271.

middle-class public's many accidental encounters with silver nitrate. One of these involved a "two-year-old Miss" who decided to pay her father a visit at his gallery. Wandering into his darkroom, the toddler found what she assumed to be a "crock of water" on the floor, but which actually contained silver waste solution; "in went one arm up to the elbow, then the other hand." The next evening, the photographer returned home to find "our little elfin with arms of a dark mulatto color, and her hands of such intense blackness that they should have put to shame a genuine son of Ham."[35] By invoking the language of race to describe the chemical staining of the young girl's body, Wilson underscores the urgency with which commercial photographers were to adopt sanitary practices in their laboratories. The photographer's filthy habit of leaving his chemicals in open dishes, after all, caused his daughter's racial blackening, which itself had become equated with dirt and disease during the Civil War.[36] What readers might dismiss as nothing more than an amusing anecdote about a mischievous toddler, both then and now, spoke to popular ideas about the pollution of "pure" whiteness in the immediate wake of black emancipation.

The emphasis in these reports on sitters' bodies is both significant and timely, given that commercial photographers were preoccupied with attracting white middle-class patrons to their studios in the 1860s, which, as we have seen, meant assuaging their anxieties about the new medium of photography and its corporeal effects. In the

decades that followed, however, the concerns about silver nitrate shifted away from this
focus on the studio public, as photographers became increasingly preoccupied with
what their own chemically ravaged bodies would convey to sitters and other aspiring
or established professionals about the social character of the commercial operator.
As Dr. Norman Bridge observed in his 1880 lecture on the "hygiene of photography,"
few photographers, physicians, or chemists thought of "removing these stains because
they think they are harmful"; they nevertheless disliked having their fingers "constantly
blackened" and were "anxious to remove the disfigurement."[37] It remained the project
of photographic literature to define this "disfigurement" in decidedly social terms and
in relation to a continually evolving professional and urban scene. The "figure cut by
the exhibitions of laboratory-stains on hands and clothing," the *Philadelphia Photographer* put it plainly in 1881, "affects not only the standing of the photographer, but has
a decided sanitary value to himself and the community."[38] A vigorous cleansing of the
body, or "lavish use of soap and water," would ensure that "ladies and children" would
be greeted with "the cleanly air and habit of a gentleman."

When soap and water were not enough to rid commercial photographers of the
"blackness" that silver nitrate introduced into their laboratories and marked upon their
bodies, they turned to cyanide of potassium, a highly toxic material that Mathew Carey
Lea repeatedly described as "the most dangerous chemical with which the photographer comes into contact." When it didn't cause actual death, he claimed, cyanide could
cause "anomalous" dermal secretions, intense physical pain, paralysis, or a breakdown
of one's "whole bodily health."[39] Lea's view was supported by numerous articles in the
photographic press describing tragic deaths and near fatalities at the hands of this
poison: a female sitter reportedly died after "taking a dose of cyanide of potassium in
mistake for rhubarb," a photographer saved his children just in time from drinking out
of a household mug that contained cyanide solution, and another, upon accidentally
ingesting cyanide when eating some cloves on his darkroom shelf, "in twenty minutes
was a corpse."[40] Were these devastating outcomes what Dr. Norman Bridge had in mind
when he described photographers' use of cyanide as "a little inconvenience" they should
be willing to endure to "remove black spots and stains" from their bodies? Perhaps not.

Indeed, physical debilitation and the occasional death could be interpreted as "a
little inconvenience" only if we consider the high price members of the commercial photographic community feared they would pay for allowing silver nitrate to "disfigure," or
blacken, their bodies. Like other men of science in late nineteenth-century Philadelphia,
whose adoption of sanitary practices in hospitals and laboratories coincided with their
professionalization, photographers understood that embracing the social codes of the
respectable classes, including those concerning personal hygiene, was required of anyone who aspired to be seen as "professional."[41] What is more, reliable scientific knowledge in this period—with its various connotations of rationality, truth, and objectivity—
was increasingly linked to the appearance of sterility in a given operation and insisted on
the absence of the operator's contaminating bodily presence. What commercial photographers desperately sought to avoid in their use of cyanide, then, was the pollution of an
ideal vision of themselves as scientific authorities and all that this implied for the social
character and value of their operations. Arguably their most extreme laboratory practice,

in terms of its corporeal effects, photographers' embrace of cyanide ultimately shows us how and why their physical health could be deemed less important than perceptions of their social fitness.

EPIDEMIC DISEASE AND THE BODY OF THE PHOTOGRAPH(ER)

As reports of accidental poisonings and other mishaps with cyanide and silver nitrate remind us, discussions of health in the photographic laboratory in an era of vigorous sanitary reform were not concerned only with the effects of that space on photographers' bodies. They aimed to show, rather, that photographers' failures to ventilate and keep clean had important implications for *any* body in the portrait studio. While the bodies of which I speak included those of unsuspecting white ladies and their mischievous children, between the 1860s and the 1880s the Philadelphia photographic community constructed another seemingly limitless corporeal field vulnerable to their darkroom operations. Through medical metaphor, that is, photographers participated in a recurring "medical" drama in which their laboratory materials played the role of animate bodies that constantly required diagnosis and treatment.

The personification of photographic materials in the darkroom became common practice in photographers' trade literature around the time of the Civil War.[42] Shortly after the highly publicized trial of those involved in Lincoln's assassination and the final surrender of Confederate troops, Edward Wilson published a letter in the *Philadelphia Photographer* written from the perspective of a *carte de visite*. Speaking in the first person, the photographic print unspools a narrative of woe, beginning with her birth at a Prussian paper factory, where she and her "sisters" were "despised, trod upon, and maltreated" as if they were "witnesses in the conspiracy case at Washington." They then endured a "long and tedious voyage across the tempestuous ocean," like slaves bound for the New World, only to arrive at a photographic studio where they would continue to be handled in a "violent and impolite" manner. At this point in the story the *carte* enters the darkroom, where she is administered a "dose" of collodion that leaves her "sick and fainting." In an effort to resist further harmful treatment, she sticks one of her corners out of the bath, only to be punished for such transgression by being exposed and developed first. When the operations on her body are finally complete, the *carte* finds an image of three children printed upon her surface; this is not just any image, but precisely the portrait of the "dead soldier's children" that inspired the poem Wilson had published in the inaugural issue of the *Philadelphia Photographer,* discussed in chapter 2 (fig. 16). With this discovery, the story takes on a decidedly sentimental and moral tone, as its narrator asks the journal's readers, "Need I tell you more? How I was placed in the breast pocket of one of our noble heroes, as he left his darling trio and their precious mother, to go defend his flag and their homes from the invader? . . . How the relentless bullet came along, whispering death and destruction and sparing me entered his noble breast, and felled him to the earth? How his eager hands grasped me, and held me before his eyes until they lost their brightness, and until his last prayer for them was sent to heaven?"[43] To record faithfully the likeness of a mother and her children, which

would give strength to a Union soldier in battle and comfort him at the moment of his
death—this, we are to understand, is the noblest purpose to which any photograph
could be put in 1865. So noble is this service to the bourgeois family and the nation that
it ultimately justifies the physical "maltreatment" of the *carte*'s body.

The moral of "The Story of a Carte de Visite" was one that the Philadelphia photographic community would have readily embraced, because it expressed not only nation-
alist sentiments on the heels of a devastating civil war but also their desire for professional status and respect. Recalling the discourse of operations through which portrait
photography entered into dialogue with surgery and anesthesia, that message was
simple: all bodies in the studio must come under the control of the photographer. The
print herself adopts this position in the final lines of the letter, when she observes that
she is tragically "fading away." This is not the result of a "bad manipulation" on the part
of the operator, she explains, "but of my refusing to be properly washed, which causes
the fading away prematurely of many a person as well as many a carte de visite."[44] The
letter thus concludes with an analogy common in views of photography as both surgery
and phototherapy, one that likens a photographic print to a human body. More specifically, Wilson sets in relation to each other a portrait of three ideal subjects, rendered
impermanent by insufficient chemical treatment, and the body of a Civil War soldier,
whose untimely death is due less to his battle wounds than to his failure to "properly
wash," or maintain good hygiene. The soldier, then, represents the *carte*'s failure to
acknowledge the authority of the operator as nothing short of a national tragedy. Within
the social context in which the letter was written, it is hard to imagine stronger support
for the professional aspirations of Wilson and the community of operators he led. At
various points in the letter he prepares us for this conclusion by subtly undermining the
print's perception of the photographer as "a man with very black fingers" who handles
her body roughly. Appearing to break away from the voice of the *carte,* Wilson pays conspicuous attention to the sanitary condition and professional character of the darkroom,
which "seemed to be very clean and nice, and in perfect order. Bottles, and brushes, and
funnels, and other articles were there in abundance, and all properly labelled, and in a
special place where they could be found when wanted, without trouble."[45] These lines
encourage readers to ask how an operator whose laboratory so closely resembled Tissandier's ideal darkroom could be anything other than professional or produce a "sick
and fainting" photographic print. According to the logic of commercial photographic
discourse in this period, such a result was virtually unimaginable.

I dwell on the details of "The Story of a Carte de Visite" because this fictional letter
expresses many of the aims and anxieties that defined subsequent fantasies of the photographic laboratory as a space in which materials thought, felt, acted, and, significantly,
got sick. Sensitive to humidity and easily contaminated by dust and dirt, photographic
negatives were often said to contract "a sort of leprous disease," to develop "Yellow
Fever," or to become afflicted with the dreaded "green fog," once dubbed "the measles
of photographic childhood."[46] When they weren't suffering from these ubiquitous
diseases, photographic prints were plagued by a collection of pathological symptoms,
including blisters, streaks, specks, and spotting.[47] Although such medical language
was used to describe the debilitated and disordered bodies of photographic materials,

the focus of these fanciful visions, implicit or otherwise, was almost always the body of the photographer. It was he, after all, who was responsible for observing his materials' symptoms, making an early diagnosis of their disease, and administering the appropriate kind and dose of "photographic medicine." The "health" of, say, a *carte de visite* therefore depended largely on the professional expertise and character of the "doctor" responsible for its care.[48]

Wilson and his band of "doctors" repeatedly employed medical metaphors to convey a stern warning to studio operators: allowing quacks into the darkroom and, more generally, into the photographic profession, had serious consequences. Ignorant, unskilled, or simply inexperienced, they argued, these men could unleash a devastating epidemic on their materials, subject them to a dangerous chemical "overdose," or even "kill" them.[49] An editorial by Wilson in the 1871 issue of *Photographic Mosaics* made this point by summarizing the various effects that a quack operator could have on his materials:

> His paper turns yellow; his prints catch all manner of diseases, from the measles to the malignant scarlet fever, and he is in a fix to know how to clear things up. . . . His poor bath had been tantalized, and doctored, and evaporated, and corrected, until it was as weak and spiritless as a consumptive. . . . His prints would blush and refuse to change color the moment he began to stir them and turn them over, or if white and nice in the running water, enter his hands, and they would all become bilious and jaundicy. He knew the names of all these diseases and the many remedies; but not knowing which to apply, he must get up on the fence and think.[50]

Medicalized knowledge and the expert judgment to apply it properly—this, the passage suggests, is what the operator needs to save lives. Yet again, medical metaphor supports the professionalization of those who practiced studio portraiture in the 1870s. Even in this damning criticism of the unconfident photographer "on the fence," however, Wilson suggests another source of disease and disorder among the materials in his darkroom. Much like the *carte de visite* that shared its story with the readers of the *Philadelphia Photographer*, the "prints" in this passage behave disobediently and according to their own will, "refusing" to acknowledge the authority of the operator. Elsewhere in the editorial Wilson speaks of the "evil" in the operator's bath and his knowledge of its "depravities" and "gymnastic properties," which resist his best efforts to control them. While blaming photographers for the various epidemics in their laboratories might persuade them to educate themselves and adopt sanitary practices, what might we say of this other view of the aggrieved operator, burdened, even sickened, by his rebellious, depraved materials?

To answer this question we must remember that American portrait photographers were not the first to personify their materials as bodies that resisted manipulation. As the historian of science Pamela Smith has argued, sculptors, printmakers, and painters working in early modern Europe described their practices as a "bodily struggle with and against matter itself. Matter was not dead but alive, and it behaved in idiosyncratic ways, which artisans had to come to know—and master—through experience."[51] A late fourteenth-century manual for painters, for instance, described varnish as "a powerful liquid . . . and it wants to be obeyed in everything. . . . And immediately, as you spread it out on your work every color immediately loses some of its resistance, and is obliged to the varnish, and never again has the power to go on refreshing itself with its own tempera." Gold, for its part, could "be 'fastidious' about the stone upon which it is burnished," making the polishing of this metal physically challenging work for the artisan.[52] In the context of the early modern workshop, Smith demonstrates, the idea that matter was capable of acting, feeling, and generally behaving like a human being stemmed from a belief that artisans shared with alchemists of the period—that nature possessed an essentially creative power to transform itself and generate new life. By the sixteenth century, alchemy had become popularly associated with the creation of the philosopher's stone, which was believed to enable the transmutation of base metals into more valuable forms (chiefly gold) as well as to function as an *elixir vitae* that could cure all ailments. While paving the way for advances in modern chemistry and medicine, this hermetic science was founded on mystical and spiritual beliefs, insofar as alchemical operations functioned as metaphors for the purification of the degraded human body and soul. According to Smith, alchemy provided artisans with highly symbolic imagery and language in which they could represent the transformations of active matter, as well as an intimate relationship between matter and spirit on which to base their work. It also lent them an epistemological model that emphasized direct observation and imitation of nature by means of bodily involvement in the creative process.

In their personifications of laboratory materials, we find evidence of photographers' connection to the world of early modern artisans and, more specifically, to the alchemical model artisans adopted. As the historian of photography Laurie Dahlberg has observed, the ideas that photography "seemed to materialize from an invisible realm," involved "a captivating physical transformation of raw materials," and "eagerly and profoundly adopted to metaphorical interpretation" have informed connections between the photographic medium and alchemy since the mid-nineteenth century. While Dahlberg argues that explicit comparisons between the two practices were limited to the "popular imagination" in the decades immediately following the introduction of photography in the United States (given the challenges to scientific authority such associations would probably have posed), a survey of Philadelphia's early photographic literature suggests otherwise, demonstrating the importance of these ideas to discussions of health and disease in studio laboratories.[53] In an editorial published in the *Philadelphia Photographer* in 1865, for example, Edward Wilson employed figurative language reminiscent of alchemical discourse to describe an operator's bodily experience of working day and night among "depraved, patience-wearing, vicious chemicals." "Your fingers become powerless in your endeavors to control them," Wilson wrote, "your brain becomes fevered, and your good resolve all forsake you; headache brings its pangs." Wilson warned that these symptoms could develop into actual psychosis: "your collodion vial sits upon your breast in the shape of a huge owl, blinking at you, and occasionally screaming; little bromide and iodide bottles dance all over you, and your sulphuret and hyposulphate of soda unmistakably resemble and smell like his Satanic highness."[54] In 1868 Wilson published a similarly colorful description of laboratory work in which an operator's chemicals stage a "mutiny in the 'darkroom'":

> The Acid family, with no premonition, had set up a separate *independency*. The Bromides and Iodides, dwelling heretofore in peaceful community, repudiated their reputation, and regardless of consequences, plunged into difficulties, proclaiming themselves belligerents. Collodion refused to fraternize with any of his former associates, and added his tumult to the general demoralization. Comets, unheavenly, with their long relentless tails, streaked up and down the befogged and bewildered plates, and there seemed an utter wreck of resource and of shift. . . . Mind ever triumphs over matter. Order eventually came out of chaos. A little enchantment poured out from a row of peacemakers, happily united the different factions, restored fealty, reconciling them unto themselves and unto their neighbors. Harmony reigned supreme, and again the mysteries of the "black-room" developed most wonderful things.[55]

In each of these examples, the invocation of specific symbols such as the owl and the comet, the personification of inanimate materials within a discourse of good versus evil, and the conflation of material and bodily dis-ease with moral and spiritual deficiency all suggest an alchemical model.[56]

Represented in medical metaphors, this model enabled American photographers to create allegories of their chemical operations that responded to the particularities of their historical, cultural, and social context. First, the Philadelphia photographic community's fantasies of disobedient and diseased materials in the years immediately following the Civil War spoke to the generalized bodily disorder in which that professional body operated. Its visions of the photographic laboratory also echoed northern sentiments about the recent rebellion, insofar as it came to be seen as a space in which a once "peaceful community" could quickly transform itself into a band of "belligerents." Second, it mattered greatly which ailments photographers' prints, negatives, and chemicals suffered from. To publish letters from operators and photographic suppliers on how to get rid of the "measles" in albumen paper, as Edward Wilson did just after the war, for instance, was to bring to the minds of readers fresh memories of this "dreaded and well-known disease," which frequently broke out among Union troops. Associated primarily with urban childhood, the measles had particularly devastating effects on northern regiments that contained young soldiers from rural communities, maintained poor hygiene, and had limited access to drugs that could treat secondary infections.[57] Similarly, the regular mention of "blisters" in photographers' trade journals in the 1870s and '80s no doubt called to mind the outbreaks of smallpox that had plagued Philadelphia and other major American cities since the start of the war. Discussion of a less common "photographic disease," such as "La Grippe," or Russian influenza, would have spoken to readers' experience of a pandemic that took hold of Philadelphia's population at a more circumscribed moment, namely, 1889–91.[58] The city's photographic literature thus demonstrated a keen awareness of the sufferings of the local community at the same time that it implicitly acknowledged the important place of urban epidemics within the broader cultural imagination of the period.[59]

In aligning their laboratory materials with the most urgent public health crises confronting Americans in the postbellum period, professionalizing photographers constructed not only their credibility but a seemingly unrivaled authority in matters of the body. Like early modern artisans, they relied on figurative language to bring their sick and rebellious materials under control and cure them of their many afflictions, which often included the very illnesses that regular physicians had failed to cure. The idea that they did so against all odds and at great risk to their own bodies aimed to encourage public appreciation of the debilitated operator. The pathological state of an operator's body, in other words, did not have to reflect his ignorance of scientific methods and sanitary practices; in certain instances it could represent the cost of his professional commitment to remedying what Wilson once called the "ills that 'printer-flesh' is heir to."[60] While the leaders of the Philadelphia photographic community underscored the selflessness of that commitment by portraying the "photographic physician" as a kind of national hero, the interests of that group become readily apparent when one considers the economic effects of eradicating laboratory disease; the production of "healthy" or pleasing portraits for studio patrons, after all, was essential to securing an operator's commercial success.

How photographers blurred the line between human bodies and their laboratory materials can also tell us much about the construction of photographic authority in relation to that of early modern artisanship. Conflating these debilitated "bodies" through medical metaphor became, in fact, a common trope in American photographic literature in the second half of the nineteenth century, often in the form of a first-person narrative. Consider a letter published in the *Philadelphia Photographer* in 1871, in which J. Perry Elliott shared his experience with the photographic disease called the "measles." "Did you ever have a disease called the 'measles?'" he asks. "I had it, 'they say,' I did, when a 'babe' . . . at the breast; and after I was grown I am personally and painfully aware of having it again; and only last week I had a third attack, but this time it came not upon my person, but upon my pictures, my negatives, and for several days it 'got me down' badly."[61] While Elliott makes a distinction in this last line between the disease upon his "person" and the disease upon his "pictures," he complicates this distinction by claiming that the latter attack "got *me* down" (emphasis added). In this way he encourages readers to ponder the question of who is the afflicted and who requires chemical treatment. The operator, his photographs, the subject in the photograph, or all three?[62]

Written from the point of view of a "sufferer," a letter that appeared in *Wilson's Photographic Magazine* in 1890 prompted a similar question. In it, the narrator recounted his experience of catching "the late epidemic":

> *I am in quarantine.* An agent for the "La Grippe Plate Co.," called on me and induced me (very much against my will) to try his plates. Thinking them easy to work I made a two-day trial of one, and then went to the studio; but it appears the plate was not thoroughly fixed, and I am back in the hypo. Now the doctor insists on my remaining in the house another week, on a developer composed mostly of quinine, and threatens if I go out under the prescribed time he will have to reduce the plate with pneumonia, which may mean utter ruination of the plate and subject too. But as I want to devote a good many years to our art, I think I will gratefully submit to the doctor's treatment.[63]

Phrases like "I am back in the hypo" suggest that readers are meant to experience the letter as one of many examples in early photographic literature in which disordered laboratory materials speak through metaphor. We encounter, in other words, what would appear to be a photographic print with its own thoughts, wants, and "will"; but unlike the narrator in "The Story of a Carte de Visite," this one pledges that he will "gratefully submit to the doctor's treatment," acknowledging the operator's authority to treat and eradicate disease. At several points in the letter, however, the voice of the "doctor" seems to insert itself into the personal narrative. Who made a "two-day trial" of the diseased plates—the print or the operator? And who "want[s] to devote a good many years to *our* art" (emphasis added)—a print resulting from a single exposure in the darkroom, or a gentleman who makes his career of exposing and printing light-sensitive materials in the portrait studio? In addition, the letter conflates the photograph-as-body and the body in the photograph by representing the health of inanimate photographic materials as closely tied to the health of the subject before the camera. Like the human body it depicts, the photographic print is susceptible to the debilitating effects of influenza, subject to quarantine, and treated with quinine; it is also at risk of experiencing the unpredictable effects of "pneumonia"—probably a pun on *ammonia,* the common darkroom chemical used to treat the victims of the influenza pandemic in 1890. Reinforcing this connection is the narrator's concern for the serious consequences of not following the doctor's orders to remain in the developer; not only would such transgression negatively affect and likely "kill" the afflicted print, it would result in the "utter ruination of the plate and subject too."

The firsthand experience with epidemic disease detailed in these letters actively minimizes the boundaries between human bodies and laboratory materials, even if the letters were motivated by an anxious desire to shore up those boundaries. They bring the world of the commercial photographer into close dialogue with that of the early modern artisan in surprising ways, reminding us that photographic authority in nineteenth-century America depended on a variety of epistemological models, not all of which support twentieth-century theories of photography as a unique form of unmediated representation. As I suggested above, the sick photographer could present himself as a professional if his illness were seen as the result of a selfless and heroic struggle with active matter. Poor health could also serve as evidence of the photographer's intimate, embodied knowledge of the process of photographic (re)production. This scenario challenges the notion that photography derives its authority chiefly from its scientific objectivity, which requires a *disembodied* gaze—the camera operator, unlike the painter, removes his mediating presence entirely from the process of representation, enabling a portrait to be seen as a truthful, authoritative image of a subject. Philadelphia's photographic literature disturbs this fantasy by suggesting that, when it came to the studio laboratory, bodily involvement in chemical operations was simply undeniable, and perhaps not altogether undesirable.

In this respect, the medicalized personification of photographic materials in the 1870s and '80s built upon the work that Mathew Carey Lea began in the 1860s to show that photographers' chemical operations were not devoid of potential benefit. In his discussions of photography and health, Lea's objective was to transmit the knowledge and skill necessary to make a timely self-diagnosis and administer appropriate treatments (e.g., in cases when efforts to ventilate and keep clean failed to protect photographers from chemical poisoning); that he had not only witnessed the "evil results" of unsanitary practices in others but was "speaking from personal experience" enabled him to counsel photographers on such important medical matters. To put it simply, Lea's authority on photography and health required a debilitated body.[64] Later dramatizations of laboratory work, such as we see in the letters quoted above, similarly emphasized the value of photographers' personal experience with and knowledge of disease and at the same time overlaid a persuasive logic onto Lea's vision of the sick photographic body: if the photographer suffered from the same diseases that afflicted his materials, it was because the photographic medium shared a unique affinity with the human body. Indeed, fantasies of photographers' chemical operations that emerged after the Civil War sought to erode not only the *distance* but the *difference* between photography and the body, in much the same way that photographic literature of the 1870s imagined that prints and negatives shared human skin's sensitivity to light. As a result, managing corporeal boundaries in the darkroom not only became a matter of tending to chemical marks on a photographer's clothes and skin; it meant imagining laboratory work as simultaneously operating on the body of the photographer, the body of the photograph, the body in the photograph, and the social body as a whole. Medical metaphor in late nineteenth-century photographic discourse served a powerful corporeal fantasy in which these bodies could have immediate effects on one another, ultimately allowing them to be seen as interchangeable.

PRESCRIBING FROM THE "PHOTOGRAPHIC PHARMACOPOEIA"

To understand the ways in which these fantasies contributed to the construction of photographic authority in postbellum America, we may now return to the narrative with which this book began: Henry Snelling's "Doctor Photo." The similarities between this and other personifications of photography become readily apparent when one considers the ways in which Snelling enables the medium to speak through medical metaphor tinged with references to alchemy. Just as *cartes de visite*, negatives, and chemical baths were made to tell their stories of suffering on the pages of Wilson's journals, a "good little invisible sprite" appeared to Snelling in his darkroom and shared with him the chemical ingredients of a remarkable panacea. When comparing the different kinds of work these texts perform, we must keep in mind that precisely who or what speaks is integral to the message they convey. What ultimately distinguishes "Doctor Photo" from the many other medicalized fantasies of laboratory work in early photographic literature, I would argue, is the way in which it gives voice to the very *idea* of photography as a cultural practice and profession, rather than ventriloquizing its materials alone. It thus articulates a powerful vision of the medium as acting directly upon the body—not to disable but to cure.

Whether Snelling came to his conclusions about photographic chemistry's therapeutic effects through medical literature, a self-motivated pharmaceutical trial, or indeed the divine intervention of Doctor Photo, his narrative demonstrates that American photographers in the 1870s were prepared to think of photographics in relation to therapeutics. In exploring that connection, Snelling used figurative language to give new meaning to an undeniable equivalence: the materials essential to studio laboratory operations doubled as the most commonly administered medicaments of their day. Indeed, nearly every photographic chemical listed in Taylor & Wetherbee's inventory (fig. 36) had an important place in the practice of regular medicine, taken either alone or in combination with other substances. Alcohol, a basic solvent in photographic chemistry, performed the same role in pharmaceutical drugs, in addition to acting as a controversial yet popularly prescribed stimulant in the mid-nineteenth century. Bromide of potassium, a photographic sensitizer, was used as a treatment for epilepsy, nervous afflictions, and genital inflammation. As already noted, silver nitrate made photographic materials sensitive to light; it was also used widely to heal the wounds of injured soldiers as well as to alleviate

FIGURE 36 Advertisement for W. A. Wetherbee, M.D., and Taylor & Wetherbee, Analytical, Pharmaceutical, and Photographical Chemists. From M. P. Simons, *Photography in a Nutshell, or The Experience of an Artist in Photography* (Philadelphia: King and Baird, 1858).

W. A. WETHERBEE, M. D.,

No. 1099 Broadway, corner 32d Street, New York,

AND

TAYLOR & WETHERBEE,

Corner of Ninth and Chestnut Streets, Philadelphia,

Analytical, Pharmaceutical,

AND

PHOTOGRAPHICAL CHEMISTS,

Have constantly on hand and for sale, at Wholesale and Retail, every variety of Photographic and Daguerrean Chemicals, consisting, in part, of the following:

ACID, ACETIC,	GOLD CHLORIDE,
" " GLACIAL,	" HYPOSULPHITE,
" " 8d BAUME,	GUN COTTON,
" GALLIC,	IODINE,
" HYDROCHLORIC,	" BROMIDE,
" NITRIC,	" CHLORIDE,
" PYROGALLIC,	IRON, BROMIDE,
" SUCCINIC,	" IODIDE,
" SULPHURIC,	" PROTO-SULPH. CRYS.
ALCOHOL, ABSOLUTE,	POTASSIUM, BROMIDE,
AMMONIA, AQUA,	" CYANIDE, GRAN.
" HYDROSULPHATE,	" " FUSED.
" BROMIDE,	" IODIDE,
" IODIDE,	SILVER, CHLORIDE,
BARIUM, CHLORIDE,	" CYANIDE,
" NITRATE,	" IODIDE,
BROMINE,	" NITRATE, CRYS.
CADMIUM,	" OXIDE,
CADMIUM, BROMIDE,	SODA, HYPOSULPHITE,
" IODIDE,	SODIUM, BROMIDE,
DEXTRINE,	" IODIDE,
ETHER, SULPH. CONCEN.	ZINC, IODIDE.

10*

nervous and ulcerative conditions, digestive disorders, and a host of degenerative diseases.[65] In the case of "Doctor Photo," Snelling claimed to have discovered a remarkable cure in photographers' collodion formula, which typically consisted of alcohol, ether, pyroxylin (gun cotton), and iodide and bromide salts. While collodion was used as a preservative and an essential component of photographic film, it also had a wide range of applications as a therapeutic medicine, from treating dermatological abnormalities to dressing inflamed, burned, or otherwise sore skin during and after the Civil War.[66]

Since commercial photographers worked with precisely the same substances as those who prepared and dispensed medicines, considerable overlap existed between their practices. Not only did they both purchase their materials from wholesale merchants like Taylor & Wetherbee, but Philadelphia photographers also embraced the precise working methods of apothecaries and druggists, often with the aim of putting more science into their chemical operations. While an advertisement for James F. Magee & Co. suggests that this prominent Philadelphia supplier could promote its chemicals as "pure" in part by displaying them like the contents of an apothecary's cabinet in clearly labeled leak-stop bottles (fig. 37), Wilson's journals regularly acknowledged that the scientific and professional character of darkroom work was tied to representations of photographic chemicals as precisely measured, unadulterated, and compositionally invariable.[67] Such journals further promoted a connection between photographics and therapeutics by basing the classification of photographers' chemicals on the science of *materia medica,* or the branch of medicine that describes "the substances used as medicines, their origin, composition, modes of preparation and administration, [and] physiological and toxological actions."[68]

The similarities between the descriptive lists of chemicals published by Philadelphia's medical and photographic communities are perhaps best expressed in an article aptly titled "Materia Photographica," which appeared in the 1872 edition of *Photographic Mosaics.* In this eight-page "ready reference" for the commercial photographer, its author, Edward Moelling, provided "a short description of the chemicals mostly used in photography," from acetic acid to zinc iodide, "giving the principal qualities of the different substances, their symbols, specific gravity, &c."[69] Like the *United States Pharmacopoeia,* Moelling's guide describes a given chemical's unique properties—its color, smell, taste, melting and boiling points, and solubility—as well as its most common compounds. The chemical's "physiological and toxological actions," which feature in the *Pharmacopoeia,* however, are replaced by its *photographic* applications, namely, the specific process(es) or solution(s) in which it is typically used. In making this substitution, "Materia Photographica" does more than put more science into photographers' laboratory practices; it encourages readers to see the photographic indications of a given substance as analogous to its therapeutic function(s).

Following the publication of "Doctor Photo," the fantasy of a "photographic pharmacopeia" fostered this analogy by providing it with a specific goal—that is, to help convince the studio public that photographers' chemical operations were thoroughly professional, sanctioned by the medical community, and even conducive to good health. Given what we know about the perils of the nineteenth-century darkroom, this was a message in dire need of dissemination. It is thus hardly surprising, though certainly ironic, that

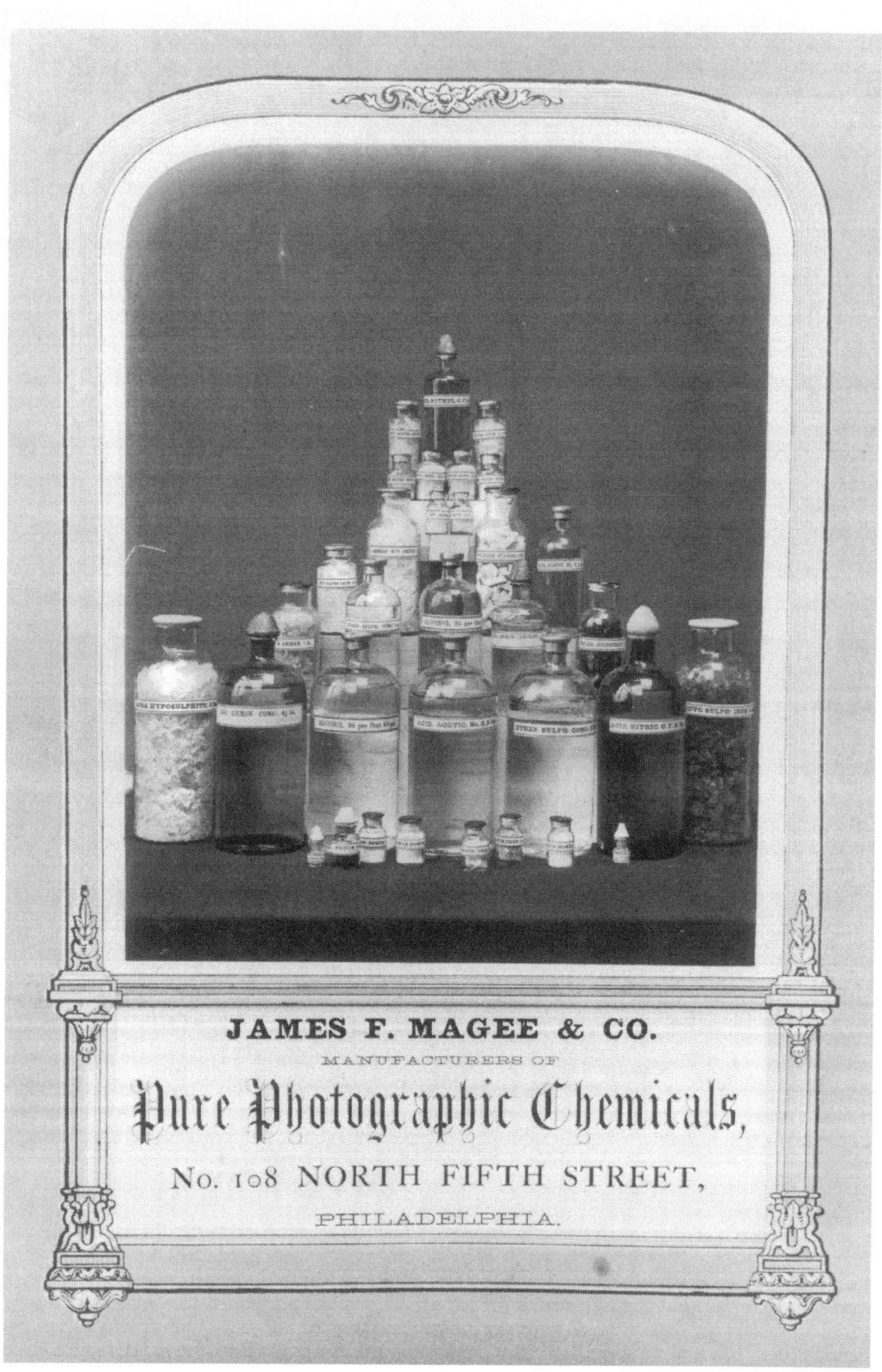

FIGURE 37 Wenderoth, Taylor & Brown, advertisement for James F. Magee & Co., Manufacturers of Pure Photographic Chemicals, 1871. Albumen print mounted on cardboard. From *The Gallery of Arts and Manufacturers Album.*

Philadelphia's photographic literature reported extensively on the curative properties of photographers' most deadly poisons, since thinking differently about the effects these toxic materials could have on the body could, if nothing else, curb the social threat they posed to commercial photographers and their practices. The same year that "Doctor Photo" appeared in the *Philadelphia Photographer,* for example, a debate over the potential benefits of cyanide of potassium as a therapeutic medicine unfolded on the pages of the *Photographic World.* In August 1871, Edward Wilson published a letter from a Frenchman, M. Eugene Ozier, who had long been afflicted with chronic pain, a violent cough, and bronchitis. Heeding his doctor's advice to take up "some light manual labor," Ozier began practicing photography, through which he was regularly exposed to cyanide. In his "reckless employment of this agent" to remove silver stains from his hands, he "paid little attention to any little scratches or ruptures of the skin produced by the plates or the pumice." Remarkably, his "inexperience" and resulting carelessness with photographic cyanide allowed Ozier to make an important medical discovery: "At the end of a fortnight's work in this manner, I found the pains in my back diminish, the sweats which troubled me at night ceased altogether, and the cough itself slackened in its intensity. . . . In a couple of months the serious symptoms with which I had been troubled had passed away, and now for three years I have enjoyed, relatively speaking, perfect health."[70] Wilson was initially quite skeptical about this use of cyanide as a medical cure, warning readers of the *Photographic World* to be cautious about taking Ozier's advice; yet two months after first publishing this report, he returned to the results with optimism. Revising his initial apprehension concerning photography's impact on health, Wilson acknowledged that much could be gained from reconfiguring not only his photographic audience as medical authorities *and* patients but also poisonous photographic chemicals as therapeutic medicine.

Like Snelling, whose stated aim in "Doctor Photo" was to "present a [new] phase . . . of photography as a physician," Wilson anticipated that findings like Ozier's would endow the fledgling profession and medium of photography with considerable, and perhaps unequaled, social value. "If the practice of photography and the individual action or combined action of any of the agents employed be found of value to consumptive patients," he predicted, "a new phase of interest will be found in the art."[71] For both Snelling and Wilson, this "new phase" of photography involved a radical revision of its relationship to the body. In cases where photographic chemistry was discovered to have therapeutic physiological effects, the mediating distance between the materials of photography and the subjects it aims to represent was erased, such that the site of the medium's transformative effects shifted from the image (the photographic negative or print) to the body itself. To put it another way, the medium of representation in these reports *becomes* the human body, which literally ingests or absorbs photography. Along with that fantasy of photography's direct somatic access came important claims about the medium's social power. Snelling and Wilson (via Ozier) could assert that the ability to cure the most deadly chronic and epidemic diseases plaguing urban Americans lay not with the medical profession, whose system of therapeutics had proved ineffectual in treating these ailments, but in the unlikely hands of studio photographers.

Modern readers may recognize the continued importance of highlighting photography's unmediated relationship to the body in twentieth-century critical theory, which generally describes that relationship in terms of an equivalence between a photographic portrait and the body of its subject. That the idea of photography as an immediate medicine had to be generated through analogies to surgery, phototherapy, and pharmacy, however, suggests that the technology's presumed lack of mediation was not as natural or seamless as the leaders of the Philadelphia photographic community, and those who later theorized their practices, have encouraged us to believe. The central problem that arose when photographers attempted to represent their chemicals as therapeutic drugs in the nineteenth century is perhaps self-evident: these substances were designed to treat other photographic materials and not intended for consumption by photographers or their sitters. As a result, the substitution of photographic chemicals for medicinal drugs frequently raised the issue of the former's adverse effects on human subjects when actually put into practice. According to the *American Journal of Photography*, one unsuspecting gentleman, upon receiving a "bottle of medicine" from a chemist, had the unfortunate experience of "being knocked out of his chair" when "it exploded with great violence, shattering a number of articles in his vicinity." Apparently there "had been an error; [his] medicine had gone to the photographer and the photographer's bottle to the patient, the contents being a *'preparation of a very sensitive kind'*"—a kind clearly unsuited to human consumption.[72] Members of the American Pharmaceutical Association expressed similar concerns about the interchangeability of photographic and pharmaceutical materials in their 1872 "Report on Adulterations and Sophistications." The preparation of ether for photographic purposes, they explained, yielded an undesirable and potentially dangerous contamination of this anesthetic agent, which was also a common ingredient in medical prescriptions. A doctor or patient could easily find himself in possession of "photographic" ether, a solution that contained a high concentration of alcohol, which was necessary to dissolve collodion properly but could potentially poison human subjects.[73] This report reminds us, in fact, that studio photographers routinely employed vast quantities of chemicals, quantities that would have constituted a potentially lethal overdose if prescribed by practitioners of irregular medicine or by doctors who administered controversial "heroic" therapies. It would seem, then, that the studio laboratory was not a proper therapeutic environment, nor was the use of photographic chemistry as medicine a proper application of photography, given that what ensured the health of photographic materials was very likely to make human bodies sick. Here again we run up against the old problem of matter being out of place in the photographic laboratory.

While these practical concerns are significant, insofar as they could ensure or prevent real material effects on the body, the aim of the cultural historian should not be to determine whether representations of photography as medicine belonged to the realm of fact or fiction. Rather, as this book has aimed to do, we must approach them as strategies that performed specific and important work in early photographic discourse. The apparent incompatibility of photographic chemistry and the body, in other words, does not change the fact that photographers imagined that their darkroom materials could be consumed by a human subject and ultimately cure her disease; nor does the fact that they often relied on figurative language to do so undercut the serious implications of their vision. The idea that photography could serve as more than a medium of representation was indeed a powerful fantasy that shaped perceptions of virtually every aspect of studio practice in nineteenth-century America. Motivated by the photographic community's professional aims and fueled by a middle-class desire for a technology of the body that could immediately cure all, that idea remains one of the most significant artifacts of the construction of photographic authority.

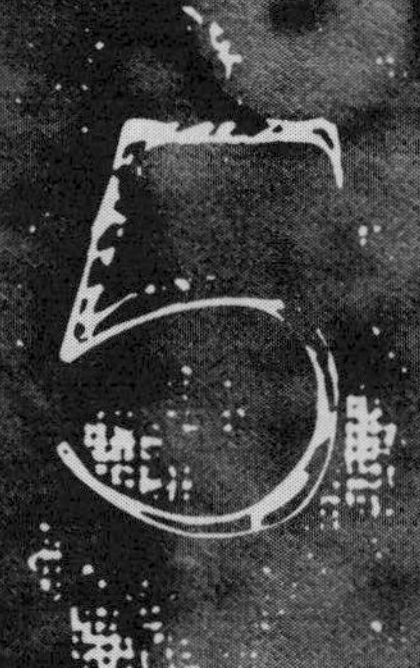

PHOTO DOCTORS AND PIXEL SURGEONS
The Medicine of Photography in the Digital Age

In May 2008 the *New Yorker* published a feature article on "the premier retoucher of fashion photographs," Pascal Dangin, whose high-profile work has graced the pages of *Vogue, Vanity Fair, Harper's Bazaar,* and countless other magazines. The author of the article, Lauren Collins, had observed and interviewed the French-born Dangin extensively in an effort to understand the man behind the computer, the man who spends long days and nights digitally manipulating the bodies of models and actresses with the help of Adobe Photoshop. The result of this process was a barrage of colorful metaphors. For many people, Collins explained, Dangin is "a translator, an interpreter, a conductor, a ballet dancer articulating choreographed steps," although she preferred to think of him as "a building superintendent . . . [who] knows how to do a lot of jobs," or as "a consigliere for a generation of photographers uncomfortable with, or uninterested in, the details of digital technology."[1]

Additional associations, including repeated comparisons to the fine arts, emerged as Collins described what Dangin actually does to the images on his computer screen. His "digital brushstrokes can be as deliberate as Jasper Johns's or John Currin's are on canvas," she wrote; he can "smooth a blemish or a blip" on a subject's face "with painterly subtlety." The work Dangin showed Collins in his "basement laboratory" suggests greater affinities, however, between his manipulations and surgical practices. Using Photoshop, Dangin "minimized [an] actress's temples, which bulged a little, tightened the skin around her chin, and excised a fleshy bump from her forehead." On another occasion "he had restructured the chest—higher, tighter—of an actress who, to his eye, seemed to have had a clumsy breast enhancement." In this case, Collins observed, "virtual plastic surgery cancelled out real plastic surgery, resulting in a believable look."[2]

The idea that manipulating a body with digital technology is akin to a medical procedure, specifically one that belongs to the now thriving field of cosmetic medicine, is not exclusive to the story of Pascal Dangin. Indeed, we needn't look far to find similar characterizations of digital retouching in American culture, given that they have been the subject of a number of controversies surrounding celebrity photographs in the popular media. Take the infamous reconstruction of Oprah Winfrey that appeared on the cover of *TV Guide* in August 1989. Often referred to as Oprah's "body transplant," the cover featured the head of the star superimposed, by means of Photoshop, on the photographic body of Ann-Margret, taken from a 1979 publicity shot of the model-actress. Performed without the knowledge of either subject, this amalgamation was presumably a quick and easy way for the magazine to slim down Oprah's body and force it to adhere to an ideal norm of white feminine beauty. More than a decade later, as Collins herself recalls, the British edition of *GQ* "doctored" photographs of Kate Winslet in a similarly liberal fashion by lengthening her legs, flattening her stomach, and generally concealing her "womanly" curves. Winslet objected to this radical operation, asserting that her body and her identity were not truthfully represented by the published photographs. The British and American press, in turn, expressed both excitement and (mild) dismay over *GQ*'s treatment of Winslet's photographs, using the incident as an opportunity to proclaim a new era in photography. "No diet, no exercise, no surgery, no pills. Just a little digital wizardry," reported the *Miami Herald* in the wake of the Winslet scandal. "Point and click here, point and click there, and unwanted pounds magically melt away—from your photographic image, that is."[3]

The discussions sparked by the Winslet pictures point to a connection between medical and photographic discourse with a long history, one with which readers of this book are familiar. There is nothing new, after all, about equating retouching with the practices of cosmetic medicine, or about the potential for a photograph to be "doctored" to the extent that a sitter no longer recognizes herself. In fact, many of the aesthetic and ethical questions raised by the now ubiquitous techniques of digital manipulation in fashion and celebrity photography recapitulate debates first waged in early American photographic circles. As in the 1870s, "doctors" of photography today disagree about whether extreme digital manipulation is a valuable tool or an unwelcome threat to the photographic body and the human subject it represents. Recalling Henry Snelling's vehement opposition to radical retouching when it was first introduced in the

United States, Pascal Dangin defines digital doctoring as "excessive" when it becomes anatomically "disfiguring." In fashion magazines, he remarks, "girls [have] their legs slimmed and they no longer have tibias and femurs, and it's weird." Explaining his refusal to correct an "endearingly crooked bottom row of teeth" on a well-known actress, he remarks, "I don't want her to become someone else."[4]

We must do more, of course, than simply acknowledge that the metaphorical language and concept of "doctoring" photographs *have* a history; we must examine the cultural work they have performed *in* history. And so I propose the following questions by way of concluding this study. In what ways has the medicalization of retouching expressed historically specific ideas about photography's cultural identity, its social function, and its perceived relationship to the body in American culture, first in the decades after the medium's invention and subsequently in the wake of its so-called digital reinvention? If medical models and metaphors helped establish the professional character of commercial photographic practices in the nineteenth century, represented the portrait studio as a space that promoted physical and social rehabilitation in a period marked by civil war and epidemic disease, and defined the "healthy" American body as white and middle class when those markers of social identity were seen as increasingly threatened by the emancipation of blacks and the steady influx of European immigrants, what might they do today for digital photography?

To begin, we might observe that the *medicine of photography* has come into being at historical moments when the medium is perceived to be facing a crisis of identity. Beginning in the late 1980s, many critics and image makers anticipated a "digital revolution" that would have far-reaching, even catastrophic, effects on the practices and culture of photography. Digital technologies, they observed, have fundamentally transformed the material characteristics of the medium we once knew; optical lenses, chemicals, and silver-based film have been replaced by electronic sensors, data processors, and computer monitors, resulting in new possibilities for the capture, storage, and transmission of images. With such changes, these observers predicted, much would be lost, including the physical space of the darkroom, the skills required to operate within it, and the tonal range and resolution one had come to expect of photographic prints. The business of photography would also be radically altered, they alleged, insofar as the materials and techniques once controlled by professional operators and marketed by corporations like Kodak and Polaroid were rendered obsolete by the personal computer. The most significant change forecast, however, concerned photography's perceived relationship to objectivity and truth. As Fred Ritchin wrote in 1990, the fact that computer technologies enabled photographs to be infinitely manipulated—and even wholly invented without reference to a preexisting physical reality—challenged popular assumptions about such images as "relatively unmediating and trustworthy."[5] Although photographs have always been material and social constructions, Ritchin argued, the camera in the digital age has acquired a new capacity to lie—what W. J. T. Mitchell would call a "temptation to duplicity"—that informs the new means of seeing, knowing, and shaping the world that it offers photojournalists, art photographers, and snapshooters.[6]

Reports of the death of photography and the advent of a "post-photographic" age continue to circulate in both the popular press and artistic circles, even though media

historians and theorists have been quick to challenge those assumptions. Contributors to the edited volume *The Photographic Image in Digital Culture* (1995) mounted an
early critique of the progressivism, technological determinism, and ahistoricism they
identified in such narratives. According to Kevin Robins, the idea of a digital revolution promoted by Mitchell and others is predicated on the problematic "belief that the
future is always superior to the past, and . . . that this superior future is a spontaneous
consequence of technological development" rather than the result of a gradual process
through which technologies are shaped by any number of social, political, and economic
factors. By "intensify[ing] contrasts between past (bad) and future (good)," moreover,
those who speak of revolution "obscure the nature and significance of very real conti-
nuities."[7] Martin Lister framed this critique in his introduction to the book, observing
that "the new image technologies are in an active relation, of some dependence and
continuity, with a 150-year-old photographic culture," having never made a "clean break"
from the "cultural forms, institutions and discourses" of this culture.[8] Without denying
its novelty, Lister and Robins acknowledged that much of what we say about digital photography once applied to analogue photography in the nineteenth century, including the
rhetoric of image revolution and debates about the medium's reality and artifice.[9] Much
of the subsequent scholarship on the emergence of new media has remained commit-
ted to understanding the digital in relation to older photographic and visual technologies, speaking in terms of adaptation, imitation, transformation, and rivalry.[10]

Significantly, it was precisely as these discussions were unfolding that medical
metaphor reemerged in the ideas about and practices of portrait photography. I speak of
reemergence not to suggest that the *medicine of photography* disappeared entirely from
photographers' trade literature or from popular writing on the medium after 1890—a
year roughly coincident with the mass marketing of photography in the United States
by companies like Eastman Kodak—but rather to point to important changes in its fre-
quency and use in these texts, of which I hope to encourage further study. For evidence
of this shift, we might look at the scattered references to "doctors of photography" in
early twentieth-century photographic journals, where they refer to any "learned and
skilled photographer," including the amateur, rather than function exclusively as instruments of professionalization.[11] Similarly, we can observe comparisons of the instruments of photography and those of medicine in the same period—as in the misappre-
hension of a boxlike Kodak camera for a doctor's leather bag—as commenting on and
contributing to something other than photographic authority in matters of the body; in
the comical illustration in figure 38, medicine functions as nothing more than a prop,
drained of the multifarious cultural meanings it once held for American studio photographers and their middle-class public, indicating only the ubiquity of amateurs and their
cameras. Admittedly, these are oversimplifications. I offer them nevertheless as a way
of framing a pressing question for scholars of new media and readers of this book: how
are we to account for the pervasive, purposeful, and at times anxious medicalization of
digital photographic practices in recent decades, and what light might it shed on both
prophetic and critical discussions of a digital revolution?

Recent reflections on that revolution suggest one possibility. In the case of representations of digital manipulation as cosmetic medicine, we might say that they redefine

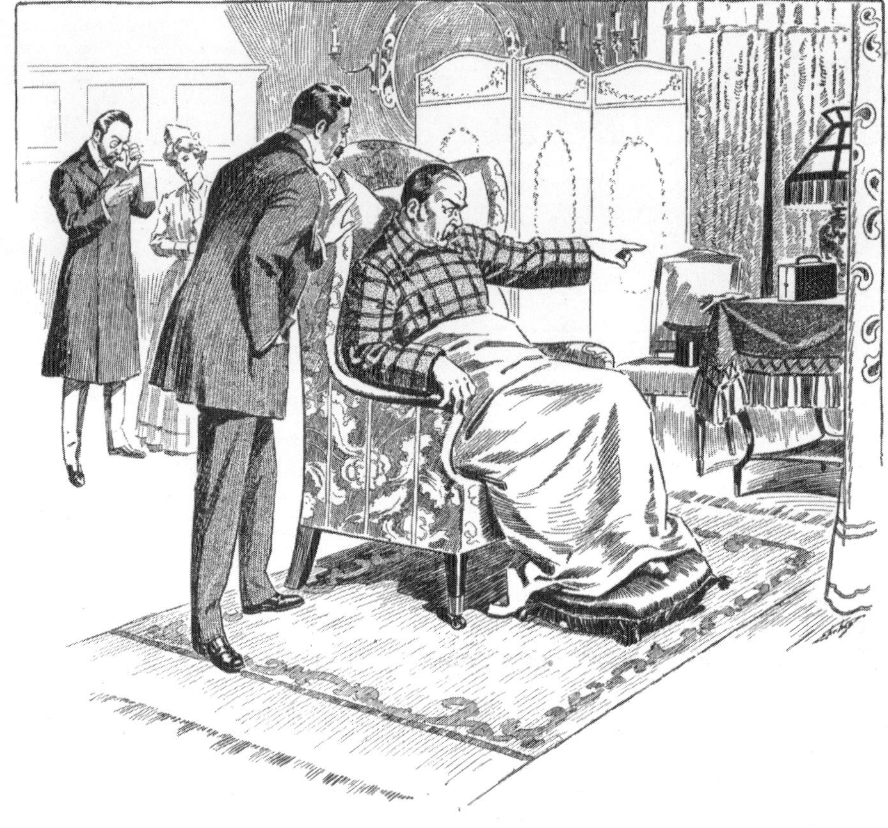

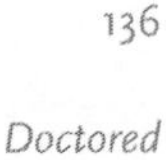

INSTINCT.

SICK MAGNATE *(feebly)*. — What is that on the table there?
SECRETARY. — That? That is the doctor's medicine-case.
SICK MAGNATE *(relieved)*. — Thanks. I — er — thought it was a camera.

FIGURE 38 *Instinct,* ca. 1910. Wood engraving. From *Puck* 67, no. 1742 (July 20, 1910): 5.

photographic authority by pointing to the digital camera's capacity to transform bodies in visible and highly mediated ways. While the promise of virtual rehabilitations that rival medicine in their transformative potential contributed to the social value of studio portraits in the nineteenth century, the idea that the authority of photography can be constructed exclusively through a self-conscious denial of its perceived relationship to the real—variously understood in terms of its immediacy, indexicality, automaticity, objectivity, or simply truth—is a novel feature of digital photographic discourse. Such an idea serves us well when considering the work of artists who make little effort to conceal the disjunction between the "real" body and the digitally manipulated photographic body, producing obvious, seemingly infinite, and often bizarre transformations of the latter. In this group we would locate Keith Cottingham, a California-based art photographer described as working "in the manner of a plastic surgeon" in the 1996 exhibition catalogue *Photography After Photography.* An "expert in digitized skin grafts," Cottingham creatively constructs new body surfaces based on a personal and at times fantastical vision of what they should look like; he "sutures selected textures from his personal color chart, and uses these to dress his 3D models captured on computer screen."[12] We might also place in Cottingham's company the thirty "cutting-edge" fashion photographers that Martin Dawber labels "pixel surgeons" in his 2005 book by that title. Influenced by cultural practices as disparate as avant-garde theater and genetic engineering, their cyborgs, aliens, vamps, and goddesses suggest that digital photography constitutes an entirely new medium of expression that mocks the apparent limits of the "real."[13]

But does this reading of medical metaphor strictly in terms of its ability to signal, if not directly facilitate, the new creative capacities and imaginative qualities of photography since the advent of the digital help us comprehend the many comparisons between digital portraiture and cosmetic medicine outside of these artistic circles? Does it allow us to make sense of such representations, that is, in image-manipulation software programs, instructional literature for amateur photographers, and commercial (predominantly Internet-based) photographic services? Can established narratives of media transitions fully account, moreover, for the *social* motivations and implications of the *medicine of photography* in contemporary American culture?

THE PHOTO DOCTOR IS IN

To offer a preliminary answer, I turn the reader's attention to two popular photographic manuals published in 2006, both intended for American snapshooters unfamiliar with the workings of Adobe Photoshop. The more self-consciously "straight-talking" of the two, Tim Daly and David Asch's *Digital Photo Doctor* promises readers "simple steps to diagnose, rescue, and enhance your images." On the cover, a stylized mark of an electrocardiogram intersects the title, a stethoscope drapes itself around a digital camera, and a series of portraits, before and after digital retouching, forms a band across the bottom (fig. 39). Inside, various chapter headings—from "Doctor, I Keep Being Exposed!" to "Doctor, I Need Assistance!"—portray the digital photograph (and sometimes the digital camera) as a sick patient that requires the medicine of Photoshop, recalling the personification of photographic materials we saw in discussions of the nineteenth-century darkroom. Illustrated with a series of pre- and postoperative photographs, each chapter in *Digital Photo Doctor* presents "symptoms" of and step-by-step "treatments" for common photographic problems. Most of these address technical problems related to composition, color, detail, lighting, and exposure that stem from the requirements of the digital camera, the insufficient skills of its amateur operator, or both.

In a chapter titled "Doctor, I Want Plastic Surgery!" the authors acknowledge the negative effects of such problems on desired body images. The first section of this chapter teaches readers how to use a Photoshop retouching tool called the "spot healing brush" (itself a conflation of artistic and medical metaphors) to remedy the "uneven skin tone and minor blemishes" of a pale-complexioned twenty-something man who is smartly dressed in coat and tie and appears to suffer from a mild case of acne. Accentuated by the camera's flash, the authors explain, "patchy skin tone . . . can turn a potentially flattering portrait into the picture you quickly flip past in the family

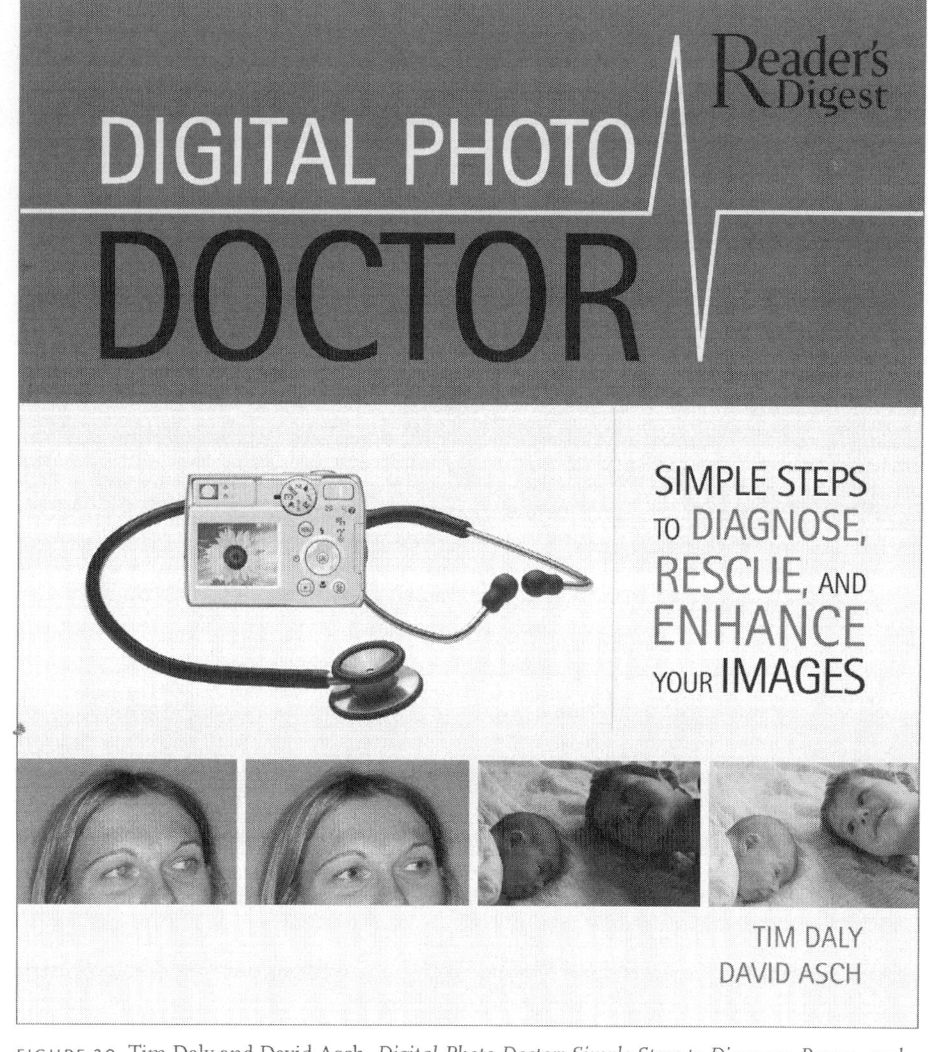

FIGURE 39 Tim Daly and David Asch, *Digital Photo Doctor: Simple Steps to Diagnose, Rescue, and Enhance Your Images* (Pleasantville, N.Y.: Reader's Digest Association, 2006), cover.

album."[14] Several pages later we are shown how to treat the "bulky body" of a young woman in an oversized T-shirt using different layers (images that can be laid on top of one another) along with the "clone stamp" and "healing brush" tools; these effectively remove the wrinkles in her shirt and reduce the appearance of fat beneath them, resulting in a body that looks "thin." While the book's claim that "photographs capture and preserve a moment—however good or bad the subject looked at the time" suggests that the apparently overweight sitter makes such treatments necessary, its observation that "harsh lighting and poor composition can change a person's appearance, often for the worst [*sic*]," puts the blame back on the technology that renders her likeness unattractive. Despite this ambivalence, the authors of *Digital Photo Doctor* remain unequivocal about the positive aesthetic and sanitary potential of digital retouching, which "can be used to straighten, tidy, and hide the features you'd rather not repeatedly see."[15]

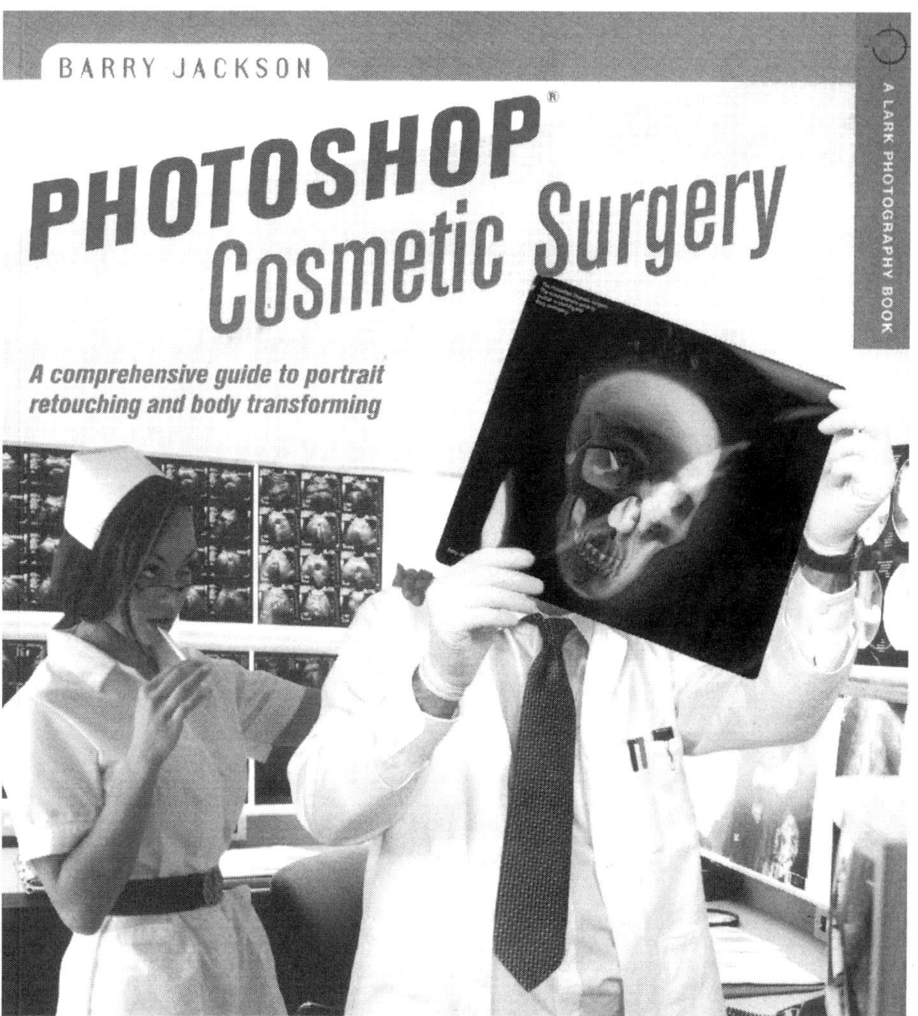

FIGURE 40 Barry Jackson, *Photoshop Cosmetic Surgery: A Comprehensive Guide to Portrait Retouching and Body Transforming* (New York: Lark Books, 2006), cover.

Also written for a lay audience, Barry Jackson's *Photoshop Cosmetic Surgery: A Comprehensive Guide to Portrait Retouching and Body Transforming* employs medical metaphor as it explores the corporeal possibilities and limits of digital photographic manipulation (fig. 40). The book's author adopts the guise of "Dr. Jackson," a middle-aged bald man dressed in either surgical scrubs or a white lab coat who variously holds up a scalpel, a paintbrush, an examination light, and an X-ray. Working alongside a provocatively clad nurse aptly named Jane Peg (J. Peg), he appears in a series of playful scenarios that illustrate each chapter; in one, Jane Peg applies a liposuction tool to Dr. Jackson's cheek as she gazes coyly at the reader, while in another he lifts the seductively posed nurse above his head in a feat of strength obviously mismatched with his modest build. Combining light humor and sexual fantasy, these illustrations encourage readers to laugh, and perhaps even turn them on, as the book's "surgical case studies" outline a wide range of "doctoring" skills.

The case studies consist of a series of letters from potential "patients" who have questions regarding particular "cosmetic" and "surgical" procedures. Jane Peg fields the former, explaining how to make a woman look like a "supermodel" not only by digitally removing pimples and freckles but also by virtually perfecting the symmetry of her face, changing her eye color from brown to blue, straightening and whitening her teeth, and treating her to a manicure. The doctor responds to the "surgical" cases by describing how to perform Photoshop "face lifts" that tighten the skin of "haggard" women and beer-drinking men over forty, construct a more prominent jaw line in a teenage boy, or create ideal noses on subjects of all ages. He also teaches his male "patients" how to build and define their muscles without leaving their computers, while women learn how to graphically alter the size of their breasts and put themselves on a "digital diet" that will slim their waists, arms, and thighs. Many of the patients who supposedly wrote to Dr. Jackson claim that they have been thinking about actually having one of these medical procedures, not because of any technical fault of the camera but because they simply don't like what they see in the mirror. Rather than go under the knife or subject themselves to harsh chemical treatments, however, they are invariably advised to opt for the relatively quick, inexpensive, painless, and risk-free operations that Photoshop offers them. Unlike *Digital Photo Doctor,* which is careful not to "overdo it," *Photoshop Cosmetic Surgery* represents these operations as seemingly limitless by including sex changes and human-to-animal transformations alongside more popular surgical procedures.

These books nevertheless share an important point of connection: they offer eager snapshooters professional knowledge and skills that they can apply to their own ailing portraits. For Daly and Asch, this means training readers to take technically superior photographs that will require as little retouching as possible, as well as teaching them how to use "state-of-the-art digital photo technology" like Adobe Photoshop when such efforts fail. Their goal, in other words, is to transform the reader into a "photo doctor" who can effectively practice both preventive and emergency medicine at home. *Photoshop Cosmetic Surgery* also promises to educate the amateur so that he can "retouch, enhance, improve, and manipulate digital photographs like a professional." In making that claim, however, another important difference from *Digital Photo Doctor* arises, for Jackson does not assume that everyone who picks up a camera can become a "photo doctor"; he chooses to reserve that title for "a distinguished Photoshop surgeon" like himself.[16] While his antics with Jane Peg are undoubtedly incongruous with traditional notions of the medical professional, which lends some comic relief to the book's otherwise technical discussions, Jackson's cultivation of the "photo doctor" persona as an embodiment of photographic authority is not to be taken lightly, given the ubiquity and social importance of this figure in contemporary commercial circles.

In fact, a staggering number of digital photographers across the United States now advertise their businesses on the Internet using the name "Photo Doctor" or variants thereof, including Photo Doctor 911, The Photo Physician, Photo Physician Rx, The Photo Surgeon, and (unlikely as it sounds) Miss Photo Surgeon.[17] Littered with scalpels, first-aid kits, ambulances, and Aesculapian staffs, their online marketing materials also draw heavily from medical models. According to her website, Dr. Louise Lutz (The Photo Doctor) of Tully, New York, "can bring your 'sick' photos back to health by performing the necessary digital 'surgery,'" which encompasses "professional digital photo repair, restoration, retouching and enhancements." Others offer a list of variously priced medicalized procedures ranging from a "basic check-up" or "Botox injection" that might include the removal of a tear in the print, a facial blemish, or other small details, to the more expensive "major reconstructive surgery" involving larger-scale manipulations to produce a desired body image, not unlike those promoted by popular magazines and *Photoshop Cosmetic Surgery.*

Much of this medical discourse may strike Internet surfers as mere entertainment, but the example of Allen Showalter—known as "The Photo Doctor" in Harrisonburg, Virginia—reminds us that such metaphor making can be instrumental to commercial success. In 2001 Showalter purchased his family's photofinishing business in the city and established the Showalter Imaging Group, which owns several retail stores as well as an Internet-based photographic printing service for local newspapers. Shortly thereafter, sporting a white lab coat and stethoscope, he began offering a "free camera clinic and checkup" in front of his King 1 Hour Photo store in Harrisonburg's Valley Mall, where he would test shoppers' photographic equipment, perform minor repairs, and "diagnose" their photographic problems. Showalter explained to *Digital Imaging Digest* and later to *PMA Magazine*—both trade publications of "the world's largest photo marketing group," on whose board he currently serves—that he first created "The Photo Doctor" in order to set King 1 Hour Photo apart from its competition, which meant attracting more customers and increasing sales.[18] Now making regular appearances on a call-in radio show as well as on the morning news program of a local television station, "The Photo Doctor" tells potential customers that he can offer them valuable, trustworthy—in a word, professional—advice about photography (see fig. 41).[19] This medical persona "helps enhance our image as photo experts," he observed frankly in 2002. "It differentiates what we offer from the mass merchants."[20] Prominently displayed on his television segment and on the King 1 Hour Photo website, Showalter's extensive credentials, which include "the area's only Certified Photofinishing Engineer

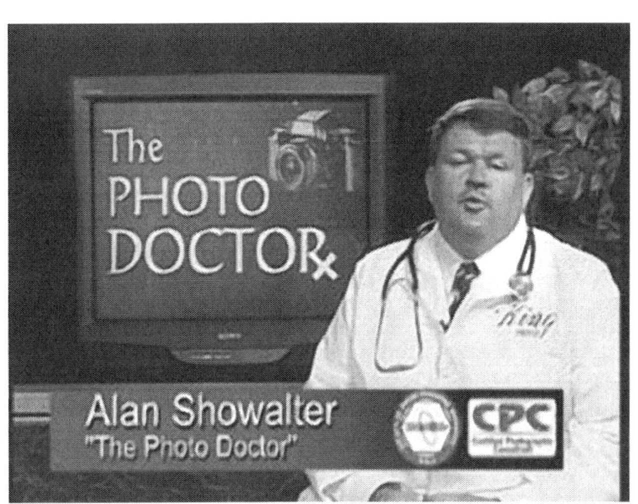

FIGURE 41 Allen Showalter as "The Photo Doctor" on WHSV-TV, Harrisonburg, Va.

and Certified Photographic Consultant," perform a similar function, attesting not only to his standing in the field but also to the high quality of his work.[21]

As Showalter has acknowledged, the performances of authority by contemporary "photo doctors" are largely responses to the social and economic effects of massive technological changes in the field of commercial photography. "It's not news to anyone there are fewer photos being printed at the retail level than 4 years or 5 years ago," he observed in 2008. "Ten years ago, we were at the start of the digital transition. This transition was warned about for such a long time—and then it came faster, harder, and more completely than I believe anyone predicted."[22] Now that seemingly anyone can take, manipulate, and share a photograph equipped with little more than a cell phone and a home computer, in other words, business owners like Showalter are struggling to adjust to the evolving market, a market in which they compete not only with others in their trade but increasingly with the public they once served. In this way, the now ubiquitous figure of the "photo doctor" in commercial photographic discourse works against the aims of popular manuals like *Digital Photo Doctor,* which tout the knowledge and skills of the "pro" only to place them in the hands of the amateur snapshooter.

Higher-profile photographers like Pascal Dangin who have embraced digital technologies are, unsurprisingly, less concerned in their public discourse with a perceived threat from amateurs. They nevertheless continue to express fear of amateurs' *perceptions,* particularly the old idea of commercial operators as "mere" manual laborers, which has been given new life now that they rely so heavily on computers. The *New Yorker* article on Dangin makes clear that this anxiety is precisely what motivates the author's and her subject's embrace of metaphor, which they use to demonstrate that the master retoucher is much more than his machine. While Lauren Collins observes candidly that Dangin's "clients are paying for his eye, and his mind, as much as for his hand," Dangin finds in the model of plastic surgery a more fitting means of describing the secret of his success. "Why is there a Mr. Lips and a Mr. Hips and a Mr. Buttocks out there? Why do they exist?" he asks. "Because people have an idea about what they don't want but not an idea about what they do. A doctor will do a million noses because he has a flair for what noses should be."[23]

In many ways, then, history seems to be repeating itself. Just as a proliferation of unskilled operators and a boom in amateur photography fueled nineteenth-century portrait photographers' self-promotion as authorities on physical and social health, a perceived need to reassert the uniquely professional character of photography in the face of the "digital revolution" informs commercial photographers' self-fashioning as "photo doctors" today. If we see such medical metaphors as a feature of early photographic discourse, then we might interpret this continuity as evidence of remediation, or the process through which a "new" medium (digital photography) and its operators make reference to the forms of an "older" medium (analogue photography). This is not the remediation traditionally described in narratives of media transition, which emphasize the adaptation of visual epistemologies; rather, it deploys established rhetorical strategies in periods of technological and professional (re)invention. But we must qualify our premise here, since medical metaphor never belonged exclusively to nineteenth-century portrait photography, just as the proliferation of "auto doctors," "shoe doctors," and "hair doctors" in the United States reminds us that its contemporary use is hardly limited to digital imaging practices.[24] As this study has aimed to show, photographers borrowed their figurative language and concepts from another profession; these, in turn, have been constructed in relation to a social context outside the portrait studio or the digital laboratory and shared by a variety of other cultural practices. In examining the intersection of digital photography and medicine, it is therefore not enough to observe that the material changes in photographic technology develop alongside social changes in the body of operators that control it; we must also attend to the ways in which that intersection enters into close dialogue with other forms of professional and popular culture that emerge at the same time.

DIGITAL PHOTOGRAPHY AND MAKEOVER CULTURE

More specifically, the discourse of "digital cosmetic surgery" sketched briefly above participates in a now pervasive "makeover culture" that incorporates national myths of transformation and reinvention as old as the United States. As the growing body of scholarship on this set of practices has observed, its texts have historically included progress narratives in American literature and advice columns in popular magazines.[25] Most recently it has taken the form of makeover-themed television shows that promise to "improve" the lives of "average" Americans by materially altering their homes, cars, clothes, and bodies. Over the past decade, many of these shows have offered cosmetic surgery as a primary means of transformation, among them ABC's highly influential *Extreme Makeover* (2002–5), the controversial and short-lived *The Swan* (2004–5, Fox) and *I Want a Famous Face* (2004–5, MTV), and the remarkably long-running *Dr. 90210* on E! (2004–).[26] While Brenda Weber and others have studied the differences across this body of programming in terms of plotlines, they have also identified a consistent assumption within it: by subjecting her body to a scrutinizing public gaze that brands it as "ugly" or "ordinary," and allowing "medical" authorities to perform an often radical reconstruction of her outward appearance, paid for (in most cases) by the network, the makeover subject can and indeed must achieve a "better" self. According to Weber, makeover programs construct this wished-for made-over self, showcased in a spectacular final unveiling, as "worthy, sexy, empowered, confident, gender congruent, and stable." This is a self, she argues, that belongs to a "good and proper citizen . . . who is self-aware, an active participant in consumer culture, marked as racially normative, and willing to alter the material signifiers of subject status to more fully assimilate into a dominant model of 'American' citizenry."[27]

There are a number of striking connections between the assumptions that makeover television makes about the surgically remade body/self/identity and those expressed in contemporary discussions and practices of digital photographic doctoring. At a basic level, the procedures outlined in popular Photoshop manuals and on the websites of "photo doctors" similarly conceive of (predominantly female) bodies as always-already operable and represent health as synonymous with a "beautiful" external appearance achieved through technological intervention. What is more, they promise that such intervention, enabled by the purchase of software for one's home computer or photographic services on the Internet, will produce only positive, happy results. Manuals like *Photoshop Cosmetic Surgery* focus primarily, though not exclusively, on "average" Americans: working men and women who can't afford gym memberships or fancy photographic equipment, let alone expensive cosmetic surgery, but seek some form of upward social mobility.[28] That many of these subjects hope someday to succeed in modeling, acting, or the music industry speaks to the fact that the ideal of beauty promoted by digital cosmetic surgery is defined largely in relation to celebrity culture and is thus subject to strict corporeal and social limits.

Those limits are articulated through the doctored bodies themselves, which are invariably made to appear thin and youthful, contributing to perceptions of their femininity (or masculinity) as well as their respectability, since physical "excess" and aging are generally seen as signs of "letting yourself go" associated with the lower class. The digital removal of tattoos similarly works to normalize bodies economically marked as "other," while tools used to hide freckles, lighten skin, and generally "balance" skin pigmentation idealize "pure" whiteness as the desired norm. While *Digital Photo Doctor* enables this social homogenization in part by choosing not to depict a single person of color in its illustrations—a conspicuous omission also common to "photo doctor" websites—*Photoshop Cosmetic Surgery* includes multiple races and ethnicities in its surgical case studies, only to pathologize their nonwhite skin. Justine, for instance, explains in a letter to Dr. Jackson, "I love to look through my women's magazines and daydream about being a famous model with perfect skin."[29] To that end, the doctor helps her create a modeling portfolio of photographs that use Photoshop filters to create "a soft-focus, glowing kind of skin." The "before" portrait of Justine's face, however, reveals not a single blemish. It is only in examining her doctored "after" shot, in which her seemingly flawless complexion is lightened dramatically, that we discover the source of dis-ease for both doctor and patient: Justine's light brown flesh tones. In another case, a woman of color named Denise, who hates the dark circles under her eyes, asks Dr. Jackson to recommend a "cream or lotion that would banish them permanently." He kindly offers Photoshop as the "perfect product" for achieving the desired results, before crudely suggesting that if she's not convinced she can "give Michael Jackson a call—he may have some tips on lightening skin."[30]

Although the language used in these "diagnoses" makes specific reference to contemporary popular culture (to the King of Pop, no less!), on the whole there is little difference between their idealization of whiteness as respectability and that enacted by early retouching practices, like those used to treat Mlle. Artot (fig. 21). What we might see as new about the discourse of digital doctoring therefore lies elsewhere. One difference between nineteenth-century and twenty-first-century practices is found in the emphasis the latter places on extreme, and often distinctly gendered, emotional distress as the primary motivation for remaking the photographic body. In *Photoshop Cosmetic Surgery*, explicit discussion of such anxiety abounds. The women in the book are generally hypersensitive to what they take as an omnipresent male gaze; they believe men only when they say their bodies are "ugly" or "too fat," and they imagine that their husbands and boyfriends are "losing interest" in them because of their big noses or small breasts.

This hypersensitivity contributes to dysfunctional relationships, low self-esteem, and the unhealthy behavior employed to cope with both.

One of the most tragic of the book's case studies concerns Suzanne, who admits to Dr. Jackson that she has "a real hang-up about my calves" because, she says, "they are really solid and muscular, which I feel is very unattractive in a woman." This poor self-image leads her to spend the whole evening at her sister's wedding "trying to find things to stand behind so that nobody could see my legs." Instead of providing Suzanne with the mental health support she clearly needs, the doctor assures her that "nobody will remember how big your lower legs are" and recommends that she wear pants in the future, after doctoring the wedding photos. The men in *Photoshop Cosmetic Surgery* are by no means emotionally fit, but they are not as consistently demeaned or mocked by the "authority" to whom they have turned for treatment. Most are presented as "very self-conscious" about their bodies and want to look more attractive to the women they work with or meet via the Internet, who all seem to desire "beefy" men with mops of hair. The most extreme of these cases would have to be Peter, whose "weak chin," as he puts it, has "affect[ed] my mental well-being. . . . I can't bear to look at myself in photographs or reflective surfaces because my appearance upsets me too much." Dr. Jackson suggests that Peter Photoshop all of his portraits and "paste them over every mirror and reflective surface of your home. It will then only be a matter of time before you begin to believe what you see and your mental well-being will greatly improve."[31] While these narratives of anxiety and self-loathing have important precedents in the history of photography—Hugh Diamond and Jean-Martin Charcot prescribed similar photographic treatments for their hysterical patients in the mid-nineteenth century—they will be all too familiar to contemporary viewers of medical makeover television, whose extreme surgical reconstructions are predicated on the emotional distress of their subjects. Even subjects who initially claim that they "wouldn't change a thing" about their appearance end up submitting to the knife, or trying some digital cosmetic surgery, if only to explore for themselves the relationship between outward looks and inner well-being.

Generated out of private feelings of inferiority, inadequacy, or an abstract malaise, the images of health that extreme makeovers (digital or otherwise) produce are, ironically, intended for public consumption, which seems to confirm their significant social effects. In the case of televised makeovers, their public nature is underscored by the requisite big "reveal," which marks the subject's transition from "ugly" social outcast to "beautiful" socialized self. Digital cosmetic surgery has a close equivalent in the posting of doctored photographs on social networking, online dating, or photosharing websites that aim to facilitate users' successful entrance into a variety of social relations. Many "photo doctors" target customers looking to beautify themselves through this new genre of portraiture; others offer to preserve or enhance the social function of more traditional portraits, such as the family photograph, school picture, or wedding portrait. In the majority of cases, these doctors seek to create "healthy" public images for their subjects that reproduce narrowly defined ideas about what it means to belong to an "American" social group, whether it be a marriage, a nuclear family, or the nation itself. Their home pages are littered, in fact, with a sea of ideal citizens: smiling brides in white dresses, children on Santa's lap, and an increasing number of soldiers in uniform. These, we are told repeatedly, are the "cherished moments" that deserve to be brought "back to life" or surgically altered to "look their best."

A PERFECT LIE?

Despite their many similarities, the distinctions between digital and televised cosmetic surgery should not be overlooked, for they speak to the unique character of photography in contemporary makeover culture. Significantly, the corporeal transformations achieved by photographic doctoring are promoted as relatively quick, cheap, easy, and never painful. They also produce seemingly permanent reconstructions of virtual bodies that will not be compromised by the environmental or temporal effects on physical bodies. Digitally doctoring a portrait, in other words, uniquely produces an "after" that will exist and circulate "forever." As I argued in the case of nineteenth-century retouching, this is not to say that the surgical makeover is a less powerful tool than its photographic counterpart; popular shows like *Dr. 90210,* after all, continue to remind American viewers that it is through cosmetic surgery alone that "the media image finds flesh and physically imprints itself on the subject." [32]

The discourse of digital cosmetic surgery not only acknowledges this view but works hard to manage its implications for the relative value of the doctored photograph. It does so in part by consistently entertaining the idea that digitally manipulating a photographic portrait is somehow equivalent to surgically altering the subject's body itself. The personal narratives in *Photoshop Cosmetic Surgery* make this imagined equivalence explicit; most of the correspondents quoted in the book write to Dr. Jackson for his "expert" advice because they are considering undergoing a cosmetic medical procedure, such as rhinoplasty or a chemical peel, and end up receiving a Photoshop tutorial. Never is the strangeness of this result acknowledged in the text, other than through the book's lightly comic frame; in fact, patients and readers alike are encouraged to see the doctor's virtual procedures as a logical substitute for, even an improvement upon, the "real thing." Rather than disrupt this fantasy, insistent claims in the popular press that changes in one's digital photograph are not indicative of changes to one's "actual" body can likewise be read as promoting it. In the case of the *Miami Herald*'s comments on the Kate Winslet scandal, the newspaper's mention that a click of the mouse can make "unwanted pounds magically melt away—*from your photographic image, that is*" registers the fact that the digitally doctored photograph is imagined to be coextensive with the physical body, despite its apparent hypermediation.

This idea, of course, is an old one, constructed in part through references to medicine in the nineteenth century and subsequently instrumental to conceptions of (analogue) photographic truth. What is both surprising and largely unacknowledged in current scholarship is the challenge it poses to theories of image revolution, which see the advent of the digital as affecting photography's relationship to the real. The idea of digital cosmetic surgery obviously does not deny that doctored photographs are the products of intention and technological intervention. But is it fair to say that "digitization abandons even the rhetoric of truth," as Geoffrey Batchen once put it, when Photoshop becomes the medicine of choice for subjects who seek body-altering procedures? Or when Pascal Dangin uses "virtual plastic surgery" to create a "believable look" on the photographic body of a model who has already gone under the knife?[33] Can we further mourn the loss of the traditional hallmark of photography's authority—the idea that the referent adheres to the photographic image—when medical metaphors for digital manipulation guarantee the existence of a true and natural body in the untouched photograph? What, after all, does Kate Winslet's outrage at *GQ*'s liberal doctoring do if not confirm the indexicality of her (digital) "before" portraits, or photography's status as a sign of the real before medicalized intervention? To look at it in a different way, why would Winslet need so vehemently to protest the operations performed on her photographic body if digital technologies have indeed caused the image's referent to become "unstuck," as W. J. T. Mitchell claimed? Wouldn't *GQ*'s readers assume that its illustrations are ontologically severed from the bodies they represent and therefore never mistake them for Winslet "as she is"?

Likewise, the medium of photography has hardly lost its perceived truth-telling capacity in medical makeover television, in which photographs routinely make visible patients' desired body images. Digital photographic "previews" of postoperative bodies are routinely represented on these TV shows as the most reliable indicators of surgical results, much as they are in contemporary surgical practices. In the case of MTV's controversial *I Want a Famous Face*, subjects also rely heavily on photographs of their favorite celebrities to guide the transformation of their own bodies. In no case does the show or its participants question the truth of these images, whose means of technological production are not disclosed; whether analogue or digital, the fetishized photographs are simply presented as faithful likenesses of Brad Pitt, Pamela Anderson, or Jessica Simpson—real bodies to emulate. Absent from such programming, in other words, is the anxiety expressed in the early twentieth century in the literature of public health, which warned middle-class Americans of the photograph's power to lie in the culture of cosmetic medicine. In 1934, for instance, the American Medical Association illustrated that power in its popular journal *Hygeia* by staging a surgical consultation in a world of artifice, one replete with lavish furniture and framed artwork and populated by two figures in fashionably angular dress: a "beauty specialist" and his "prospective patient." But the most artful objects of all, the very things that enable the female patient's "last qualms" about undergoing a body-altering operation to be "dispelled," the caption tells us, are the "carefully retouched photographs of previous victims" that the face-lifter holds out for her to examine.[34] For the AMA, this was the image of a dangerous quack who used the American public's misplaced faith in the authority of the photograph to increase his revenue; in contemporary makeover culture, by contrast, it is almost always the photograph that speaks the truth and offers hope to an unfaithful physical body.

With the exception of the provocative drama *Nip/Tuck* (2003–10, FX), known for its simultaneously critical and celebratory vision of cosmetic surgery, popular medical television has rarely drawn attention to, let alone problematized, this privileged status of the portrait photograph. The final episode of the second season, for instance, begins with a surgical consultation in the office of the show's protagonists, Dr. Christian Troy and Dr. Sean McNamara. Addressing their potential new patient, actress-comedian Joan Rivers, Dr. Troy opens with a much-rehearsed invitation that sparks a witty exchange punctuated by moments of sentimentality:

CHRISTIAN TROY   Tell me what you don't like about yourself.

JOAN RIVERS   Are you kidding? Everything. My body's dropping so fast my gynecologist needs a hard hat. But seriously, I was sent to you by Barbara Busberger. She told me you're the best surgeons in Miami . . .

SEAN MCNAMARA   So, what exactly . . .

RIVERS (*picking up a framed black-and-white photograph*)   I wanna look like her. Joan Alexandra Molinsky. Born in Brooklyn, raised in Larchmont. Graduated from Barnard Phi Beta Kappa.

MCNAMARA (*looking at the portrait*)   This is you?

RIVERS   That's me. Unretouched. The face and the photograph. I want you to make me look just like that.

TROY   Like a four-year-old girl?

RIVERS (*pointing to McNamara*)   I think I want you to do the surgery.

MCNAMARA   You haven't said what it is yet . . .

RIVERS (*after requiring the pair to sign a confidentiality agreement, she continues*)   Okay. Here it is. I've always wanted to have a twin because I wanted to see what I would look like if I had never had plastic surgery. But I don't have a twin. I just have me. So I want you to put me back the way I would look if I had never been Joan Rivers.

TROY   I'm confused. Are you asking us to do a complete makeover that would restore your natural appearance?

RIVERS   Yes, yes. It'll be career Viagra. I mean, I can bring back all those jokes I used to do about myself before plastic surgery . . .

MCNAMARA   Ms. Rivers, with all the work that you've had done it seems like a pretty extreme thing to do for the sake of your career.

RIVERS   Well, it's not *just* my career. It's also my grandson, Cooper. We have the most amazing relationship. It's probably the most honest relationship I've ever had with anybody in my whole life. He loves me exactly the way I am.

MCNAMARA   So why change?

RIVERS   I'm a goddamn lie . . .

It is through the vintage photograph in this scene that *Nip/Tuck* explores its central ontological question: where does one locate truth and beauty in a world of lies? On the face of things, it would appear that both can be found in that portrait, which Rivers describes as if it were her "real" self. Within the picture frame, viewers see the face of a young girl—her smile subtle and sweet, her collared dress simple, her complexion soft and clear, her wavy, light-colored hair tamed by a single barrette. A shot of Rivers holding the photograph up to her face encourages us to recognize a striking contrast between this image of her past and what we observe of her body in the present (see fig. 42 a–c). Through this juxtaposition, the lines of Rivers's cheekbones and nose appear noticeably

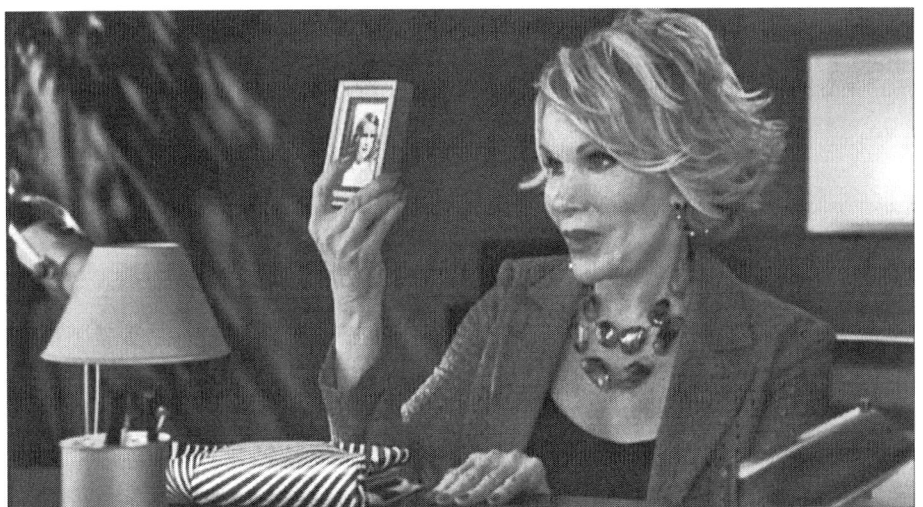

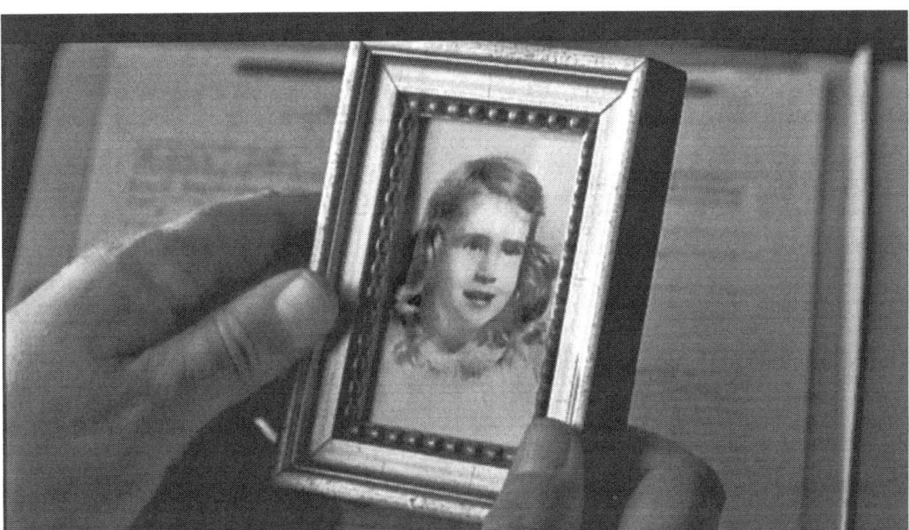

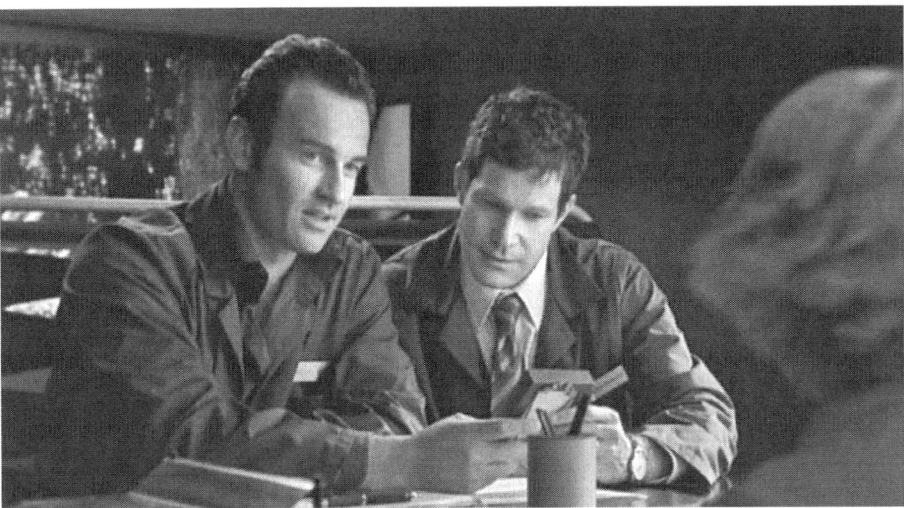

FIGURE 42a–c Screen shots from *Nip/Tuck*, season 2, episode 29 (originally aired October 5, 2004, on FX).

angular; her forehead, eyes, and lips, apparently the result of various injections and lifts, seem capable of only the most forced expressions, while her hair, a combination of bleached blonde and browner tones, is arranged in an impossibly regular pattern of upturned waves. Significant changes in costume and makeup, accentuated by the predominance of the color red in her appearance at Troy and McNamara's office, further contribute to our perception of radical difference between the "real" four-year-old child and the surgically constructed woman. We would appear to be presented, then, with a rather naïve notion of the photographic portrait as an embodiment of the subject "as she was," and not as the highly constructed performance of that subject's identity that cultural historians of photography understand it to be. In the context of the scene, however, this idealization of photography as a truth-telling medium has its limits; as Rivers herself acknowledges, the vintage photograph, much like the human face, can be "retouched," or artistically manipulated, to produce a desired image that conforms to ideals of beauty. While she is probably mistaken in assuming that the photograph of young Joan Alexandra Molinsky has *not* been doctored, given the ubiquity of retouching practices since the 1870s, her commitment to seeing it as such supports a reading of her present face as "a goddamn lie."

Much like the participants on American reality makeover television, Rivers seeks to arrive at the "truth" embodied by the untouched photograph through highly artificial technological means. The irony of this scenario and its implications for photographic authority are underscored later in the episode when Troy and McNamara reveal a digital construction of what Rivers will look like after surgery provides her with a more aged appearance. Horrified by the wrinkled, sagging face staring back at her from the computer screen, Rivers decides not to go through with her extreme makeover, proclaiming that cosmetic surgery should be embraced as a "natural" evolutionary advancement. In this spectacular display of new media, obviously presented as a machine-made fantasy of what can/will be, Rivers and her doctors thus find another, and more compelling, truth *in the digital image*, rendering the vision of the analogue photographic portrait—as a marker of the real that initially framed the episode—ambivalent at best. Through this gesture, *Nip/Tuck* nevertheless poses a challenge to both the prophets and the critics of the digital revolution by imagining that analogue photography *and* digital imaging technologies can still connote truth in a hypermediated makeover culture; it is the operable body that lies, the show suggests, and not its medium of representation.

What the examples in this chapter suggest is precisely what many working photographers today acknowledge, implicitly or otherwise—that is, the need to rethink digital photographic authority in relation to contemporary medical culture. This book has sought to begin that process by recognizing the different ways in which the intersection of photography and medicine has constructed the cultural identity of both technologies in relation to the human body for more than 150 years; this, in turn, enables us to read medical models and metaphors as one of the many aspects of digital photographic culture that invokes the medium's chemical past. As the specific forms of the *medicine of photography* continue to evolve in twenty-first-century America, they thus remain indebted to, and at times haunted by, the legacy of Doctor Photo.

The following periodicals are organized chronologically according to their earliest date of publication. With noted exceptions, they were all published in Philadelphia and distributed to other urban centers in the United States.

Philadelphia Photographer, 1864–88. Edited by Edward L. Wilson. Published in Philadelphia by Benerman and Wilson (1864–87) and in New York by Edward L. Wilson (1887–88).

The *Philadelphia Photographer* was the first photographic periodical published in Philadelphia and quickly became America's premier journal of its kind, an honor it held for the duration of its existence. It began as a monthly publication but was issued bimonthly between 1886 and 1888. From the start, the journal served as the official organ of the Philadelphia Photographic Society (est. 1862), and later of the National Photographic Association (est. 1868) and the Photographic Association of America (est. 1880), printing the proceedings of their meetings and conventions. In the 1870s the *Philadelphia Photographer* absorbed two other photographic periodicals, the *Photographic World* (1871–72) and the *Photographer's Friend* (published in Baltimore, 1871–74). When Wilson's partnership with Benerman ended in 1887, Wilson moved his editorial offices to New York and began publishing the *Philadelphia Photographer* himself. In 1889 the journal was replaced by *Wilson's Photographic Magazine.*

In the journal's first issue, Wilson described its aim as the education of novice and experienced photographers as well as the studio public. The articles in the *Philadelphia Photographer* addressed a range of technical, aesthetic, cultural, and entertaining aspects of photography. Their authors included Wilson himself, American commercial photographers, foreign correspondents, authorities on the fine arts and sciences, and occasionally amateurs and other members of the public.

Each issue began with an "actual" photographic specimen produced by a North American photographer, often a studio portrait, the technical and artistic merit of which was discussed in an editorial comment under the heading "Our Picture." The pages that followed contained primarily original contributions in the form of commissioned essays, letters to the editor, and regular columns, although the journal also reprinted excerpts from other photographic periodicals as well as from the local and scientific press. Each issue concluded with a section titled "Salad for the Photographer" or "Editor's Table," which offered advice to practicing photographers and reported miscellaneous "photographic" news, such as a notable studio fire or the introduction of a new photographic apparatus. Commercial advertisements for photographic equipment and supplies were circulated with the *Philadelphia Photographer,* although modern bindings of the journal do not contain identical selections of ads.

Photographic Mosaics, 1866–1901. Edited by Edward L. Wilson. Published in Philadelphia by Benerman and Wilson (1866–87) and in New York by Edward L. Wilson in cooperation with Mathew Carey Lea (1887–1901).

Issued annually, *Photographic Mosaics* published articles held over from the *Philadelphia Photographer,* other original essays, excerpts from current photographic literature, and items from the foreign photographic press. At the beginning of each issue, Wilson included a review of the major "photographic news" from the previous year. This review and many of the articles published in the journal emphasized the technical and cultural "progress" of photography. The journal concluded with an advice column, "Many Mites from Many Minds," in which Wilson offered practical and professional tips for commercial photographers.

Like the *Philadelphia Photographer, Photographic Mosaics* was published in New York by Wilson after 1887. Wilson also enlisted the editorial assistance of Mathew Carey Lea, whose contributions to the study of photographic chemistry and its impact on health are considered in chapter 4 of this book.

Photographic Review of Medicine and Surgery, 1870–72. Edited by Dr. Louis Adolphus Duhring and Dr. Frank Fontoire Maury. Published in Philadelphia by J. B. Lippincott and Co.

This journal represents one of the earliest published uses of photography in American medicine and a rare artifact in the history of both practices. Both native Philadelphians, Duhring was a renowned dermatologist and Maury a surgeon. They intended to publish the *Photographic Review* on a monthly basis, describing two medical cases in each issue and illustrating these with original, tipped-in photographs. Publication of the journal ceased after two years, however, presumably owing to a lack of funding; a total of forty-eight photographs were printed. These photographs, attributed to Philadelphia photographer John L. Gihon, illustrate cases of unusual and extreme disease, the majority of which were gross deformities associated with cancer, birth defects, or syphilis.

Photographic World, 1871–72. Edited by Edward L. Wilson. Published in Philadelphia by Benerman and Wilson.

The contents and format of this monthly periodical closely resemble those of the journal that later absorbed it, the *Philadelphia Photographer.*

Magic Lantern, 1874–85. Edited by Edward L. Wilson. Published in Philadelphia by Benerman and Wilson.

The *Magic Lantern* was issued in connection with the *Philadelphia Photographer* and was directed primarily at practitioners of this branch of photography. It contained technical discussions of lantern slide production and projection, with suggestions for illustrated lectures.

American Journal of Photography, 1879–1912. Edited by Thomas H. McCollin (1879–90) and by Julius Sachse (1890–97). Published in Philadelphia by Thomas H. McCollin.

A typical issue of this journal included approximately eight pages of text. It was published monthly by Thomas McCollin, owner of a photographic supply company in Philadelphia and an original member of the Philadelphia Photographic Society. It was edited in the 1890s by Julius Sachse, a "serious" amateur photographer from Philadelphia who was also active in the society and was one of the first historians of American photography. Under the direction of McCollin and Sachse, the *American Journal of Photography* placed a greater emphasis on amateur practices than other early photographic periodicals, though it also printed many articles of interest to the commercial photographic community. McCollin included a current price list of photographic materials in each issue.

Science of Photography at Home and Abroad, 1888–89. Edited by Joseph J. Fox. Published in Philadelphia by James W. Queen and Co.

This publication described itself as "a monthly review of current progress, outings, and practical applications of photography." It aimed to describe improvements in photographic apparatuses and processes, publish the proceedings of several photographic societies, and review and illustrate new patents related to the improvement of photography. Although the journal claimed to focus on the "science" of photography, Fox also addressed the artistic composition of photographs and compared it to the conventions of painting and drawing.

Wilson's Photographic Magazine, 1889–1914. Edited by Edward L. Wilson (1889–1903) and L. W. Wilson (1903–14). Published in New York by Edward L. Wilson.

Issued bimonthly, this successor to the *Philadelphia Photographer* largely maintained the format and content of its predecessor. The discontinuation of the *Philadelphia Photographer* coincided with Wilson's establishment of a new publishing company based in New York. *Wilson's Photographic Magazine* continued to be published after its founder's death in 1903, and in 1915 was renamed the *Photographic Journal of America.*

NOTES

INTRODUCTION

1.   H. H. Snelling, "Doctor Photo," *Philadelphia Photographer* 8, no. 92 (August 1871): 271. (The *Philadelphia Photographer* is cited hereafter by the abbreviation *PP.*)

2.   Born in 1817, Snelling was a longtime resident of New York State and a major figure in the history of American photography. In addition to his business contributions to the photographic firm of E. & H. T. Anthony, he is best known for publishing *The History and Practice of the Art of Photography, or The Production of Pictures Through the Agency of Light, Containing all the Instructions Necessary for the Complete Practice of the Daguerrean and Photogenic Art, Both on Metallic Plates and on Paper* (New York: G. P. Putnam, 1849), and for subsequently editing the *Photographic Art Journal* (1851–53) and the *Photographic and Fine Art Journal* (1854–60). For a summary of Snelling's life and career, see A. J. Olmstead, "Snelling: The Father of Photographic Journalism," *Camera* 47 (December 1933): 391–94.

3.   Snelling, "Doctor Photo," 270.

4.   J. Perry Elliott, "Our Profession: What Is It?" *PP* 9, no. 100 (April 1872): 106.

5.   On this point historians of American photography differ. Beaumont Newhall and, more recently, Paul Spencer Sternberger have argued that the proliferation of amateur photography was the driving force behind photography's legitimization as art. See Newhall, *The History of Photography: From 1839 to the Present Day* (New York: Museum of Modern Art, 1939); and Sternberger, *Between Amateur and Aesthete: The Legitimization of Photography as Art in America, 1880–1900* (Albuquerque: University of New Mexico Press, 2001).

6.   Although he was born in Ohio in 1808 and worked in at least seven states before his death in 1888, Root is considered a Philadelphian, as he spent much of his adult life there. He opened one of the city's best-known daguerreotype galleries at 140 Chestnut Street in the mid-1840s and lent his name to another at Fifth and Chestnut a decade later.

7.   Marcus Aurelius Root, *The Camera and the Pencil, or The Heliographic Art* (1864; reprint, Pawlet: Helios, 1971). Despite its historical importance, Root's text has received relatively little critical attention from photographic historians of the last century. One notable exception is Allan Sekula, who discusses the book at length in "Photography Between Labour and Capital," in *Mining Photographs and Other Pictures, 1948–1968: A Selection from the Negative Archives of Shedden Studio, Glace Bay, Cape Breton*, ed. Benjamin H. D. Buchloh and Robert Wilkie (Halifax: Press of the Nova Scotia College of Art and Design, 1983), 193–268. See also Anthony W. Lee, "American Histories of Photography," *American Art* 21, no. 3 (2007): 2–9.

8.   See Charles H. Caffin, *Photography as a Fine Art: The Achievements and Possibilities of Photographic Art in America* (New York: Doubleday, Page, 1901); Sadakichi Hartmann, *The Valiant Knights of Daguerre: Selected Critical Essays on Photography and Profiles of Photographic Pioneers* (Berkeley and Los Angeles: University of California Press, 1978); Newhall, *History of Photography;* and John Szarkowski, *Photography Until Now* (New York: Museum of Modern Art, 1989). Joel Eisinger provides an overview of this historiography in *Trace and Transformation: American Criticism of Photography in the Modernist Period* (Albuquerque: University of New Mexico Press, 1995).

9.   See the essays in Martha A. Sandweiss, ed., *Photography in Nineteenth-Century America* (New York: Harry N. Abrams, 1991), especially Barbara McCandless, "The Portrait Studio and the Celebrity: Promoting the Art" (48–75); Peter Bacon Hales, "American Views and the Romance of Modernization" (204–57); and Sarah Greenough, "'Of Charming Glens, Graceful Glades, and Frowning Cliffs': The Economic Incentives, Social Inducements, and Aesthetic Issues of American Portrait Photography, 1880–1902" (258–81). Reiterations of photography's legitimization story appear in Marshall Battani, "Organizational Fields, Cultural Fields, and Art Worlds: The Early Effort to Make Photographs and Make Photographers in the Nineteenth-Century United States of America," *Media, Culture, and Society* 21, no. 5 (1999): 601–26; and Sternberger's *Between Amateur and Aesthete*. There have been several recent challenges to that narrative in studies of early, and predominantly British, photography. While Steve Edwards "complicates the story of art" by observing photography's associations with the "crudest form[s] of mechanical labor," Jennifer Tucker and Kelley Wilder explore the importance of scientific discourses and institutions to the development of photography's cultural identity and authority. See Edwards, *The Making of English Photography: Allegories* (University Park: Pennsylvania State University Press, 2006), 1–2; Tucker, *Nature Exposed: Photography as Eyewitness in Victorian Science* (Baltimore: Johns Hopkins University Press, 2005); and Kelley Wilder, *Photography and Science* (London: Reaktion Books, 2009).

10.   See Allan Sekula, "The Body and the Archive," *October* 39 (Winter 1986): 3–64; and John Tagg, *The Burden of Representation: Essays on Photographies and Histories* (Amherst: University of Massachusetts Press, 1988; reprint, Minneapolis: University of Minnesota Press, 1993).

11.   Discussions of the photograph as coexistent with the "thing itself" are indebted to the work of André Bazin, who proposed that photography derives its "quality of credibility" and "essentially objective character" from its automatic nature. As Roland Barthes would later famously argue, the authority of the photograph is its intrinsic guarantee of an object's "having been there." See Bazin, "Ontology of the Photographic Image," in *What Is Cinema?* vol. 1, trans. Hugh Gray (Berkeley and Los Angeles: University of California Press, 1967), 9–16; Barthes, *Camera Lucida: Reflections on Photography*, trans. Richard Howard (New York: Hill and Wang, 1981); Barthes, "Rhetoric of the Image," in *Image/Music/Text*, trans. Stephen Heath (New York: Hill and Wang, 1977), 32–51; Rudolf Arnheim, "On the Nature of Photography," *Critical Inquiry* 1 (September 1974): 149–61; and Susan Sontag, *On Photography* (New York: Farrar, Straus and Giroux, 1977).

12.   Examples of this scholarship include Shawn Michelle Smith, *American Archives: Gender, Race, and Class in Visual Culture* (Princeton: Princeton University Press, 1999); Andrea Volpe, "Cartes de Visite Portrait Photographs and the Culture of Class Formation," in *The Middling Sorts: Explorations in the History of the American Middle Class*, ed. Burton J. Bledstein and Robert D. Johnston (New York: Routledge, 2001), 157–69; and Elspeth H. Brown, *The Corporate Eye: Photography and the Rationalization of American Commercial Culture, 1884–1929* (Baltimore: Johns Hopkins University Press, 2005).

13.   Scholars in the field of science and technology studies have similarly assumed that perceptions of a scientist's body and discourse necessarily inform perceptions of his materials and the authority of his work; the reverse is also true, such that trust in things almost always guarantees trust in people. See Steven Shapin, *A Social History of Truth: Civility and Science in Seventeenth-Century England* (Chicago: University of Chicago Press, 1994); Christopher Lawrence and Steven Shapin, eds., *Science Incarnate: Historical Embodiments of Natural Knowledge* (Chicago: University of Chicago Press, 1998); Bruno Latour and Steve Woolgar, *Laboratory Life: The Construction of Scientific Facts* (Princeton: Princeton University Press, 1986); and Michael Lynch, *Art and Artifact in Laboratory Science: A Study of Shop Work and Shop Talk in a Research Laboratory* (London: Routledge and Kegan Paul, 1985).

14.   See William H. Helfand, *Quack, Quack, Quack: The Sellers of Nostrums in Prints, Posters, Ephemera, and Books* (New York: Grolier Club, 2002).

15.   Serious scholarly interest in the history of medical photography in the United States began in the 1960s and '70s with the publication of Alison Gernsheim's "Medical Photography in the Nineteenth Century," *Medical and Biological Illustration* 11 (1961): 85–92; Robert

Ollerenshaw, "Medical Illustration: The Impact of Photography on Its History," *Journal of the Biological Photographic Association* 36 (1968): 3–12; Leonard A. Julin, "A History of Still Photography in the Operating Room," *Journal of the Biological Photographic Association* 39 (1971): 129–43; and Sander L. Gilman, *The Face of Madness: Hugh Welch Diamond and the Origin of Psychiatric Photography* (Secaucus: Citadel Press, 1976). Since then, the collector Stanley B. Burns has contributed to the largely descriptive study of the genre through numerous publications that showcase his private collection, including *Early Medical Photography in America (1839–1883)* (New York: Burns Archive, 1983); *A Morning's Work: Medical Photographs from the Burns Archive and Collection, 1843–1939* (Santa Fe: Twin Palms, 1998); and Joel-Peter Witkin, *Masterpieces of Medical Photography: Selections from the Burns Archive* (Pasadena: Twelvetrees Press, 1987). For critical discussion of photography's role in the development of Anglo-American medicine, see Charles E. Rosenberg, "Representing Medicine: Philadelphia, Health, and Photography, 1860–1945," in *Pictures of Health: A Photographic History of Health Care in Philadelphia, 1860–1945*, ed. Janet Golden and Charles E. Rosenberg (Philadelphia: University of Pennsylvania Press, 1991), xxi–xxix; Daniel M. Fox and Christopher Lawrence, *Photographing Medicine: Images and Power in Britain and America Since 1840* (New York: Greenwood Press, 1988); Jennifer Green-Lewis, *Framing the Victorians: Photography and the Culture of Realism* (Ithaca: Cornell University Press, 1996); and Rachelle A. Dermer, "Photographic Objectivity and the Construction of the Medical Subject in the United States" (PhD diss., Boston University, 2002).

16. Warner has developed this idea of the medical marketplace throughout his work. See in particular *The Therapeutic Perspective: Medical Practice, Knowledge, and Identity in America, 1820–1885* (Cambridge: Harvard University Press, 1986); *Against the Spirit of System: The French Impulse in Nineteenth-Century American Medicine* (Baltimore: Johns Hopkins University Press, 2003); and "Image-Making, Identity, and the Aesthetic Grounding of Modern American Medicine," paper delivered at "The Art of Medicine: Image-Making and Communication" symposium, Yale University, April 15–17, 2004.

17. Jennifer Tucker has similarly argued that photography's authority had to be constructed in order for the medium to "work for" science. According to Tucker, neither photography's apparent "indexicality" nor its ties to discourses of social regulation could guarantee its presentation of reliable facts; rather, the medium's status as a credible witness depended upon the social and material conditions surrounding the production and consumption of a given image. Tucker, *Nature Exposed*.

18. See Erin O'Connor, "Camera Medica: Towards a Morbid History of Photography," *History of Photography* 23, no. 3 (1999): 232–44; Chris Amirault, "Posing the Subject of Early Medical Photography," *Discourse* 16, no. 2 (1993–94): 51–76; Lisa Cartwright, *Screening the Body: Tracing Medicine's Visual Culture* (Minneapolis: University of Minnesota Press, 1995); Sekula, "Body and the Archive"; and Tagg, *Burden of Representation*.

19. George Lakoff and Mark Johnson, *Metaphors We Live By*, 2d ed. (Chicago: University of Chicago Press, 2003), 154, 5. On metaphor's mapping across conceptual domains, see also Lakoff, "The Contemporary Theory of Metaphor," in *Metaphor and Thought*, 2d ed., ed. Andrew Ortony (New York: Cambridge University Press, 1993), 202–51.

20. Many of the essays in Ortony's edited volume demonstrate that the distinctions between metaphor and other kinds of figurative language have been the subject of much debate in literary studies, linguistics, philosophy, and psychology. While acknowledging that each term traditionally posits a different relationship between the objects it concerns—whether of correspondence, resemblance, coincidence, substitution, and so on—I align myself with scholars who see those differences as matters of degree and view metaphor itself as a broad category that encompasses all of these structural mappings. As Dedre Gentner and Michael Jeziorski argue in "The Shift from Metaphor to Analogy in Western Science," for example, "analogy is a special case of metaphor, one based on a purely relational match" between two objects rather than on any similarities in their appearance or description (452).

21. Geoffrey Batchen, "The Naming of Photography: 'A Mass of Metaphor,'" *History of Photography* 17, no. 1 (1993): 22–32.

22. Alan Trachtenberg, "Mirror in the Marketplace: American Responses to the Daguerreotype, 1839–1851," in *Lincoln's Smile and Other Enigmas* (New York: Hill and Wang, 2007), 13.

23. See ibid.; and Melissa Miles, "The Burning Mirror: Photography in an Ambivalent Light," *Journal of Visual Culture* 4, no. 3 (2005): 329–49. Lakoff discusses what he calls the "experiential basis" and "realizations" of metaphor in "Contemporary Theory of Metaphor," 239–44.

24. On the ways in which metaphors serve as a "guide for further action," see Lakoff and Johnson, *Metaphors We Live By*, 156.

25. Tom Gunning, "Re-Newing Old Technologies: Astonishment, Second Nature, and the Uncanny in Technology from the Previous Turn-of-the-Century," in *Rethinking Media Change: The Aesthetics of Transition*, ed. David Thorburn and Henry Jenkins (Cambridge: MIT Press, 2003), 39.

26. See Mary Douglas, *How Institutions Think* (Syracuse: Syracuse University Press, 1986); and JoAnne Brown, *The Definition of a Profession: The Authority of Metaphor in the History of Intelligence Testing, 1890–1930* (Princeton: Princeton University Press, 1992).

27. Brown, *Definition of a Profession*, 23.

28. See Michel Foucault, *The Order of Things: An Archeology of the Human Sciences* (New York: Pantheon Books, 1970); and Foucault, *The Archaeology of Knowledge*, trans. A. M. Sheridan Smith (New York: Pantheon Books, 1972).

29. Foucault, *Order of Things*, xi.

30. Mary Douglas, *Natural Symbols: Explorations in Cosmology* (New York: Pantheon Books, 1970), 65, 70.

31. Michel Foucault, *History of Sexuality: An Introduction*, trans. Robert Hurley (New York: Vintage Books, 1978); and Foucault, *The Birth of the Clinic: An Archeology of Medical Perception*, trans. A. M. Sheridan Smith (New York: Pantheon Books, 1973). My understanding of disordered bodies as tied to social structures has also been shaped by Peter Stallybrass and Allon White, *The Politics and Poetics of Transgression* (Ithaca: Cornell University Press, 1986).

32. Martha Banta, "Medical Therapies and the Body Politic," *Prospects: An Annual Journal of American Culture Studies* 8 (1983): 63. See also Heather Renee Beatty, "The Body Politic: Medical Metaphor in the Age of the American Revolution" (honors thesis, College of William and Mary, 2002).

33. Thomas Jefferson, *Notes on the State of Virginia* (1781–82; reprint, New York: Library of America, 1984), 291, quoted in Banta, "Medical Therapies and the Body Politic," 68. For a discussion of dismembered bodies as political metaphors in American visual culture of the late eighteenth and nineteenth centuries, see William H. Helfand, *Medicine and Pharmacy in American Political Prints, 1765–1870* (Madison: American Institute of the History of Pharmacy, 1978); and Martin A. Berger, "The Anatomy of the Early Republic," *Early Popular Visual Culture* 7, no. 3 (2009): 231–52.

34. Quoted in Banta, "Medical Therapies and the Body Politic," 67. On Lincoln's prolific use of figurative language, see James M. McPherson, "How Lincoln Won the War with Metaphors," in McPherson, *Abraham Lincoln and the Second American Revolution* (New York: Oxford University Press, 1990), 93–112.

35. On Philadelphia's importance in the history of the American medical profession, see Leo O'Hara, *An Emerging Profession: Philadelphia Doctors, 1860–1900* (New York: Garland, 1989); and Rosenberg, "Representing Medicine."

36. This is by no means an exhaustive list. One might also include Wills Eye Hospital (1832), the first American hospital devoted to the practice and study of ophthalmology, and the Children's Hospital of Philadelphia (1855), the first devoted to the care of children.

37. Julius F. Sachse, "Philadelphia's Share in the Development of Photography," *Journal of the Franklin Institute* 135, no. 4 (1893): 285. For a more recent discussion of Philadelphia's unparalleled contributions to early photography, see Kenneth Finkel, *Nineteenth-Century Photography in Philadelphia: 250 Historic Prints from the Library Company of Philadelphia* (New York: Dover Publications 1980); Mary Panzer, "Romantic Origins of American Realism: Photography, Arts, and Letters in Philadelphia, 1850–1875" (PhD diss., Boston University, 1990); Philadelphia Museum of Art, *Legacy in Light: Photographic Treasures from Philadelphia Area Public Collections* (Philadelphia: Photography Sesquicentennial Project, 1990); and Linda Ries, "Photography," in

Pennsylvania: A History of the Commonwealth, ed. Randall Miller and William Pencak (University Park: Pennsylvania State University Press, 2002), 501–26.

38. See Sachse, "Philadelphia's Share in the Development of Photography." Philadelphia was also the home of America's first museum devoted to photography. Founded by Louis Walton Sipley in 1940, the museum operated on South Fifteenth Street until Sipley's death in 1968. In 1977 this collection was transferred from the 3M Company to the George Eastman House, International Museum of Photography and Film, in Rochester, New York.

39. William and Marie Brey have done the important and laborious work of compiling a list of nineteenth-century Philadelphia photographers based on the city business directories at the Historical Society of Pennsylvania and the Free Library of Philadelphia. The Breys name photographic establishments along with their street locations and dates of operation. See Brey and Brey, *Philadelphia Photographers, 1840–1900: A Directory with Biographical Sketches* (Cherry Hill: Willowdale Press, 1992). See also Linda A. Ries and Jay W. Ruby, *Directory of Pennsylvania Photographers, 1839–1900* (Harrisburg: Pennsylvania Historical and Museum Commission, 1999).

40. According to U.S. Census records, Philadelphia's population jumped from 80,462 in 1830, to 565,529 in 1860 (at which time approximately 30 percent of its inhabitants were foreign born and 4 percent were black), to 1,046,964 in 1890. See Russell F. Weigley, Nicholas B. Wainwright, and Edwin Wolf, eds., *Philadelphia: A 300-Year History* (New York: W. W. Norton, 1982); and John Thomas Scharf and Thompson Westcott, *History of Philadelphia, 1609–1884*, 3 vols. (Philadelphia: L. H. Everts and Co., 1884).

41. Stuart M. Blumin, *The Emergence of the Middle Class: Social Experience in the American City, 1760–1900* (Cambridge: Cambridge University Press, 1985); and John Henry Hepp IV, *The Middle-Class City: Transforming Space and Time in Philadelphia, 1876–1926* (Philadelphia: University of Pennsylvania Press, 2003).

42. Blumin, *Emergence of the Middle Class*, 297.

43. See Smith, *American Archives;* Volpe, "Cartes de Visite Portrait Photographs"; Shirley Teresa Wajda, "The Commercial Photographic Parlor," in *Shaping Communities: Perspectives in Vernacular Architecture,* ed. Carter L. Hudgins and Elizabeth Collins Cromley (Knoxville: University of Tennessee Press, 1997), 216–30; Wajda, *"Social Currency": Commercial Portrait Photography and the Fashioning of an American Middle Class, 1839–1889* (Philadelphia: Temple University Press, forthcoming); and Susan Annette Newberry, "Commerce and Ritual in American Daguerrean Portraiture, 1839–1859" (PhD diss., Cornell University, 1999).

44. J. Matthew Gallman, *Mastering Wartime: A Social History of Philadelphia During the Civil War* (New York: Cambridge University Press, 1990), 35.

45. Elizabeth Milroy, "Avenue of Dreams: Patriotism and the Spectator at Philadelphia's Great Central Sanitary Fair," in *Making and Remaking Pennsylvania's Civil War,* ed. William Blair and William Pencak (University Park: Pennsylvania State University Press, 2001), 23.

46. Henry Whitney Bellows, *Speech of the Rev. Dr. Bellows . . .* (Philadelphia: C. Sherman, Son and Co., 1863), 7. The U.S. government also published pocket guides for soldiers passing through the city that included information on transportation, the house numbering system, and specific instructions on how and where the wounded could find medical care. See *The Soldiers' Guide in Philadelphia* (Philadelphia: Geo. H. Ives, n.d. [ca. 1861–65]).

47. For detailed histories of Philadelphia's medical contributions during the Civil War, see Frank H. Taylor, *Philadelphia in the Civil War, 1861–1865* (Philadelphia: City of Philadelphia, 1913); Gallman, *Mastering Wartime;* and Gary B. Nash, *First City: Philadelphia and the Forging of Historical Memory* (Philadelphia: University of Pennsylvania Press, 2002).

48. See Joan Burbick, *Healing the Republic: The Language of Health and the Culture of Nationalism in Nineteenth-Century America* (New York: Cambridge University Press, 1994); Erin O'Connor, *Raw Material: Producing Pathology in Victorian Culture* (Durham: Duke University Press, 2000), chapter 3; Lisa A. Long, *Rehabilitating Bodies: Health, History, and the American Civil War* (Philadelphia: University of Pennsylvania Press, 2004); Robert I. Goler, "Loss and the Persistence of Memory: 'The Case of George Dedlow' and Disabled Civil War Veterans," *Literature and Medicine* 23, no. 1 (2004): 160–83; and Laura L. Behling, *Gross Anatomies: Fictions of the Physical in American Literature* (Selinsgrove: Susquehanna University Press, 2008).

49. S. Weir Mitchell, "The Case of George Dedlow," *Atlantic Monthly*, July 1866, 5.

50. Oliver Wendell Holmes, "Doings of the Sunbeam," *Atlantic Monthly*, July 1863, 1–15. See Alan Trachtenberg, *Reading American Photographs: Images as History, Matthew Brady to Walker Evans* (New York: Hill and Wang, 1989), 91; and Burbick, *Healing the Republic*, 294.

51. See Timothy Sweet, *Traces of War: Poetry, Photography, and the Crisis of the Union* (Baltimore: Johns Hopkins University Press, 1990); James T. H. Connor and Michael G. Rhode, "Shooting Soldiers: Civil War Medical Images, Memory, and Identity in America," *Invisible Culture: An Electronic Journal for Visual Culture* 5 (Winter 2003), http://www.rochester.edu/in_visible_culture/Issue_5/ConnorRhode/ConnorRhode.html (accessed January 15, 2010).

52. Gallman, *Mastering Wartime*, 257. Gallman cites the data published in Edwin T. Freedley, *Philadelphia and Its Manufacturers* (Philadelphia: Edward Young & Co., 1867), which show that the total output for photographs and materials increased from $180,000 in 1860 to $1,000,000 in 1866. This amounts to a percentage shift of 454.9, the fourth largest among the sixty-nine manufacturing industries Freedley selected for study, which Gallman claims had "no apparent relationship to the war."

53. For a summary of Wilson's many contributions to American photography, see John A. Tennant, "In Memoriam: Edward L. Wilson," *Wilson's Photographic Magazine* 40, no. 559 (July 1903): 289–304.

54. Edwards, *Making of English Photography*, 4, 7. Jennifer Tucker is one of the few other scholars to undertake extensive critical readings of early photographic trade journals, which she describes as "a crucial and hitherto overlooked source." *Nature Exposed*, 41.

55. Edwards, *Making of English Photography*, 10.

CHAPTER 1

1. Pierre Bourdieu, *Photography: A Middle-Brow Art*, trans. Shaun Whiteside (Stanford: Stanford University Press, 1990), 96–97.

2. Ibid., 173. While Bourdieu is not specific about the precise historical period he discusses, his references point primarily to sources from the 1930s through the early 1960s.

3. Ibid., 152.

4. William Heighway, "Our Noble Selves," *PP* 10, no. 109 (January 1873): 21.

5. H. H. Snelling, "Photographic Instruction," *PP* 9, no. 103 (July 1872): 246–47.

6. On the importance of education to the legitimization of a profession in nineteenth-century America, see Burton J. Bledstein, *The Culture of Professionalism: The Middle Class and the Development of Higher Education in America* (New York: W. W. Norton, 1976); Samuel Haber, "The Professions and Higher Education in America: A Historical View," in *Higher Education and the Labor Market*, ed. Margaret S. Gordon (New York: McGraw-Hill, 1974), 237–80; Haber, *The Quest for Authority and Honor in the American Professions, 1750–1900* (Chicago: University of Chicago Press, 1991); Magali Sarfatti Larson, *The Rise of Professionalism* (Berkeley and Los Angeles: University of California Press, 1977); Thomas Haskell, ed., *The Authority of Experts: Studies in History and Theory* (Bloomington: Indiana University Press, 1984); and Mary N. Woods, *From Craft to Profession: The Practice of Architecture in Nineteenth-Century America* (Berkeley and Los Angeles: University of California Press, 1999). For Bourdieu's conception of education in relation to social status, one can start with his *Distinction: A Social Critique of the Judgment of Taste*, trans. Richard Nice (Cambridge: Harvard University Press, 1984).

7. Only a few scholarly studies of early photographic education have been published in the United States; these have focused largely on the two decades after photography's invention and the turn of the century, leaving out the crucial period between 1860 and 1880. See Battani, "Organizational Fields, Cultural Fields, and Art Worlds"; Sternberger, *Between Amateur and Aesthete*; and Nathan Lyons, "History of Photographic Education with an Emphasis on Its Development in the United States," in *The Education of a Photographer*, ed. Charles Traub and Steven Heller (New York: Allworth Press, 2006), 177–84.

8. On the decline in doctors' professional status and the evolution of medical education in nineteenth-century America, see Ronald L. Numbers, "The Fall and Rise of the American Medical Profession," in *Sickness and Health in America: Readings in the History of Medicine and Public Health*, ed. Judith Walzer Leavitt and Ronald L. Numbers (Madison: University of Wisconsin Press, 1997), 225–26; Kenneth M. Ludmerer, *Learning to Heal: The Development of American Medical Education* (New York: Basic Books, 1985); Paul Starr, *The Social Transformation of American Medicine: The Rise of a Sovereign Profession and the Making of a Vast Industry* (New York: Basic Books, 1982); Ronald L. Numbers, ed., *The Education of American Physicians: Historical Essays* (Berkeley and Los Angeles: University of California Press, 1980); Martin Kaufman, *American Medical Education: The Formative Years, 1765–1910* (Westport, Conn.: Greenwood Press, 1976); William G. Rothstein, *American Physicians in the Nineteenth Century: From Sects to Science* (Baltimore: Johns Hopkins University Press, 1972); and Haber, *Quest for Authority and Honor*, chapters 2 and 10. Leo O'Hara focuses on Philadelphia's role in educating doctors in *Emerging Profession*.

9. "Proceedings of the National Photographic Convention," *PP* 5, no. 52 (April 1868): 138, 142. For Edward Wilson's contributions to the discussions leading up to the formation of the photographic union, see the following articles from the *Philadelphia Photographer* 5: "A National Photographic Union," no. 53 (May 1868): 169–70; "The National Photographic Union," no. 56 (August 1868): 250–52; "The National Photographic Union," no. 58 (October 1868): 347–48; and "The Union!" no. 60 (December 1868): 440–41.

10. On the relationship between industrial expositions and the NPA exhibitions of the 1870s, see Julie K. Brown, *Making Culture Visible: The Public Display of Photography at Fairs, Expositions, and Exhibitions in the United States, 1847–1900* (Amsterdam: Harwood Academic Publishers, 2001), 47–55.

11. American Medical Association, *Proceedings of the National Medical Conventions, Held in New York, May, 1846, and in Philadelphia, May, 1847* (Philadelphia: T. K. and P. G. Collins, 1847), 89.

12. Towler had also edited the *American Photographic Almanac* and published a regular series in the *Philadelphia Photographer* beginning in 1867. The latter was drawn from his widely read photographic manual *The Silver Sunbeam: A Practical and Theoretical Text-Book on Sun Drawing and Photographic Printing; Comprehending All the Wet and Dry Processes at Present Known* (New York: Joseph H. Ladd, 1864).

13. "The Lectures," *PP* 6, no. 67 (July 1869): 228–29. Other contributors to Wilson's journals and to the early work of the NPA, such as Dr. P. H. van der Weyde, were also important figures in the field of American medical education. After practicing medicine for several years, Van der Weyde held professorships in science at the Cooper Institute, New York Medical College, and Girard College in Philadelphia.

14. Ryder quoted in "The National Photographic Union," *PP* 5, no. 56 (August 1868): 252. On the aims of the AMA's 1847 code of ethics, see Robert Baker, ed., *The Codification of Medical Morality: Historical and Philosophical Studies of the Formalization of Western Medical Morality in the Eighteenth and Nineteenth Centuries*, vol. 2, *Anglo-American Medical Ethics and Medical Jurisprudence in the Nineteenth Century* (Dordrecht: Kluwer Academic Publishers, 1995).

15. Written in the hand of Louis Walton Sipley, founder of the first American museum devoted to photography, the inscription reads, "This was the group to organize the Nat'l Phot Assoc. at Phila. Abraham Bogardus—standing light suit, E. L. Wilson—seated, striped pants, E. Schreiber—bald, smooth face." That there are two men in the portrait with striped pants has caused some confusion among those who have studied this image. Julie Brown identifies Wilson as the sitter on the far right, although my communication in November 2009 with Joseph Struble, archivist at the George Eastman House, suggests that Wilson is probably seated at center. Likewise, "E. Schreiber" may refer to Gerhard Schreiber or to his father, Francis Schreiber, who ran a studio with his sons for many years in Philadelphia. Brown's other identifications include John C. Browne, Coleman Sellers, S. Fisher Corlies, and Frederick Graff. Brown, *Making Culture Visible*, 48.

16. E. K. Hough, "Photographic Rights: III," *PP* 12, no. 139 (July 1875): 205. For a summary of the external threats to photographic authority at this time and the NPA's work to combat them,

see Edward L. Wilson, "The Advantages of Association," *Photographic World* 2, no. 15 (March 1872): 94–95.

17.   Beaumont Newhall reprinted the pamphlet as "To My Patrons," in *Photography, Essays and Images: Illustrated Readings in the History of Photography*, ed. Beaumont Newhall (New York: Museum of Modern Art, 1980), 129. Wilson claimed in 1872 that he had sold one million copies of *The Photographer to His Patrons* in English, German, and Spanish editions. For discussion of the pamphlet's popularity, see "Editor's Table," *PP* 8, no. 89 (May 1871): 159; and "The Photographer to His Patrons," *PP* 9, no. 104 (August 1872): 298–99. In its code of ethics, the AMA spelled out its own position on the "obedience of a patient to the prescriptions of his physician." This, it explained, "should be prompt and explicit. He [the patient] should never permit his own crude opinions as to their fitness, to influence his attention to them. A failure in one particular may render an otherwise judicious treatment dangerous, and even fatal." American Medical Association, *Proceedings of the National Medical Conventions*, 96.

18.   The NPA's Committee on the National Price List, chaired by Wilson, published its recommendations in its *Manual of the National Photographic Association of the United States* (Philadelphia: Sherman & Co., 1873), 30–33.

19.   H. H. Snelling, "The Wants of Photography," *PP* 9, no. 100 (April 1872): 102.

20.   Pro Bono Publico, "What Shall We Do About It?" *PP* 4, no. 42 (June 1867): 163–64. For additional comparisons of the fees charged by portrait photographers and medical doctors, see Hough, "Photographic Rights: III," 206; and J. F. Ryder, "On the Business Management of Photography," *PP* 21, no. 249 (September 1884): 268.

21.   On the efforts of nineteenth-century physicians in this respect, see Charles E. Rosenberg, "Toward an Ecology of Knowledge: On Discipline, Context, and History," in *The Organization of Knowledge in Modern America, 1860–1920*, ed. Alexandra Oleson and John Voss (Baltimore: Johns Hopkins University Press, 1979), 440–55.

22.   Bruce Sinclair, *Philadelphia's Philosopher Mechanics: A History of the Franklin Institute, 1824–1865* (Baltimore: Johns Hopkins University Press, 1974); and Haber, *Quest for Authority and Honor.*

23.   Wilson, "Advantages of Association," 94; and "Talk and Tattle," *PP* 13, no. 146 (February 1876): 41.

24.   Wilson, "Many Mites from Many Minds," *Photographic Mosaics* 14 (1879): 140.

25.   Perhaps best known for his work with the Centennial Photographic Company, Gihon contributed two regular columns to the *Philadelphia Photographer* (Hints from the Record of an Artist and Photographer and Gihon's Photographic Scraps) before his death in 1878. Simpson, who was the editor of London's leading photographic trade journal, *Photographic News*, from 1861 until his death in 1880, also wrote two columns for Wilson at the same time: Practical Notes on Various Photographic Subjects and Notes in and Out of the Studio.

26.   See the following articles, all by Marcus Aurelius Root: "Heliographic School," *Photographic and Fine Art Journal* 13, no. 4 (April 1860): 111–12; "A Heliographic School—Its Importance," *Photographic and Fine Art Journal* 13, no. 5 (May 1860): 140; "Heliographic School," *American Journal of Photography* 2, no. 24 (May 15, 1860): 376–78; "A Heliographic School—Its Importance," *American Journal of Photography* 3, no. 1 (June 1, 1860): 11–14; "Heliographic Schools," *Humphrey's Journal of Photography* 12, no. 4 (June 15, 1860): 49–52, and 12, no. 5 (July 1, 1860): 70; "The Heliographic School," *American Journal of Photography* 3, no. 3 (July 1, 1860): 33–35, 41–42; "A Photography College," *Photographic and Fine Art Journal* 13, no. 8 (August 1860): 219; and "Photography in Schools," *American Journal of Photography* 3, no. 6 (August 15, 1860): 93–95.

27.   Root, "Heliographic School," *American Journal of Photography* 2, no. 24 (May 15, 1860): 376.

28.   Root, "A Heliographic School—Its Importance," *American Journal of Photography* 3, no. 1 (June 1, 1860): 13–14.

29.   Wilson, "Advantages of Association," 95.

30.   See "Report of the Committee on Apprenticeship," *PP* 8, no. 91 (July 1871): 228; and "Report of the Committee on Apprenticeship," *PP* 10, no. 117 (September 1873): 304–9.

31. "National Photographic Institute," *PP* 10, no. 112 (April 1873): 97. After Alfred C. Harmer, a representative from Pennsylvania, introduced *A Bill to Establish a National Photographic Institute*, HR 3752, 42d Cong., 3d sess., it was referred to the Committee on Appropriations on February 3, 1873. The large sum it provided for, however, was never approved.

32. Hough, "Photographic Rights: III," 204.

33. Snelling, "Photographic Instruction," 247–48.

34. Root, "Heliographic School," *American Journal of Photography* 2, no. 24 (May 15, 1860): 376–77; Root, "Heliographic School," *American Journal of Photography* 3, no. 3 (July 1, 1860): 41.

35. Root, "Heliographic School," *American Journal of Photography* 3, no. 3 (July 1, 1860): 41. Root makes the same recommendation in "Heliographic Schools," *Humphrey's Journal of Photography* 12, no. 5 (July 1, 1860): 70.

36. See Rothstein, *American Physicians in the Nineteenth Century*, chapters 3 and 5.

37. Samuel D. Gross, *Autobiography of Samuel D. Gross, M.D.* (Philadelphia: G. Barrie, 1887), 1:197–98, quoted in ibid., 55–56.

38. Root, *Camera and the Pencil*, 33.

39. On the meanings of science in the context of the professions in nineteenth-century America, see Haber, *Quest for Authority and Honor*. As John Henry Hepp IV argues in *Middle-Class City*, the middle-class conception of "science" as connoting rationality and logic informed a wide range of cultural practices in late nineteenth-century Philadelphia, including the organization of the Centennial Exhibition and the city's public transit system.

40. Samuel D. Gross, *A System of Surgery; Pathological, Diagnostic, Therapeutic, and Operative* (Philadelphia: Blanchard and Lea, 1859). For discussion of the impact of professional education and scientific rhetoric on the development of American surgery, see Courtney R. Hall, "The Rise of Professional Surgery in the United States: 1800–1865," *Bulletin of the History of Medicine* 26, no. 3 (1952): 231–62; and Gert H. Brieger, "Surgery," in Numbers, *Education of American Physicians*, 175–204.

41. See John Harley Warner, "Science, Healing, and the Character of the Physician" (143–49), and "Professional Optimism and Professional Dismay over the Coming of the New Scientific Medicine" (216–24), in John Harley Warner and Janet A. Tighe, eds., *Major Problems in the History of American Medicine and Public Health* (Boston: Houghton Mifflin, 2001); and S. E. D. Shortt, "Physicians, Science, and Status: Issues in the Professionalization of Anglo-American Medicine in the Nineteenth Century," *Medical History* 27, no. 1 (1983): 51–68.

42. "Talk and Tattle," *PP* 11, no. 125 (May 1874): 135.

43. Hermann Vogel, "German Correspondence," *PP* 12, no. 134 (February 1875): 50–51.

44. "A Photographic Educational Institution Probable," *PP* 14, no. 165 (September 1877): 276. America's first professional photographic academy, the Chicago College of Photography (est. 1881) offered a course on practical photography, another on optics and chemistry, and a third on the art of retouching; the first two were taught by a physician, Professor H. D. Garrison. See "The Chicago College of Photography," *PP* 18, no. 208 (April 1881): 113–15.

45. For discussion of these paintings as commentaries on surgery's road to professionalization, see Gert H. Brieger, "A Portrait of Surgery: Surgery in America, 1875–1889," *Surgical Clinics of North America* 67, no. 6 (1987): 1181–1216; and two articles in *Prospects: An Annual Journal of American Culture Studies* 11, section 2 (1987): Diana E. Long, "The Medical World of *The Agnew Clinic*: A World We Have Lost?" (185–98); and Margaret Supplee Smith, "*The Agnew Clinic*: 'Not Cheerful for Ladies to Look At'" (161–83).

46. Michael Fried, *Realism, Writing, Disfiguration: On Thomas Eakins and Stephen Crane* (Chicago: University of Chicago Press, 1987), 15–16.

47. In the late nineteenth century Keen gained international attention for his innovative surgical techniques, including the drainage of the cerebral ventricles and the successful removal of large brain tumors. He also co-wrote the first American surgery text based on Listerian principles, in 1892; later, his *Surgery, Its Principles and Practices* became an essential textbook and reference for American surgeons. On Eakins's relationship to Keen and their shared emphasis on anatomy in the curriculum at PAFA, see Pennsylvania Academy of the Fine Arts, *In This Academy: The Pennsylvania Academy of the Fine Arts, 1805–1976, a Special Bicentennial Exhibition*

(Philadelphia: Pennsylvania Academy of the Fine Arts, 1976); and Amy Werbel, "Body Casts and 'Anatomical Eyes': Thomas Eakins, William Williams Keen, and the Curriculum at the Pennsylvania Academy of the Fine Arts," in Werbel, *Thomas Eakins: Art, Medicine, and Sexuality in Nineteenth-Century Philadelphia* (New Haven: Yale University Press, 2007), 53–85.

48. The anatomical instruction offered at PAFA was largely modeled on that of European academies, where artists had been studying anatomy since the Renaissance; see Werbel, *Thomas Eakins.*

49. William C. Brownell, "The Art Schools of Philadelphia," *Scribner's Monthly,* September 1879, 742, 747.

50. "Editor's Table," *PP* 12, no. 134 (February 1875): 64.

51. Wilson, "Artistic Anatomy," *PP* 12, no. 135 (March 1875): 96.

52. Quoted in Brownell, "Art Schools of Philadelphia," 744–45.

53. W. H. Tipton, "Anatomy, Phrenology, and Physiognomy, and Their Relations to Photography, No. 1," *PP* 14, no. 158 (February 1877): 54.

54. Michael Sappol, *A Traffic of Dead Bodies: Anatomy and Embodied Social Identity in Nineteenth-Century America* (Princeton: Princeton University Press, 2002), 7. See also John B. Blake, "Anatomy," in Numbers, *Education of American Physicians,* 29–47.

55. Sappol, *Traffic of Dead Bodies,* 47.

56. Before the 1870s and '80s, amateur photographers in Philadelphia were primarily scientists by training who had little education in the fine arts. These gentleman-scientists, including Joseph Saxton and Paul Beck-Goddard, were instrumental in the invention of photographic portraiture and the technical development of daguerreotypy in the 1840s and '50s. On the similar role of amateur photographers in Britain and their relation to discourses of art and science, see Grace Seiberling, *Amateurs, Photography, and the Mid-Victorian Imagination* (Chicago: University of Chicago Press, 1986); and Tucker, *Nature Exposed.*

57. Quoted in Brownell, "Art Schools of Philadelphia," 744–46.

58. On Snelling's defense of photography as a fine art in the 1850s, see Trachtenberg, "Mirror in the Marketplace," in *Lincoln's Smile and Other Enigmas,* 3–25. Although Snelling celebrated photography's relationship to drawing, painting, and sculpture in his inaugural editorial for the *Photographic Art Journal,* he anticipated some of his later arguments in describing the medium as a "noble science" to distinguish it from "lesser" mechanical work. See "The Art of Photography," *Photographic Art Journal* 1, no. 1 (January 1851): 1–3.

59. Gayton A. Douglass, "The Education of Photographers," *PP* 18, no. 211 (July 1881): 209.

60. "The World's Photography Focussed," *PP* 23, no. 277 (July 3, 1886): 400.

61. Root, *Camera and the Pencil,* 417.

62. Wilson made these sets of comments in relation to two examples of clinical photography: first, the short-lived Philadelphia journal the *Photographic Review of Medicine and Surgery,* which was copiously illustrated with photographs taken by John L. Gihon, and second, the before-and-after portraits published by the prominent French physician Guillaume-Benjamin-Armand Duchenne. See "Photographic Review of Medicine and Surgery," *PP* 8, no. 95 (November 1871): 376; and "The Photographic World," *PP* 7, no. 76 (April 1870): 142. For an excellent summary of photography's instrumental relationship to science in the late 1880s, see Reynold W. Wilcox, "Photography the Handmaid of the Physical Sciences," *PP* 24, no. 289 (January 1, 1887): 2–3.

63. "The World's Photography Focussed," *PP* 25, no. 335 (December 1, 1888): 722.

64. See, for instance, Pierre Bourdieu, "The Forms of Capital," in *Handbook of Theory and Research for the Sociology of Education,* ed. J. Richardson (New York: Greenwood Press, 1986), 241–58; Bourdieu, *La noblesse d'état: Grands écoles et spirit de corps* (Paris: Les Éditions de Minuit, 1989); and Bourdieu and Loïc J. D. Wacquant, *An Invitation to Reflexive Sociology* (Chicago: University of Chicago Press, 1992). In applying Bourdieu's notion of "investment strategies" to the history of commercial photography, I am indebted to others' reflections on this concept, especially David Swartz, *Culture and Power: The Sociology of Pierre Bourdieu* (Chicago: University of Chicago Press, 1997); Timothy Lenoir, *Instituting Science: The Cultural Production of Scientific Disciplines* (Stanford: Stanford University Press, 1997); and Garry Stevens, *The Favored Circle: The Social Foundations of Architectural Distinction* (Cambridge: MIT Press, 1998).

CHAPTER 2

1. The illustration appeared in *Arthur's Home Magazine,* February 1854, and the article, "Sitting for a Daguerreotype," in ibid., March 1854, 173–74. The two parts first appeared together in an expanded version, under the byline of T. S. Arthur, as "American Characteristics No. V.—The Daguerreotypist," in *Godey's Lady's Book,* May 1849, 352–55.

2. "Sitting for a Daguerreotype," *Arthur's Home Magazine,* March 1854, 173.

3. G. Wharton Simpson, "The Management of the Studio," *Photographic World* 1, no. 2 (February 1871): 42.

4. *Dictionary of the English Language* (Philadelphia: Lippincott Press, 1883), s.v. "operation."

5. Michel Foucault, *Discipline and Punish: The Birth of the Prison,* trans. A. M. Sheridan Smith (New York: Vintage Books, 1977), 155.

6. Lev Manovich, "The Operations," in Manovich, *The Language of New Media* (Cambridge: MIT Press, 2001), 116–75.

7. Some discussion of photography's similarities to dentistry appears in historical surveys of photographic humor, including Bill Jay, *Cyanide and Spirits: An Inside-Out View of Early Photography* (Munich: Nazraeli Press, 1991); and Heinz K. Henisch and Bridget A. Henisch, *Positive Pleasures: Early Photography and Humor* (University Park: Pennsylvania State University Press, 1998). On photography's impact on the dental profession, see Richard A. Glenner, Audrey B. Davis, and Stanley B. Burns, *The American Dentist: A Pictorial History with a Presentation of Early Dental Photography in America* (Missoula: Pictorial Histories, 1990).

8. "The Humor of It," *PP* 23, no. 280 (August 21, 1886): 490.

9. R. J. Chute, "Slide V.—Apparatus," *Photographic World* 2, no. 17 (May 1872): 146.

10. Olive Branch, "The Dentist's Chair," *Arthur's Home Magazine,* February 1853, 388. On dentists' reaction to the anxiety and pain their patients experienced in the dental chair, see "Pain in Dental Operations," *Dental News Letter* 11 (January 1858): 112–13.

11. Katherine C. Grier, *Culture and Comfort: Parlor Making and Middle-Class Identity, 1850–1930* (Washington, D.C.: Smithsonian Institution Press, 1988).

12. Karen Halttunen, "Humanitarianism and the Pornography of Pain in Anglo-American Culture," *American Historical Review* 100, no. 2 (1995): 332.

13. Rev. H. J. Morton, "Photography Indoors," *PP* 1, no. 7 (July 1864): 105.

14. "Oral Surgery," *Philadelphia Medical Times* (November 1, 1873): 70. See also "Dentistry," *Philadelphia Medical Times* (May 16, 1874): 522–23. On the elevation of dentistry as a distinct profession in American culture, see "Dentistry as a Profession," *Medical and Surgical Reporter* 8, no. 2 (April 12, 1862): 46–48; and James Harvey Young's more recent account, "The Long Struggle Against Quackery in Dentistry," in Young, *American Health Quackery* (Princeton: Princeton University Press, 1992), 107–24.

15. Roland Vanweike, "Under the Skylight, X. Expression," *PP* 9, no. 97 (January 1872): 6.

16. See Jonathan Taft, *A Practical Treatise on Operative Dentistry* (Philadelphia: Lindsay and Blakiston, 1877), 144.

17. This strategy was used by Napoleon Sarony in advertisements for his posing stand, e.g., "Sarony's Universal Rest and Posing Apparatus," *PP* 3, no. 34 (October 1866): 321. Robert Chute also drew an analogy between photography and dentistry to promote the proper use of posing equipment, specifically the use of the "improved Wilson Rest" over other models; see Chute, "Slide V.—Apparatus," 146–47.

18. Elbert Anderson, *The Skylight and the Dark-Room: A Complete Text-Book on Portrait Photography* (Philadelphia: Benerman and Wilson, 1872), 197.

19. H. S. Keller, "Proverbs," *Photographic Mosaics* 19 (1884): 52.

20. Surveys of early photographic humor include Rolf H. Krauss, *Fotografie in der Karikatur* (Seebruck am Chiemsee: Heering, 1978); Jay, *Cyanide and Spirits;* Bill Jay, *Some Rollicking Bull: Light Verse, and Worse, on Victorian Poetry* (Munich: Nazraeli Press, 1996); and Henisch and Henisch, *Positive Pleasures.* My critical approach to nineteenth-century jokes about photography is indebted to the work of media historians David Thorburn and Henry Jenkins, who have observed that "often the most powerful explorations of the features of a new medium occur in comedy."

See their "Introduction: Toward an Aesthetics of Transition," in *Rethinking Media Change*, 5. Carolyn Marvin also presents a useful model for thinking critically about humor in trade literature in *When Old Technologies Were New: Thinking About Electric Communication in the Late Nineteenth Century* (New York: Oxford University Press, 1990).

21. "The Humor of It," *PP* 23, no. 276 (June 19, 1886): 379.

22. Roland Vanweike, "Under the Skylight, No. III," *PP* 7, no. 80 (August 1870): 294–95. On studio patrons' common comparisons of photographers, dentists, and hangmen, see J. H. Kent, "Suggestions on Posing," *Photographic Mosaics* 5 (1870): 30–32. In chapter 1 of his *Realism, Photography, and Nineteenth-Century Fiction* (Cambridge: Cambridge University Press, 2008), Daniel A. Novak examines the theoretical work of such comparisons in nineteenth-century British writing on portrait photography, arguing that they defined the photographic body as "generic and indefinite" and thus as the subject of artful interpretation (46). Wilson's joke recalls a report that circulated widely in photographic journals of the late 1860s and early 1870s suggesting that the removal of the sitter's head as punishment for disturbing the photographic operation was within the realm of possibility for some operators. Photographers in Arkansas, the report explained, managed to coax sitters into keeping their heads still by pointing a loaded pistol at them during exposure and uttering the threat, "I will blow your brains out!" See "Salad for the Photographer," *PP* 4, no. 47 (November 1867): 364; G. Wharton Simpson, "Head-rests: Should They Be Used or Not?" *Photographic World* 2, no. 21 (September 1872): 261–62; and Jay, *Cyanide and Spirits*, 81.

23. Foucault, *Discipline and Punish*, 104–5. For a discussion of portrait photography as a visualization of discursive practices of social regulation, including medicine and the law, see Sekula, "Body and the Archive," 7–8; and Tagg, *Burden of Representation*.

24. "What Photographers Say When Press-ed," *Wilson's Photographic Magazine* 26, no. 346 (May 18, 1889): 291–92. For discussion of the pathological physical effects of sitting before the camera, see H. P. Robinson, "How to Manage the Sitter," *Photographic Mosaics* 2 (1867): 111–13; "Stray Thoughts on Exposures," *Photographic Mosaics* 4 (1869): 50; "The Sitter Hath Trial as Well, or The Other Side," *PP* 7, no. 77 (May 1870): 171–75; Roland Vanweike, "Under the Skylight, XI. Moving Sitters," *PP* 9, no. 98 (February 1872): 55–56; and William Heighway, "A Bull in a Glass-Room," *Photographic Mosaics* 8 (1873): 36–41.

25. "Our Picture," *PP* 3, no. 36 (December 1866): 387–89.

26. In a chapter called "The Human Face—the Mirror of the Soul and the Chief Subject of Art," Root explicitly stated that photographers were "all physiognomists in practice, if not in theory." Root, *Camera and the Pencil*, 89.

27. Ibid., 439, 177.

28. Root claimed to have derived his "notes on the subject" of medical observation and bodily inscription from "Dr. S. S. Brooks of this city" (ibid., 177–78). A regularly trained physician who lectured on physiology at the Franklin Institute in the 1850s, Dr. Silas Swift Brooks held the chair of institutes and practice at the Homeopathic Medical College in Philadelphia at the time that Root was writing *The Camera and the Pencil*.

29. I borrow the term "clinical gaze" from Michel Foucault, who has identified this way of seeing as the primary characteristic of an epistemological shift that occurred in Western medicine at the beginning of the nineteenth century. According to Foucault, the physician who employs a clinical gaze "reads at a glance the visible lesions of the organism and the coherence of pathological forms." As a result, the "relation between the visible and the invisible . . . necessary to all concrete knowledge" is restructured, "revealing through gaze and language what has previously been below and beyond their domain." See Foucault, *Birth of the Clinic*, 4–5, xii.

30. While it is impossible to list all of the instances in which Philadelphia physicians used the language of the "glance" to describe the epistemological basis of their work, treatises in the library of the College of Physicians of Philadelphia that promote the art of visual observation in medical case taking include Worthington Booker, *Physician and Patient, or A Practical View of the Mutual Duties, Relations, and Interests of the Medical Profession and the Community* (New York: Baker and Scribner, 1849); Thomas Bryant, *A Manual for the Practice of Surgery* (Philadelphia: Henry C. Lea's Son and Co., 1881); and Thomas Laycock, *Lectures on the Principles and Methods of Medical Observation and Research for the Use of Advanced Students and Junior Practitioners* (Edinburgh: Adam and Charles Black, 1856).

31.   Root, *Camera and the Pencil*, 177–79. While not every photographer made the connection between photographic and medical perception as explicitly as Root does, the notion that the "glance" was the primary means by which operators could diagnose their sitters' bodies was common. See, for instance, E. T. Whitney, "The Treatment of the Sitter," *PP* 10, no. 117 (September 1873): 321; and Robinson, "How to Manage the Sitter," 112.

32.   While Foucault never specifies such a parallel, he does invoke an analogy to portraiture in *The Birth of the Clinic.* The early nineteenth century, he argues, produced a "scientifically structured discourse about an individual"; as a result, the "space of configuration of the disease and the space of localization of the illness have been superimposed." He goes on to compare the application of the premodern "nosological" approach, or "flat medicine," to painting a portrait in which the patient's body is subtracted so as to isolate its symptoms, yielding a general corporal space or order. Conversely, in the case of modern medical perception, the "patient [i.e., his body] is the rediscovered portrait of the disease; he is the disease itself" (xiv, 15). This change recalls the rise of the photographic portrait in the same period, which critical theories of photography have associated with a fundamentally new mode of representation, one in which the image represents "the thing itself."

33.   In "Joel-Peter Witkin and Dr. Stanley B. Burns: A Language of Body Parts," *History of Photography* 23, no. 3 (1999), Rachelle Dermer makes a similar claim. "Medicine defines the normal and the abnormal," she argues, "and photographic representation effectively differentiates these categories" (245).

34.   See Elizabeth Grosz, "Inscriptions and Body Maps: Representations and the Corporeal," in *Space, Gender, Knowledge: Feminist Readings,* ed. Linda McDowell and Joanne P. Sharp (New York: J. Wiley, 1997), 236–46. Grosz makes brief but specific mention of surgery as a technology of inscription. Lines of social position and rank, she argues, "are inscribed in the case of the 'civilized body' as the lines of incision of surgical and chemical intervention, sites of social and personal remaking" (242).

35.   Georges Canguilhem, *The Normal and the Pathological,* trans. Carolyn R. Fawcett (New York: Zone Books, 1989).

36.   For a discussion of portrait photography as a means of archiving pathology, see Sekula, "Body and the Archive." Lisa Cartwright proposes a similar analogy between the use of medical cinema to "analyze, regulate, and reconfigure the transient, uncontrollable field of the body" and the performance of medical operations. Cartwright, *Screening the Body,* xiii.

37.   H. B. Hillyer, "Baby Pictures," *Photographic Mosaics* 15 (1880): 53.

38.   Root, *Camera and the Pencil,* 117.

39.   K. H. W., "The Dead Soldier's Children," *PP* 1, no. 1 (January 1864): 15.

40.   Mark H. Dunkelman tells the story of this soldier and his photograph in great detail in *Gettysburg's Unknown Soldier: The Life, Death, and Celebrity of Amos Humiston* (Westport, Conn.: Praeger, 1999). It was also the subject of a series of online essays by Errol Morris, beginning with "Whose Father Was He? (Part One)," *New York Times,* March 29, 2009, http://morris.blogs .nytimes.com/2009/03/29/whose-father-was-he-part-one/.

41.   "To the Fraternity," *PP* 1, no. 4 (April 1864): 60.

42.   United States Sanitary Commission, *Great Central Fair of the Sanitary Commission: To Professional and Amateur Photographers* (Philadelphia: United States Sanitary Commission, 1864). On photographers' participation in the Great Central Fair, see "Editor's Table," *PP* 1, no. 4 (April 1864): 63; "The Photographic Department at the Great Central Fair," *PP* 1, no. 7 (July 1864): 106–8; and "Our Picture," *PP* 1, no. 10 (October 1864): 157–58. The relationship between the USSC and photographic discourse is discussed further in chapter 4.

43.   On the realities of surgery during the Civil War, see Ira M. Rutkow, *Bleeding Blue and Gray: Civil War Surgery and the Evolution of American Medicine* (New York: Random House, 2005); and Laurann Figg and Jane Farrell-Beck, "Amputation in the Civil War: Physical and Social Dimensions," *Journal of the History of Medicine and Allied Sciences* 48, no. 4 (1993): 454–75.

44.   On the social history and value of artificial limbs in Civil War and Reconstruction Philadelphia, see Lisa Herschbach, "Prosthetic Reconstructions: Making the Industry, Re-Making the Body, Modelling the Nation," *History Workshop Journal* 44 (Autumn 1997): 22–57; and O'Connor, *Raw Material,* chapter 3. Then the largest manufacturer of artificial limbs in the city, B. Franklin

Palmer sold his patented "Palmer Arm & Leg" to the U.S. government for distribution to "mutilated" soldiers; he also operated a "national studio" modeled on a commercial parlor at 1609 Chestnut Street where customers could view and be fitted with the prosthetics. The apparatus and studio are described in Palmer, *The Palmer Arm & Leg: Correspondence with the Surgeon-General U.S.A. and the Chief Bureau of Medicine and Surgery U.S.N. . . .* (Philadelphia: C. Sherman & Son, 1862); and Oliver Wendell Holmes, "The Human Wheel, Its Spokes and Felloes," *Atlantic Monthly*, May 1863, 567–80.

45. On the rise of plastic surgery during the Civil War, see Richard B. Stark, "Plastic Surgery During the Civil War," *Plastic and Reconstructive Surgery* 16, no. 2 (1955): 103–20; Blair O. Rogers and Michael G. Rhode, "The First Civil War Photographs of Soldiers with Facial Wounds," *Aesthetic Plastic Surgery* 19, no. 3 (1995): 269–83; and Blair O. Rogers, "Rehabilitation of Wounded Civil War Veterans," *Aesthetic Plastic Surgery* 26, no. 10 (2002): 498–519. According to Stark, "seventy-two percent of the wounds of the Civil War were of the extremities, eighteen percent were of the torso, and ten per cent were of the head and neck" (104). The "9,815 cases of facial wounds from all cases reported" in the Union army, moreover, led to 672 operations, thirty-two of which were considered "plastic" or reconstructive in nature (106).

46. Rev. H. J. Morton, D.D., "Photography as an Authority," *PP* 1, no. 12 (December 1864): 182.

47. Michael G. Rhode and Blair O. Rogers, "Civil War Faces: The Wounded," manuscript. For a biography of Bell that tracks his professional development as a photographer, see Terrence R. Pitts, *William Bell: Philadelphia Photographer* (master's thesis, University of Arizona, 1987).

48. "Government Photography," *PP* 3, no. 31 (July 1866): 214–15.

49. The photographs of Rowland Ward were originally bound in the eight-volume *Photographs of Surgical Cases and Specimens,* which was distributed by the Army Medical Museum between 1865 and 1882. They were also published in *Photographs of Surgical Cases and Specimens Taken at the Army Medical Museum,* reprinted as Bradley P. Bengston and Julian E. Kuz, eds., *Photographic Atlas of Civil War Injuries: Photographs of Surgical Cases and Specimens,* Otis Historical Archives (Grand Rapids: Medical Staff Press, 1996). The portraits reproduced here as figure 17 appear in volume 4. On the publication history of the Army Medical Museum photographs, see Connor and Rhode, "Shooting Soldiers"; and Rhode, "Foreword," in Bengston and Kuz, *Photographic Atlas of Civil War Injuries,* iv–ix.

50. Sander L. Gilman, *Making the Body Beautiful: A Cultural History of Aesthetic Surgery* (Princeton: Princeton University Press, 1999), 41.

51. Gutekunst took seven views of Gettysburg shortly after the battle and before Matthew Brady had arrived on the scene. He also photographed countless military subjects during the war, including the Union's highest-ranking men, in his Arch Street studio. See Bob Zeller, *The Blue and Gray in Black and White: A History of Civil War Photography* (Westport, Conn.: Praeger, 2005), 112.

52. See the advertisements for Cremer & Co. in the *West Philadelphia Hospital Register* 1, no. 15 (May 23, 1863): 67, and no. 16 (May 30, 1863): 75. Many other Philadelphia studios advertised their services in this publication, including those owned by James E. McClees, R. Richardson, C. H. Spieler, F. Keller, and J. R. Laughlin.

53. Rhode and Blair, "Civil War Faces." The authors cite two pieces of correspondence between Bell and Dr. George A. Otis, then curator of the Army Medical Museum; both letters (one undated and the other dated May 28, 1868) are in the Otis Historical Archives of the National Museum of Health and Medicine, Washington, D.C.

54. "Our Picture," *PP* 2, no. 22 (October 1865): 170; "Our Picture," *PP* 14, no. 165 (September 1877): 284–85. For discussion of other Civil War subjects illustrated in the journal, see the "Our Picture" feature in *PP* 2, no. 21 (September 1865): 152–53; *PP* 2, no. 23 (November 1865): 186; *PP* 4, no. 43 (July 1867): 231–32; and *PP* 9, no. 100 (April 1872): 124–25.

55. William H. Rau, "A Photographic Visit to Some of Our Battlefields," *PP* 22, no. 257 (May 1885): 136–37.

56.   Sarah Burns, *Painting the Dark Side: Art and the Gothic Imagination in Nineteenth-Century America* (Berkeley and Los Angeles: University of California Press, 2004), 208. Burns makes this observation to account for Philadelphia artist Thomas Eakins's postbellum paintings of "vigorous oarsmen," which "celebrat[e] their highly developed physiques, perfect coordination, and winning spirit."

57.   Roland Vanweike, "Under the Skylight, No. VIII. Peculiarities of Faces," *PP* 8, no. 90 (June 1871): 166.

58.   For a rare discussion of photographers' application of colored pigments to sitters' faces and the nineteenth-century practice of retouching photographs, see Kathy Peiss, *Hope in a Jar: The Making of America's Beauty Culture* (New York: Henry Holt, 1998).

59.   Other pairs of photographs before and after retouching appear in "Our Picture," *PP* 7, no. 75 (March 1870); J. P. Ourdan, *The Art of Retouching* (New York: E. & H. T. Anthony and Co., 1880), frontispiece; and Anderson, *Skylight and the Dark-Room*, photographs 1–4.

60.   Charles W. Hearn, "Are Our Portraits Artistic? A Few Remarks on the Lighting of the Model, and the Exposing, Developing, Fixing, and Retouching of the Negative," *PP* 16, no. 183 (March 1879): 74.

61.   See W. H. Tipton, "Anatomy, Phrenology, and Physiognomy, and Their Relations to Photography, No. 1," *PP* 14, no. 158 (February 1877): 53–54.

62.   On rare occasions, the voices of female retouchers were heard in the Philadelphia photographic press. See, by A Photographer's Wife, "Retouching the Negative," *PP* 9, no. 100 (April 1872): 101; and Jennie, "What a Retoucher Can See on This Touchy Subject," *PP* 10, no. 113 (May 1873): 139–41. I would like to thank Marni Sandweiss for encouraging me to examine the gender politics of retouching in the nineteenth century.

63.   David Prince, *Plastics: A New Classification and a Brief Explanation of Plastic Surgery* (Philadelphia: Lindsay and Blakiston, 1868), 1.

64.   H. H. Snelling, "To Touch or Not to Touch; That's the Question," *PP* 9, no. 104 (August 1872): 300. Snelling's article was written in response to a letter to the editor published in the previous issue of the journal, in which the author expressed his enthusiastic support for retouching negatives. See "To Touch or Not to Touch," letter to the editor from "A Little Photo," *PP* 9, no. 103 (July 1872): 249–50.

65.   See H. H. Snelling, "Is Photography an Art?" *Photographic World* 2, no. 19 (July 1872): 211–12, in which Snelling argues that photography's "conception and practice is based *entirely* upon scientific principles," specifically truth and objectivity, "whereas *art* has nothing to do with science." An overview of the retouching debates can be gleaned from the following discussions: W. J. Baker, "Negative Retouching," *PP* 7, no. 76 (April 1870): 126–28; Prof. J. Towler, "Retouching," *Photographic Mosaics* 6 (1871): 63–68; "The Purpose and Limits of Retouch," *Photographic World* 1, no. 6 (June 1871): 163–64; G. Wharton Simpson, "Retouching Negatives," *Photographic World* 2, no. 17 (May 1872): 138–39; and G. Wharton Simpson, "Photographic Truth and Retouching," *Photographic World* 2, no. 15 (March 1872): 75–76.

66.   "The Humor of It," *PP* 24, no. 297 (May 7, 1887): 266.

67.   H. H. Snelling, "A Touching Subject," *PP* 9, no. 107 (November 1872): 380.

68.   On the importance of the posing stand to the production of upstanding social character in early American portrait studios, see Volpe, "Cartes de Visite Portrait Photographs."

69.   On the relationship between comfort and class in the nineteenth-century portrait studio, see Grier, *Culture and Comfort,* chapter 1.

70.   Studies that examine nineteenth-century anesthetics in relation to medical authority and professionalization include Martin S. Pernick, *A Calculus of Suffering: Pain, Professionalism, and Anesthesia in Nineteenth-Century America* (New York: Columbia University Press, 1985); Mary Poovey, "'Scenes of an Indelicate Character': The Medical 'Treatment' of Victorian Women," *Representations* 14 (Spring 1986): 137–68; and David B. Morris, *The Culture of Pain* (Berkeley and Los Angeles: University of California Press, 1991).

71.   Henry Jacob Bigelow, "Insensibility During Surgical Operations Produced by Inhalation," in *Surgery in America: From the Colonial Era to the Twentieth Century,* ed. A. Scott Earle

(New York: Praeger, 1983), 196, 201. This article was first published in *Boston Medical and Surgical Journal* 35, no. 16 (November 18, 1846): 309–17.

72. Susan Buck-Morss uses the metaphor of anesthesia to define a similarly "uncanny sense of self-alienation" that modern subjects experience. See her "Aesthetics and Anaesthetics: Walter Benjamin's Artwork Essay Reconsidered," *October* 62 (Fall 1992): 31. On the redistribution of power in the surgical operating theater, see also Stefan Hirschauer, "The Manufacture of Bodies in Surgery," *Social Studies of Science* 21, no. 2 (1991): 279–319.

73. "An Hour with Mr. Sarony—Our Picture," *PP* 4, no. 39 (March 1867): 83.

74. For a discussion of the daguerreotypes made of early administrations of ether at Massachusetts General Hospital, see Bates Lowry and Isabel Lowry, "Simultaneous Developments: Documentary Photography and Painless Surgery," in *Young America: The Daguerreotypes of Southworth & Hawes,* ed. Grant B. Romer and Brian Wallis (New York: International Center of Photography, 2005).

75. On the history of instantaneous photography, see Phillip Prodger, *Time Stands Still: Muybridge and the Instantaneous Photography Movement* (New York: Oxford University Press, 2003).

76. Rev. H. J. Morton, "Instantaneous Photography," *PP* 3, no. 35 (November 1866): 334.

77. A. A. Pearsall, "Instantaneous Portraiture," *PP* 8, no. 96 (December 1871): 385.

78. Charles King, "Sitter and Operator," *PP* 16, no. 189 (September 1879): 283.

79. See Root, *Camera and the Pencil,* 389; and Kent, "Suggestions on Posing."

80. Robinson, "How to Manage the Sitter," 112.

81. Frank P. W. Bellew [Chip, pseud.], *How to Sit for Your Photograph* (Philadelphia: Benerman and Wilson, 1872), 17.

82. Vanweike, "Under the Skylight, X. Expression," 5–6.

83. Pernick, *Calculus of Suffering,* chapter 7.

84. See "Surgery and Different Races," *Medical and Surgical Reporter* 49, no. 19 (November 10, 1883): 527.

85. "Some Thoughts About Cartes de Visite," *Godey's Lady's Book,* September 1862, 303.

86. On the prevalence of medical metaphor in photographic history and theory, see O'Connor, "Camera Medica."

87. Benjamin writes, "The surgeon represents the polar opposite of the magician. The magician heals a sick person by the laying on of the hands; the surgeon cuts into the patient's body. . . . Magician and surgeon compare to painter and cameraman. The painter maintains in his work a natural distance from reality, the cameraman penetrates deeply into its web." See Walter Benjamin, "The Work of Art in the Age of Mechanical Reproduction," in *Illuminations,* ed. Hannah Arendt (New York: Schocken Books, 1969), 233. Benjamin's brief comment on the epistemological similarities between photographic media and surgery has been substantiated in Terri Kapsalis's study of the filmic nature of surgical procedures and Giuliana Bruno's examination of film's anatomical and surgical roots. See Kapsalis, *Public Privates: Performing Gynecology from Both Ends of the Speculum* (Durham: Duke University Press, 1997); and Bruno, "Spectatorial Embodiments: Anatomies of the Visible and the Female Bodyscape," *Camera Obscura* 28 (January 1992): 239–62.

88. For a discussion of pain as a marker of the real, see Elaine Scarry, *The Body in Pain: The Making and Unmaking of the World* (New York: Oxford University Press, 1985).

89. Manovich, *Language of New Media,* 106–7; and Barthes, *Camera Lucida,* 13, 57.

90. See Sontag, *On Photography;* and Sontag, *Regarding the Pain of Others* (New York: Farrar, Straus and Giroux, 2003).

CHAPTER 3

1. Augustus J. Pleasonton, *The Influence of the Blue Ray of the Sunlight and of the Blue Color of the Sky, in Developing Animal and Vegetable Life; in Arresting Disease, and in Restoring Health in Acute and Chronic Disorders to Human and Domestic Animals* (Philadelphia: Claxton, Remsen and Haffelfinger, 1876), 24.

2. Augustus J. Pleasonton, "Blue and Sunlights, Their Influence in Developing Animal and Vegetable Life, in Arresting Disease and Restoring Health in Acute and Chronic Disorders to Human and Domestic Animals" (Philadelphia: Claxton, Remsen and Haffelfinger, 1877), 3. This four-page circular was distributed with the 1877 reprint of Pleasonton's treatise.

3. For an overview of the popular applications of blue glass in the nineteenth century, see Robert Means Lawrence, *Primitive Psycho-Therapy and Quackery* (New York: Houghton Mifflin, 1910); and Paul Collins, *Banvard's Folly: Thirteen Tales of Renowned Obscurity, Famous Anonymity, and Rotten Luck* (New York: Picador USA, 2001).

4. Little is now known about the blue-glass treatments administered at Markoe House, beyond what H. M. Beidler published in *Blue Glass Sun-Baths as a Curative* (Philadelphia: H. M. Beidler, 1877).

5. A number of book-length defenses of Pleasonton's theories were published after 1876, including T. Ormsbee, *The Influence of Blue and Sun-Light upon the Unbalanced Human System* (Chicago: Jameson and Morse, 1877); and William Channing, *Blue Glass: Its Influence upon Life and Disease, with a Large Number of Cases Showing Its Remarkable Salutary Effect* (Philadelphia: Commercial Pub. Co., n.d. [ca. 1878–90]). Edward B. Foote Jr., a New York physician who coined the phrase "panes curing pains," also published prolifically on blue glass in his monthly journal and collected his many public lectures on the subject in *The Blue Glass Cure: How and When It Originated; Why It Has Been Ridiculed . . . etc.* (New York: Murray Hill, 1880). Other phototherapists expanded upon Pleasonton's system of therapeutics by accounting for the healing and spiritual powers of colored light. See Seth Pancoast, *Blue and Red Light, or Light and Its Rays as Medicine . . .* (Philadelphia: J. M. Stoddard and Co., 1877); and Edwin Babbitt, *The Principles of Light and Color . . .* (New York: Babbitt and Co., 1878). According to Pleasonton, the electrophysiologist S. W. Beckwith and the University of Pennsylvania surgeon David Hayes Agnew regularly administered his therapy to their patients with much success (Pleasonton, *Influence of the Blue Ray of the Sunlight*, 10–14, 28). Although Agnew never publicized his use of blue light, the *Philadelphia Medical Times* did report (albeit critically) that by 1877 blue glass had been introduced into Philadelphia's hospitals. See "Blue Light in Therapeutics," *Philadelphia Medical Times* (January 30, 1875): 282.

6. Popular satires on blue glass include John Carboy [John A. Harrington], *Blue Glass, a Sure Cure for the Blues* (New York: J. B. Collin, 1877); and Samuel C. Upham, *The Wonders of Blue Glass as Seen Through a Blue Glass Bluely* (Philadelphia: Samuel C. Upham, 1877). Augustin Daly also wrote and presented a play in New York at the height of the blue-glass craze titled simply *Blue Glass!* While the plot strayed far from the subject of the blue-glass craze, the story turned on a man's failed and foolish investment in blue glass "stock." For other satirical images and musical scores inspired by the blue-glass craze, see Helfand, *Quack, Quack, Quack*.

7. Some discussion of Pleasonton's cure appears in histories of quackery. See Lawrence, *Primitive Psycho-Therapy and Quackery*; James J. Walsh, *Cures: The Story of Cures That Fail* (New York: D. Appleton, 1924); Collins, *Banvard's Folly*; and Helfand, *Quack, Quack, Quack*. Harvey Green has also studied light therapeutics in the context of health and fitness trends that emerged in late nineteenth-century America; see Green, *Fit for America: Health, Fitness, Sport, and American Society* (New York: Pantheon Books, 1986).

8. For an overview of these discussions, see Carolyn Thomas de la Peña, "'Slow and Low Progress,' or Why American Studies Should Do Technology," *American Quarterly* 58, no. 3 (2006): 915–41; and Elspeth H. Brown, "Technology, Culture, and the Body in Modern America," *American Quarterly* 56, no. 2 (2004): 449–60, which reviews de la Peña's *The Body Electric: How Strange Machines Built the Modern American* (New York: New York University Press, 2003) and Joel Dinerstein's *Swinging the Machine: Modernity, Technology, and African American Culture Between the World Wars* (Amherst: University of Massachusetts Press, 2003).

9. Pleasonton, *Influence of the Blue Ray of the Sunlight*, 26. Pleasonton does not explicitly name Shove but refers to him as the author of "Life Under Glass." Shove had published an article in the *Atlantic Monthly* and a book by this title in 1873 and 1874, respectively.

10. "The Glass-House," *PP* 3, no. 30 (June 1866): 162. The same illustration of Henszey's "model" studio appeared as figure 7 in Hermann Vogel, *The Chemistry of Light and Photography* (New York: D. Appleton, 1875), 24.

11. "Glass for the Studio," *PP* 3, no. 34 (October 1866): 302.

12. Ibid. See also the following, all in *Photographic Mosaics:* T. R. Williams, "Portraiture—Hints on Lighting," 3 (1868): 122–26; A Practical Man, "Studio Hints," 4 (1869): 53–54; and Old Argentum, "How to Build the Very Best Skylight," 7 (1872): 91–93.

13. R. J. C., "Health and Actinism," *PP* 14, no. 162 (June 1877): 161–62.

14. "The Insane Department of the Philadelphia Almshouse," *Philadelphia Illustrated,* December 5, 1874, 2, 5.

15. See William A. Hammond, *Treatise on Hygiene with Special Reference to the Military Service* (Philadelphia: J. B. Lippincott, 1863), 210.

16. On photographers' use of blue glass to soothe the eyes of their sitters, see "Blue Glass Blindness," *Scientific American,* June 23, 1877, 384; and "Danger to the Eyes in Using Flash Powder," *PP* 25, no. 318 (March 17, 1888): 184.

17. On the relationship between gender, class, and nervousness, see Anson Rabinach, *The Human Motor: Energy, Fatigue, and the Origins of Modernity* (New York: Basic Books, 1990); and Poovey, "'Scenes of an Indelicate Character.'"

18. Babbitt, *Principles of Light and Color,* 360.

19. *Scientific American* was consistently critical of Pleasonton's supposed cure, running articles in 1877 with the following titles: "The Blue Glass Deception," "More Blue Glass Skeptics," "The Blue Glass Epidemic," and "Blue Glass Blindness." Even irregular physicians who advocated the use of blue light observed that Pleasonton's theories did not warrant the authority with which the American public had invested them. The general, they argued, crucially failed to account for the fact that the blue ray is already present at its full strength in unfiltered sunlight. Blue glass simply blocks the harmful effects of the yellow, orange, and red rays of the sun on human skin, thus acting as a shade or filter that allows individuals to absorb the healthful rays of the sun for longer periods of time without damaging the skin or eyes.

20. See in particular the prolific writings of the Boston glass manufacturer Thomas Gaffield, who was also a lifetime member of the National Photographic Association: *Action of Sunlight on Glass* (New Haven: Tuttle, Morehouse and Taylor, 1867); *Glass for the Studio and Darkroom* (Philadelphia: Benerman and Wilson, 1876); "Glass for Photographers' Use," *Photographic Mosaics* 12 (1877): 21–24; "The Uses of Glass in Photography," *PP* 18, no. 213 (September 1881): 277; and the four-part series titled "The Blue Glass Mania: Notes on General Pleasonton's Book," which appeared in the *Boston Evening Transcript* in 1877: February 12 (part I), February 20 (part II), March 7 (part III), and March 14 (part IV).

21. Gaffield, "Blue Glass Mania," part II (February 20, 1877), 6.

22. See, for instance, "Society Gossip," *PP* 16, no. 185 (May 1879): 147–51, which provides the transcript of a meeting in which members of the Chicago Photographic Association debated the professional implications and material benefits of using blue glass.

23. On the cultural authority of popular science and technologies of the body in this period, see de la Peña, *Body Electric;* Green, *Fit for America;* Charles E. Rosenberg, *Right Living: An Anglo-American Tradition of Self-Help Medicine and Hygiene* (Baltimore: Johns Hopkins University Press, 2003); Rosenberg, *No Other Gods: On Science and American Social Thought* (Baltimore: Johns Hopkins University Press, 1976); and Arthur Wrobel, ed., *Pseudo-Science and Society in Nineteenth-Century America* (Lexington: University Press of Kentucky, 1987).

24. See Isaac Parrish, "Report on the Sanitary Condition of Philadelphia," *Transactions of the American Medical Association* 2 (1849): 461–62.

25. Forbes Winslow, *Light: Its Influence on Life and Health* (New York: Moorhead, Simpson and Bond, 1868), 3, 6.

26. Ibid., 4.

27. Henry S. Taylor, *The Family Doctor: A Counselor in Sickness, Pain, and Distress, for Childhood, Manhood, and Old Age . . .* (Philadelphia: John E. Potter, 1860), 31.

28. Hammond quoted in "Sanitary Value of Light," *Philadelphia Medical Times* (May 17, 1873): 519.

29. There have been several studies in the past decade on the social politics of scientific discourse on climate, including Gary Robert McKee, "Climate, Science, and Politics in Victorian

Britain" (PhD diss., Queen's University of Belfast, 2002); Roxann Wheeler, *The Complexion of Race: Categories of Difference in Eighteenth-Century British Culture* (Philadelphia: University of Pennsylvania Press, 2000); and Mart A. Stewart, "'Let Us Begin with the Weather?' Climate, Race, and Cultural Distinctiveness in the American South," in *Nature and Society in Historical Context*, ed. Mikuláš Teich, Roy Porter, and Bo Gustafsson (New York: Cambridge University Press, 1997), 240–56. Discussions of race and climate in the American context are indebted to Winthrop D. Jordan's *White Over Black: American Attitudes Toward the Negro, 1550–1812* (Chapel Hill: University of North Carolina Press, 1968).

30. Robley Dunglison, *Human Health, or The Influence of Atmosphere and Locality. . . .* (Philadelphia: Lea and Blanchard, 1844), 52.

31. Hammond, *Treatise on Hygiene*, 295. The idea that racial character is tied to the size and shape of certain physical features, particularly the cranium, had become popular in American scientific circles by the mid-nineteenth century. It was articulated famously by Josiah C. Nott and George R. Gliddon in *Types of Mankind, or Ethnological Researches. . . .* (Philadelphia: J. B. Lippincott, Grambo, 1854), which expanded upon earlier work published by the Philadelphia physician Samuel George Morton. For a critical discussion of these studies, see William R. Stanton, *The Leopard's Spots: Scientific Attitudes Toward Race in America, 1815–1859* (Chicago: University of Chicago Press, 1960); Stephen J. Gould, *The Mismeasure of Man* (New York: W. W. Norton, 1981); and Robyn Wiegman, *American Anatomies: Theorizing Race and Gender* (Durham: Duke University Press, 1995).

32. Winslow, *Light*, 23.

33. Ibid., 15–16.

34. Decades after the scientific community had refuted the idea that the black pigmentation of "Negro" skin was a symptom of illness, the pathologizing of blackness remained an important feature of American scientific thought and popular culture. The distinguished Philadelphia physician Benjamin Rush had advocated this idea at the turn of the century; see Rush, "Observations Intended to Favor a Supposition that the Black Color (as It Is Called) of the Negroes Is Derived from Leprosy," *Transactions of the American Philosophical Society* 4 (1799): 289–97. On the racist politics underlying American scientific inquiries into skin color, see Jordan, *White Over Black;* George M. Frederickson, *The Black Image in the White Mind: The Debate on Afro-American Character and Destiny, 1817–1914* (New York: Harper and Row, 1971); Ronald Takaki, *Iron Cages: Race and Culture in Nineteenth-Century America* (New York: Oxford University Press, 2000); and the secondary sources cited in note 31.

35. George A. Shove, *Life Under Glass: Containing Suggestions Toward the Formation of Artificial Climates* (Boston: James R. Osgood, 1874), 29.

36. Ibid., 47.

37. See David R. Roediger, *The Wages of Whiteness: Race and the Making of the American Working Class* (London: Verso, 1991); and Matthew Frye Jacobson, *Whiteness of a Different Color: European Immigrants and the Alchemy of Race* (Cambridge: Harvard University Press, 1998).

38. Michael B. Katz and Thomas J. Sugre, eds., *W. E. B. Du Bois, Race, and the City: The Philadelphia Negro and Its Legacy* (Philadelphia: University of Pennsylvania Press, 1998), 10. Bounded east–west by 7th and 25th streets and north-south by Spruce and South streets, the Seventh Ward famously became the focus of Du Bois's *The Philadelphia Negro: A Social Study* (Philadelphia: published for the University of Pennsylvania, 1899). In recent decades numerous historical studies of the nonwhite populations in nineteenth-century Philadelphia have appeared, many of which have paid special attention to the social development of the black community. See Allen F. Davis and Mark H. Haller, eds., *The Peoples of Philadelphia: A History of Ethnic Groups and Lower-Class Life, 1790–1940* (Philadelphia: Temple University Press, 1973); Theodore Hershberg, ed., *Philadelphia: Work, Space, Family, and Group Experience in the Nineteenth Century* (New York: Oxford University Press, 1981); Gary B. Nash, *Forging Freedom: The Formation of Philadelphia's Black Community, 1720–1840* (Cambridge: Harvard University Press, 1988); Roger Lane, *Roots of Violence in Black Philadelphia, 1860–1900* (Cambridge: Harvard University Press, 1986); and Roger Lane, *William Dorsey's Philadelphia and Ours: On the Past and Future of the Black City in America* (New York: Oxford University Press, 1991).

39.   Pleasonton's *Diary, 1838–1844* (Historical Society of Pennsylvania), quoted in Nash, *First City*, 169. Studies of the antebellum race riots in Philadelphia include Sam Bass Warner Jr., "Riots and the Restoration of Public Order," in his *Private City: Philadelphia in Three Periods of Its Growth* (Philadelphia: University of Pennsylvania Press, 1968), 125–57; Michael Feldberg, *The Philadelphia Riots of 1844: A Study of Ethnic Conflict* (Westport, Conn.: Greenwood Press, 1975); Russell F. Weigley, "'A Peaceful City': Public Order in Philadelphia from Consolidation Through the Civil War," in Davis and Haller, *Peoples of Philadelphia*, 155–74; and Emma Jones Lapansky, "'Since They Got Those Separate Churches': Afro-Americans and Racism in Jacksonian Philadelphia," in *African Americans in Pennsylvania: Shifting Historical Perspectives*, ed. Joe William Trotter Jr. and Eric Ledell Smith (University Park: Pennsylvania State University Press, 1997), 93–120.

40.   For an overview of black Philadelphians' struggles for social equality in the Civil War and Reconstruction periods, see Gallman, *Mastering Wartime*; Lane, *Roots of Violence in Black Philadelphia;* and Nash, *Forging Freedom.*

41.   Henry C. Silcox, "Nineteenth-Century Philadelphia Black Militant: Octavius V. Catto (1839–1871)," in Trotter and Smith, *African Americans in Pennsylvania*, 198–219.

42.   Pleasonton, "Blue and Sunlights," 4.

43.   See "Colored Glass in Insanity," *Philadelphia Medical Times* (April 29, 1876): 383; and Augustus Barnes, *New and Important Discovery! Marks and Discolorations, Both Natural and Artificial, of Every Shade and Color, Entirely Taken Away* (Southington, Conn.: A. Barnes, 1867).

44.   Carboy, *Sure Cure for the Blues*, 50.

45.   Ibid., 31. That the general's black patient suffered from "softening of the brain" was meant to be read as humorous, given that this degeneration of the mind was commonly associated in the nineteenth century with men who overtaxed their brains through intellectual work. For popular descriptions of the disease, see "Softening of the Brain," *Lady's Home Magazine,* April 1859, 208; and A Family Doctor, "Plain Advice to Brain-Workers," *Arthur's Home Magazine,* April 1882, 260–62.

46.   Carboy, *Sure Cure for the Blues*, 33.

47.   On cultural anxieties concerning racial mixing after emancipation, see Elise Lemire, *"Miscegenation": Making Race in America* (Philadelphia: University of Pennsylvania Press, 2002); and Carolyn Sorisio, *Fleshing Out America: Race, Gender, and the Politics of the Body in American Literature, 1833–1879* (Athens: University of Georgia Press, 2002).

48.   Saidiya V. Hartman, *Scenes of Subjection: Terror, Slavery, and Self-Making in Nineteenth-Century America* (New York: Oxford University Press, 1997), 185. Contemporary treatises, such as Benjamin P. Hunt's *Why Colored People in Philadelphia Are Excluded from the Street Cars* (Philadelphia: Merrihew & Son, 1866), make explicit the close relationship between infringements on black freedom in postbellum Philadelphia—such as segregation in streetcars, homes for orphans and disabled veterans, schools, and public baths—and white fears of miscegenation.

49.   Carboy, *Sure Cure for the Blues*, 34. For discussion of the social and political importance of the "white Negro" in the era of the Civil War and Reconstruction, see Charles D. Martin, *The White African American Body: A Cultural and Literary Exploration* (New Brunswick: Rutgers University Press, 2002); and Mary Niall Mitchell, "'Rosebloom and Pure White,' or So It Seemed," *American Quarterly* 54, no. 3 (2002): 369–410.

50.   Vogel, *Chemistry of Light and Photography*, 2–3.

51.   Ibid., 129.

52.   On the privileging of white skin in twentieth-century photographic technologies, see Richard Dyer, *White* (London: Routledge, 1997); and Brian Winston, "A Whole Technology of Dyeing: A Note on Ideology and the Apparatus of the Chromatic Moving Image," *Daedalus* 114, no. 4 (1985): 105–23.

53.   Williams, "Portraiture—Hints on Lighting," 123.

54.   R. J. Chute, "Hints Under the Skylight: The Light and the Subject," *PP* 11, no. 130 (October 1874): 313–14.

55.   Deborah Willis, *Reflections in Black: A History of Black Photographers, 1840–1999* (New York: W. W. Norton, 2000), ix. See also Brian Wallis and Deborah Willis, *African American Vernacular Photography: Selections from the Daniel Cowin Collection* (New York: International

Center of Photography, 2005), which I review in "African American Vernacular Photography: Selections from the Daniel Cowin Collection," *Journal of American History* 93, no. 3 (2006): 815–19.

56. F. N. Blake, "Photographing Groups of Persons of Different Complexions," *Photographic Mosaics* 13 (1878): 129. See also F. Leyde, "Concerning Illumination," *Photographic Mosaics* 19 (1884): 118–23.

57. H. J. Rodgers, *Twenty-Three Years Under a Sky-Light, or Life and Experiences of a Photographer* (Hartford: H. J. Rodgers, 1872), 175–76.

58. For a description of this lighting method, see Blake, "Photographing Groups of Persons," 130.

59. For a discussion of this genre and its contributions to white sentimental discourse, see Laura Wexler, *Tender Violence: Domestic Visions in an Age of U.S. Imperialism* (Chapel Hill: University of North Carolina Press, 2000).

60. Roland Vanweike, "Under the Skylight, No. V. Groups," *PP* 8, no. 85 (January 1871): 8.

61. Gretchen A. Condran and Jennifer Murphy, "Defining and Managing Infant Mortality: A Case Study of Philadelphia, 1870–1920," *Social Science History* 32, no. 4 (2008): 473–513. As these authors note, the Philadelphia Board of Health counted 85,957 births in the city and 19,227 deaths in children under the age of one between 1865 and 1870, "producing a mortality rate of 22.36 percent during the first year of life" (481).

62. Dr. Andrew Winslow, quoted in Winslow, *Light*, 164–65; and Babbitt, *Principles of Light and Color*, 332.

63. See Winslow, *Light*, 163. Winslow makes this observation about the health of "savage" children alongside the proposal for "photographic" nurseries, promoting a connection between the two.

64. On baby pictures and constructions of whiteness in the late nineteenth century, see Smith, *American Archives*.

65. J. C. Leake Jr., quoted in Mathew Carey Lea, ed., *Newman's Manual of Harmonious Coloring* (Philadelphia: Benerman and Wilson, 1866), 137.

66. Vogel, *Chemistry of Light and Photography*, 46.

CHAPTER 4

1. See Gaston Tissandier, *History and Handbook of Photography*, ed. and trans. John Thompson (London: S. Low, Marston, Low, and Searle, 1876), 90–91; and Edward L. Wilson, *Wilson's Photographics; A Series of Lessons, Accompanied by Notes, on All the Processes Which Are Needful in the Art of Photography* (Philadelphia: Edward L. Wilson, 1881), 91. The American edition of Tissandier's book was published by the Scovill Manufacturing Company of New York in 1877.

2. Wilson, *Wilson's Photographics*, 91.

3. See David A. Hollinger, "Inquiry and Uplift: Late Nineteenth-Century American Academics and the Moral Efficacy of Scientific Practice," in Haskell, *Authority of Experts;* and Rosenberg, *No Other Gods*.

4. Edward L. Wilson, "Dirt," *Photographic Mosaics* 5 (1870): 59–60.

5. Mary Douglas, *Purity and Danger: An Analysis of Concepts of Pollution and Taboo* (London: Routledge and Kegan Paul, 1966; reprint, New York: Routledge, 2002), 44.

6. Ibid.

7. Wilson, "Dirt," 58–59.

8. David Armstrong, "Public Health Spaces and the Fabrication of Identity," *Sociology* 27, no. 3 (1993): 393.

9. Isaac Parrish, "Report on the Sanitary Condition of Philadelphia," *Transactions of the American Medical Association* 2 (1849): 471.

10. "Minutes of the Proceedings of the Quarantine Convention," *Medical News and Library* 15, no. 174 (June 1857): 95–103.

11. Ibid., 101.

12.   Authorities on public health commonly compared foul vessels to filthy cities throughout the second half of the nineteenth century. See, for instance, John M. Woodworth's postbellum reflections on the cholera epidemic of 1854, "The General Subject of Quarantine, with Particular Reference to Cholera and Yellow Fever," in *Transactions of the International Medical Congress of Philadelphia, 1876*, ed. John Ashhurst Jr. (Philadelphia: International Medical Congress: 1877), 1059–71.

13.   Sam Alewitz, *"Filthy Dirty": A Social History of Unsanitary Philadelphia in the Late Nineteenth Century* (New York: Garland, 1989), 19.

14.   Parrish, "Report on the Sanitary Condition of Philadelphia," 466, 462.

15.   See Alewitz, *"Filthy Dirty"*; and Michael A. Flannery, *Civil War Pharmacy: A History of Drugs, Drug Supply and Provision, and Therapeutics for the Union and Confederacy* (New York: Haworth Press, 2004).

16.   United States Sanitary Commission, *An Appeal to the People of Pennsylvania for the Sick and Wounded Soldiers* (Philadelphia: United States Sanitary Commission, 1861), 12, 1, 10–11.

17.   Henry Bowditch, *Public Hygiene in America: Being the Centennial Discourse Delivered Before the International Medical Congress, Philadelphia, September, 1876* (Boston: Little, Brown, 1877), 1, 2. For a discussion of Bowditch's lecture as part of a larger effort to promote public health reform in American cities at the time of the Centennial Exhibition, see Julie K. Brown, *Health and Medicine on Display: International Expositions in the United States, 1876–1904* (Cambridge: MIT Press, 2009).

18.   Surveys of the American public health movement after the war include Howard D. Kramer's two-part article, "Agitation for Public Health Reform in the 1870s," *Journal of the History of Medicine and Allied Sciences* 3, no. 4 (1948): 473–88 (part I), and 4, no. 1 (1949): 75–89 (part II); Wilson G. Smillie, *Public Health: Its Promise for the Future; a Chronicle of the Development of Public Health in the United States, 1607–1914* (New York: Macmillan, 1955); and John Duffy, *The Sanitarians: A History of American Public Health* (Urbana: University of Illinois Press, 1990).

19.   Lewis W. Leeds, *A Treatise on Ventilation: Comprising Seven Lectures Delivered Before the Franklin Institute, Philadelphia, 1866–1868* (New York: J. Wiley & Son, 1871), 3, 82–83.

20.   Representative of this vast body of literature are Henry Hartshorne, *Our Homes* (Philadelphia: Presley Blakiston, 1880); George R. Moore, *Ventilation in Our Homes* (Philadelphia: George S. Harris and Sons, 1882); and a six-part series by Felix L. Oswald titled "Healthy Homes" published in *Lippincott's Magazine* in 1884. For critical surveys of this literature, see Gavin Townsend, "Airborne Toxins and the American House, 1865–1895," *Winterthur Portfolio* 24 (Spring 1989): 29–42; Maureen Ogle, "Domestic Reform and American Household Plumbing, 1840–1870," *Winterthur Portfolio* 28 (Spring 1993): 33–58; and Nancy Tomes, "The Private Side of Public Health: Sanitary Science, Domestic Hygiene, and the Germ Theory, 1870–1900," in Leavitt and Numbers, *Sickness and Health in America*, 506–28.

21.   Alan C. Braddock, "Bodies of Water: Thomas Eakins, Racial Ecology, and the Limits of Civic Realism," in *A Keener Perception: Ecocritical Studies in American Art History*, ed. Alan C. Braddock and Christoph Irmscher (Tuscaloosa: University of Alabama Press, 2009), 129–50. On water pollution and disease in late nineteenth-century Philadelphia, see also Alewitz, *"Filthy Dirty"*; and Michael P. McCarthy, *Typhoid and the Politics of Public Health in Nineteenth-Century Philadelphia* (Philadelphia: American Philosophical Society, 1989).

22.   Bowditch, *Public Hygiene in America*, 2.

23.   "Editor's Table," *PP* 23, no. 272 (April 17, 1886): 255.

24.   Mathew Carey Lea, "Photography vs. Health," *PP* 5, no 52 (April 1868): 133.

25.   Mathew Carey Lea, *A Manual of Photography* (Philadelphia: Benerman and Wilson, 1868), 45. Lea also published his observations concerning photographic chemistry and health in "The Hygiene of Photography," *PP* 1, no. 8 (August 1864): 123–26; and "Photography and Disease," *PP* 5, no. 59 (November 1868): 392–93.

26.   Robert J. Chute, "Things New and Old," *PP* 11, no. 122 (February 1874): 40. In addition, see, also by Chute, "Things New and Old," *PP* 11, no. 123 (March 1874): 68–69, and "Photography vs. Health," *PP* 5, no. 52 (April 1868): 133; Chas. Wager Hull, "Ventilation of Dark-Rooms," *PP* 5, no. 50 (February 1868): 43; and J. H. Fitzgibbons, "Health," *Photographic Mosaics* 10 (1875): 34–35.

27. Nelson K. Cherrill compared the photographic laboratory to a poorly ventilated home in "A Suggestion for the Better Ventilation of Dark-Rooms," *PP* 4, no. 48 (December 1867): 377–80.

28. "Photography and Health," *PP* 10, no. 110 (February 1873): 38–39.

29. Dr. Norman Bridge, "Hygiene of Photography," *PP* 28, no. 202 (October 1880): 305–6.

30. The subject of exercise in late nineteenth-century photographic discourse and its relationship to the physical culture movement is an important one that I intend to take up in a future study. On the "movement cure" and its benefits to commercial photographers in this period, see Lea, *Manual of Photography*, 392–93; Chute, "Slide V.—Apparatus," *Photographic World* 2, no. 17 (May 1872): 146–47; "The Health Lift," *PP* 11, no. 126 (June 1874): 190; M. P. Brown, "Good Health," *PP* 20, no. 229 (January 1883): 13–14; M. P. Brown, "Getting Ahead," *PP* 21, no. 242 (February 1884): 44–45; Irving Saunders, "Health of Photographers," *Photographic Mosaics* 19 (1884): 110–11; and the following three articles in *Wilson's Photographic Magazine*: "The World's Photography Focussed," 26, no. 346 (May 18, 1889): 309; "Health and Art," 26, no. 357 (November 2, 1889): 667–69; and "Art and Athletics," 27, no. 362 (January 18, 1890): 45–47.

31. "Can You Tell?" *PP* 18, no. 209 (May 1881): 153.

32. For a discussion of the nineteenth-century emigrant car, see Anthony J. Bianculli, *Trains and Technology: The American Railroad in the Nineteenth Century*, vol. 2 (Newark: University of Delaware Press, 2001), 34–35.

33. Leeds, *Treatise on Ventilation* (2d ed., 1876), 48–49.

34. Samuel V. Allen, "That Chemical Room," *Photographic Mosaics* 15 (1880): 130.

35. "Salad for the Photographer," *PP* 3, no. 34 (October 1866): 319–20. See also "Salad for the Photographer," *PP* 3, no. 26 (February 1866): 62. These reports followed the publication in Philadelphia of the memoir of Sarah Edmonds, a white woman who claimed to have used silver nitrate to pass as a black slave during the Civil War. See S. Emma E. Edmonds, *Nurse and Spy in the Union Army: Comprising the Adventures and Experiences of a Woman in Hospitals, Camps, and Battle-Fields* (Hartford: W. S. Williams & Co., 1865).

36. On the relationship between blackness, filth, and disease in Civil War writings on sanitation, see Long, *Rehabilitating Bodies*, chapter 3.

37. Bridge, "Hygiene of Photography," 305.

38. "Can You Tell?" 153.

39. Lea, *Manual of Photography*, 324.

40. "Editor's Table," *PP* 4, no. 48 (December 1867): 403; "Sad Death of a Young Photographer," *Photographic World* 2, no. 17 (May 1872): 160. For a summary of the health effects of working with photographic cyanide, see Lea, *Manual of Photography*, 325. Historian Bill Jay has conducted extensive primary research on the subject of cyanide and other chemical poisonings based on photographic literature of the period. See Jay, "Dangers in the Dark," in his *Cyanide and Spirits*, 145–88.

41. On the social value of cleanliness in nineteenth-century American culture, see Suellen Hoy, *Chasing Dirt: The American Pursuit of Cleanliness* (New York: Oxford University Press, 1995); and Richard L. Bushman and Claudia L. Bushman, "The Early History of Cleanliness in America," *Journal of American History* 74, no. 4 (1988): 1213–38.

42. For examples, see "The Story of a Carte de Visite," *PP* 2, no. 20 (August 1865): 127–30; Julie, "A Visit to a Country Gallery, and What It Prevented," *PP* 5, no. 49 (January 1868): 9–12; and Helios, "Some Recollections of a Developing Glass," *American Journal of Photography* 9, no. 12 (December 1, 1888): 335.

43. "Story of a Carte de Visite," 128, 130. Although an ambrotype was found in the hands of Amos Humiston, the dead Union soldier to whom this passage refers, readers commonly mistook it for a *carte de visite* after copies of the portrait circulated in this paper format in 1865. See Dunkelman, *Gettysburg's Unknown Soldier*.

44. "Story of a Carte de Visite," 130.

45. Ibid., 129, 128.

46. "A Persistent Evil: Trouble in the Darkroom," *PP* 14, no. 165 (September 1877): 266; and "Measles, How to Get Them, and How to Get Rid of Them," *PP* 3, no. 28 (April 1866): 105. For discussion of yellow fever, see "The Open Corner," *PP* 23, no. 265 (January 2, 1886): 20. On the

"green fog" disease, see Lyonel Clark, "Green Fog," *Wilson's Photographic Magazine* 26, no. 357 (November 2, 1889): 657–58.

47.   In the last quarter of the nineteenth century, speculation about the causes of and remedies for blisters occupied more pages of Philadelphia's photographic journals than any other photographic ailment. See, for instance, L. W. Crawford, "A Cure for Blisters, and a Few Good Ideas," *Photographic Mosaics* 14 (1879): 84–85; and C. F. Krauss, "Blisters! Blisters! Blisters!" *Wilson's Photographic Magazine* 26, no. 355 (October 5, 1889): 601.

48.   I would make a distinction here between photographers' medical self-treatment and the popular middle-class practice of administering home remedies in nineteenth-century America on the basis of the scientific authority that photographers sought to gain through their laboratory work. On the varieties and cultural importance of self-care in this period, see Guenter B. Risse, Ronald L. Numbers, and Judith Walzer Leavitt, eds., *Medicine Without Doctors: Home Health Care in American History* (New York: Science History Publications, 1977); and Anita Clair Fellman and Michael Fellman, *Making Sense of Self: Medical Advice Literature in Late Nineteenth-Century America* (Philadelphia: University of Pennsylvania Press, 1981).

49.   For examples of such language, see J. F. Ryder, "Killed by Overdose," *PP* 24, no. 306 (September 17, 1887): 567–68; and Mathew Carey Lea, "A Word on Cleanliness," *PP* 6, no. 70 (October 1869): 325.

50.   Wilson, "The Photographer on the Fence," *Photographic Mosaics* 6 (1871): 72.

51.   Pamela H. Smith, *The Body of the Artisan: Art and Experience in the Scientific Revolution* (Chicago: University of Chicago Press, 2004), 114.

52.   Cennino d'Andrea Cennini, *The Craftsman's Handbook: The Italian 'Il libro dell'arte,'* trans. Daniel V. Thompson Jr. (New York: Dover, 1960), 99, 83, quoted in ibid., 115.

53.   Laurie Dahlberg, "The Material Ethereal: Photography and the Alchemical Ancestor," in *Art and Alchemy,* ed. Jacob Wamberg (Copenhagen: Museum Tusculanum Press, 2006), 86. Dahlberg does acknowledge the presence of alchemical language and symbolism in the writings of Nathaniel Hawthorne and Oliver Wendell Holmes.

54.   "The Total Depravity and Gymnastics of Inanimate Things Photographic," *PP* 2, no. 22 (October 1865): 157.

55.   Quoted in Julie, "Visit to a Country Gallery," 12.

56.   On the importance of alchemical symbols in American arts and culture, see David Bjelajac, *Washington Allston, Secret Societies, and the Alchemy of Anglo-American Painting* (Cambridge: Cambridge University Press, 1997); and Randall A. Clack, *The Marriage of Heaven and Earth: Alchemical Regeneration in the Works of Taylor, Poe, Hawthorne, and Fuller* (Westport, Conn.: Greenwood Press, 2000).

57.   See "Measles, How to Get Them," 105; J. Perry Elliott, "Measles," *PP* 8, no. 87 (March 1871): 76–77; and A. St. Clair, "Measles," *Photographic World* 1, no. 4 (April 1871): 122. On the enormous challenges that measles posed to the medical community during the Civil War, see Flannery, *Civil War Pharmacy,* 133.

58.   References to these photographic diseases include Crawford, "Cure for Blisters"; Krauss, "Blisters! Blisters! Blisters!"; and Alexander L. Pach, "Photography and 'La Grippe,'" *Wilson's Photographic Magazine* 27, no. 365 (March 1, 1890): 156–57. Roland G. Curtin and Edward W. Watson describe "La Grippe" and its effects on the city of Philadelphia in "Epidemic of Influenza in Philadelphia in 1889, '90, '91," *Transactions of the American Climatological and Clinical Association* 8 (1892): 109–26.

59.   On the cultural history of epidemics in the United States, see Charles E. Rosenberg, *The Cholera Years: The United States in 1832, 1849, and 1866* (Chicago: University of Chicago Press, 1987); and Rosenberg, *Explaining Epidemics and Other Studies in the History of Medicine* (New York: Cambridge University Press, 1992).

60.   "System," *Wilson's Photographic Magazine* 26, no. 358 (November 16, 1889): 697–98.

61.   Elliott, "Measles," 76.

62.   In his 1871 letter to the *Photographic World,* A. St. Clair omitted Elliott's loose distinction altogether by using the first person to describe a "severe attack of the measles." "I have been

making photographs on albumen paper since 1858," he wrote, "and never suffered from this disease. . . . About two weeks ago I caught it."

63. Pach, "Photography and 'La Grippe,'" 156–57.

64. See Lea, *Manual of Photography*, 323, 328.

65. The medical bibliography on each of these chemicals is extensive. Good summaries of their therapeutic functions are available in any handbook of *materia medica* or in the *United States Pharmacopoeia* of the period. For discussion of their therapeutic properties, see also "Alcohol: Its Therapeutical Uses, Internally and Externally," *Philadelphia Medical Times* 11 (July 16, 1881): 647–52; "Physiological Action of the Bromide of Potassium," *Philadelphia Medical Times* 3 (September 6, 1873): 770–73; and John Higginbottom, *A Practical Essay on the Use of the Nitrate of Silver, in the Treatment of Inflammation, Wounds, and Ulcers* (London: John Churchill and Sons, 1865).

66. On collodion's uses in photography and medicine, see Wilson, *Wilson's Photographics;* "Collodion Instead of Court-plaster," *PP* 25, no. 332 (October 20, 1888): 615; "Applications of Collodion," *Medical and Surgical Reporter* 1, no. 24 (March 12, 1859): 432; "Collodion," *Druggists' Circular and Chemical Gazette* 10, no. 7 (July 1866): 162; and "Gun Cotton and Its Preparations," *Philadelphia Medical Times* 2 (September 2, 1872): 456–57. Although Snelling implies that he was the first to discover collodion's powers as a remedy for toothache, the professional medical community actually beat him to that discovery by at least three years. As Philadelphia's *Medical and Surgical Reporter* noted in 1868, the premier British medical journal the *Lancet* "says toothache can be cured by one drachm of collodion to two drachms of Calvert's carbolic acid." See "News and Miscellany," *Medical and Surgical Reporter* 19, no. 26 (December 26, 1868): 522.

67. See "Science for the Photographer," *PP* 17, no. 193 (January 1880): 13–14.

68. Samuel O. L. Potter, *A Compend of Materia Medica and Therapeutics, with Especial Reference to the Physiological Actions of Drugs* (Philadelphia: P. Blakiston, Son and Co., 1883).

69. Edward Moelling, "Materia Photographica," *Photographic Mosaics* 7 (1872): 120.

70. Quoted in G. Wharton Simpson, "Cyanide as a Cure for Consumption," *Photographic World* 1, no. 8 (August 1871): 245.

71. "Cyanide of Potassium as a Cure for Consumption," *Photographic World* 1, no. 10 (October 1871): 299. In this second article, the editors reprinted Ozier's original letter, which is signed "E. P. Ogier, St. Helier's, Jersey, June 7, 1871," in its entirety. It is unclear which is the proper spelling, although the journal does consistently refer to the author as "Ogier" in this second report.

72. *American Journal of Photography* 4, no. 9 (September 1883): 4.

73. Quoted in "Adulteration of Chemicals," *Druggists' Circular and Chemical Gazette* 16, no. 8 (August 1872): 135. Pharmacists expressed similar concerns about using photographic collodion for medicinal purposes, noting that the collodion preferred by photographers at high temperatures "is not so good for pharmaceutical purposes as that prepared at a lower temperature." See William Silver Thompson, "Remarks on Collodion and Cantharidal Collodion," *American Journal of Pharmacy* 42 (1870): 115–16.

CHAPTER 5

1. Lauren Collins, "Pixel Perfect: Pascal Dangin's Virtual Reality," *New Yorker*, May 12, 2008, 94, 96.

2. Ibid., 96–97, 94, 100.

3. "Beauty Not Just Smaller Than Life," *Miami Herald*, January 31, 2003, 1B. For discussion of these and other well-known examples of digital doctoring in the media, see Geoffrey Batchen, "Ectoplasm," in *Each Wild Idea: Writing, Photography, History* (Cambridge: MIT Press, 2001), 128–43; and W. J. T. Mitchell, *The Reconfigured Eye: Visual Truth in the Post-Photographic Era* (Cambridge: MIT Press, 1992).

4. Quoted in Collins, "Pixel Perfect," 100.

5. Fred Ritchin, *In Our Own Image: The Coming Revolution in Photography* (New York: Aperture Foundation, 1990), 2.

6.   Mitchell, *Reconfigured Eye,* 19. See also Anne-Marie Willis, "Digitisation and the Living Death of Photography," in *Culture, Technology, and Creativity in the Late Twentieth Century,* ed. Philip Hayward (London: John Libbey, 1990), 197–208. For a critical summary of the discourse on photography's death, see Batchen, "Ectoplasm."

7.   Kevin Robins, "Will Image Move Us Still?" in *The Photographic Image in Digital Culture,* ed. Martin Lister (New York: Routledge, 1995), 30.

8.   Martin Lister, "Introduction," ibid., 8.

9.   See ibid., 9; Robins, "Will Image Move Us Still?" 32.

10.   See Lev Manovich, "The Paradoxes of Digital Photography," in *Photography After Photography: Memory and Representation in the Digital Age,* ed. Hubertus von Amelunxen, Stefan Iglhaut, and Florian Rötzer (Amsterdam: G and B Arts, 1996), 57–65; Sarah Kember, *Virtual Anxiety: Photography, New Technologies, and Subjectivity* (Manchester: Manchester University Press, 1998); Jay David Bolter and Richard Grusin, *Remediation: Understanding New Media* (Cambridge: MIT Press, 1999); Manovich, *Language of New Media;* Thorburn and Jenkins, *Rethinking Media Change;* Lauren Rabinovitz and Abraham Geil, eds., *Memory Bytes: History, Technology, and Digital Culture* (Durham: Duke University Press, 2004); and Gail Baylis, "Remediations: Or When Is a Boring Photograph Not a Boring Photograph?" *Photographies* 1, no. 1 (2008): 29–48.

11.   Geo. D. Jopson, "A Standard of Excellency," *American Annual of Photography* 22 (1908): 207. At the same time, trade journals made self-conscious efforts to distance studio portraiture from the discourse of operations that shaped photographic authority in the nineteenth century. A 1915 editorial in *Studio Light,* for example, encouraged portrait photographers not to call themselves "operators" or their studios "operation rooms" for fear that these terms would revive old associations between photography, surgery, dentistry, and torture. Likewise, it explained, the financially successful photographer was one who avoided scientific rhetoric and references to his "modern apparatus." Instead, he emphasized only the pleasures of portrait taking, inviting comparisons to shopping. See "Is There a Better Name?" *Studio Light* 7, no. 8 (October 1915): 3–4, 8.

12.   See James Clayseen, "Digital (R)evolution," in Amelunxen, Iglhaut, and Rötzer, *Photography After Photography,* 78.

13.   Martin Dawber, *Pixel Surgeons: Extreme Manipulation of the Figure in Photography* (London: Octopus Publishing Group, 2005).

14.   Tim Daly and David Asch, *Digital Photo Doctor: Simple Steps to Diagnose, Rescue, and Enhance Your Images* (Pleasantville, N.Y.: Reader's Digest Association, 2006), 138.

15.   Ibid., 144.

16.   Barry Jackson, *Photoshop Cosmetic Surgery: A Comprehensive Guide to Portrait Retouching and Body Transforming* (New York: Lark Books, 2006), dust jacket.

17.   In January 2010, at the time of this writing, this list included but was by no means limited to the following businesses: Photo Doctor (Goleta, California), http://www.photodoctor .com/; The Photo Doctor (Tully, New York), http://www.cnyphotodoc.com/; The Photo Doctor (Boston, Massachusetts), http://www.thephotodoctor.org/; Photo Doctor 911 (Tampa, Florida), http://www.photodoctor911.com/; Photo Doctor Graphics (San Francisco, California), http://www.photodoctorgraphics.com/; Miss Photo Surgeon (Golden, Colorado), http:// www.missphotosurgeon.com/; The Photo Physician (New Haven, Connecticut), http://www .thephotophysician.com/; The Photo Surgeon (Brooklyn, New York), http://www.photosurgeon .com/; Photo Physician Rx (Cleveland, Tennessee), http://www.photophysicianrx.com/.

18.   Gary Pageau, "Presidential Profile: PMA President Allen Showalter Talks About Growing Up in the Photo Industry," *PMA Magazine* 83 (March 2008): 44–45; and Ken Beer, "The Secrets of Their Success: Industry Leaders Share Unique Promotions," *Digital Imaging Digest,* June 1, 2002.

19.   The TV image in fig. 41 misspells Showalter's first name.

20.   Quoted in Beer, "Secrets of Their Success."

21.   See http://www.king1hourphoto.com/ (accessed January 15, 2010).

22.   Quoted in Pageau, "Presidential Profile," 45.

23.   Quoted in Collins, "Pixel Perfect," 101.

24. For a critical analysis of the "hair doctor" as a metaphorical construction of African American hairstylists' professional knowledge and authority, see Lanita Jacobs-Huey, "'We Are Like Doctors: Socializing Cosmetologists into the Discourse of Science," in *From the Kitchen to the Parlor: Language and Becoming in African American Women's Hair Care* (New York: Oxford University Press, 2006): 29–46.

25. See Dana Heller, ed., *The Great American Makeover: Television, History, Nation* (New York: Palgrave Macmillan, 2006); Heller, *Makeover Television: Realities Remodelled* (New York: I. B. Tauris, 2007); Toby Miller, *Makeover Nation: The United States of Reinvention* (Columbus: Ohio State University Press, 2008); and Brenda R. Weber, *Makeover TV: Selfhood, Citizenship, and Celebrity* (Durham: Duke University Press, 2009).

26. In addition to the work of Heller and Weber cited in the previous note, see the 2007 two-part special issue of *Configurations* (vol. 15, nos. 1–2), which includes critical essays on medical makeover television by Bernadette Wegenstein, Pamela Orosan-Weine, Virginia L. Blum, Kimberly Jackson, Brenda R. Weber, Julie M. Albright, Joanna Zylinska, Mark Poster, and William Egginton.

27. Weber, *Makeover TV*, 6, 39.

28. Jackson does include two female authors, one of whom worked as a missionary in Africa, as well as several women who claim that they had consultations with plastic surgeons and presumably the financial means to do so. These women are exceptions to the rule, however, and figure in the manual as tokens of female "success."

29. Jackson, *Photoshop Cosmetic Surgery*, 54.

30. Ibid., 92.

31. Ibid., 86.

32. Heller, *Great American Makeover*, 167.

33. Batchen, "Ectoplasm," 134.

34. See Jacques W. Maliniak, "Facts and Fallacies of Cosmetic Surgery," *Hygeia* 12, no. 3 (1934): 200–202. I regret that I was unable to reproduce the illustration discussed here, which appears on the first page of this article.

SELECTED BIBLIOGRAPHY

NONPERIODICAL LITERATURE FIRST PUBLISHED BEFORE 1900

American Medical Association. *Proceedings of the National Medical Conventions, Held in New York, May, 1846, and in Philadelphia, May, 1847.* Philadelphia: T. K. and P. G. Collins, 1847.

Anderson, Elbert. *The Skylight and the Dark-Room: A Complete Text-Book on Portrait Photography.* Philadelphia: Benerman and Wilson, 1872.

Babbitt, Edwin. *The Principles of Light and Color: Including Among Other Things the Harmonic Laws of the Universe, the Etherio-atomic Philosophy of Force, Chromo Chemistry, Chromo Therapeutics, and the General Philosophy of the Fine Forces, Together with Numerous Discoveries and Practical Applications.* New York: Babbitt and Co., 1878.

Barnes, Augustus. *New and Important Discovery! Marks and Discolorations, Both Natural and Artificial, of Every Shade and Color, Entirely Taken Away.* Southington: A. Barnes, 1867.

Beidler, H. M. *Blue Glass Sun-Baths as a Curative.* Philadelphia: H. M. Beidler, 1877.

Bellew, Frank P. W. [Chip, pseud.]. *How to Sit for Your Photograph.* Philadelphia: Benerman and Wilson, 1872.

Bellows, Henry Whitney. *Speech of the Rev. Dr. Bellows, President of the United States Sanitary Commission, Made at the Academy of Music, Philadelphia, Tuesday Evening, Feb. 24, 1863, Philadelphia Agency of the United States Sanitary Commission, 1307 Chestnut Street.* Philadelphia: C. Sherman and Son, 1863.

Booker, Worthington. *Physician and Patient, or A Practical View of the Mutual Duties, Relations, and Interests of the Medical Profession and the Community.* New York: Baker and Scribner, 1849.

Bowditch, Henry. *Public Hygiene in America: Being the Centennial Discourse Delivered Before the International Medical Congress, Philadelphia, September, 1876.* Boston: Little, Brown, 1877.

Bryant, Thomas. *A Manual for the Practice of Surgery.* Philadelphia: Henry C. Lea's Son and Co., 1881.

Carboy, John [John A. Harrington]. *Blue Glass, a Sure Cure for the Blues.* New York: J. B. Collin, 1877.

Cennini, Cennino d'Andrea. *The Craftsman's Handbook: The Italian 'Il libro dell'arte.'* Translated by Daniel V. Thompson Jr. New York: Dover, 1960.

Channing, William. *Blue Glass: Its Influence upon Life and Disease, with a Large Number of Cases Showing Its Remarkable Salutary Effect.* Philadelphia: Commercial Pub. Co., n.d. [ca. 1878–1890].

Du Bois, W. E. B. *The Philadelphia Negro: A Social Study.* Philadelphia: published for the University of Pennsylvania, 1899.

Dunglison, Robley. *Human Health, or The Influence of Atmosphere and Locality; Change of Air and Climate; Seasons; Food; Clothing; Bathing and Mineral Springs; Exercise; Sleep;*

Corporeal and Intellectual Pursuits; &c. &c. on Healthy Man; Constituting Elements of Hygiene. Philadelphia: Lea and Blanchard, 1844.

Edmonds, S. Emma E. *Nurse and Spy in the Union Army: Comprising the Adventures and Experiences of a Woman in Hospitals, Camps, and Battle-Fields.* Hartford: W. S. Williams & Co., 1865.

Foote, Edward B., Jr. *The Blue Glass Cure: How and When It Originated; Why It Has Been Ridiculed; Gen. Pleasonton Not a Success as an Experimental Philosopher; His Facts and Theories; What They Are Worth; the Light of Science Brought to Shine on Blue Glass; Panes Curing Pains; Real Merits Made Plain, and the Cob-webs Brushed Away; The Sun the Source of All Power; Its Beneficial and Its Baneful Influences; Absence of Sun-light Injurious; Why It Is Avoided; the Properties of Sun-light; How They Are Modified by Blue-glass; a Few Practical Hints; etc.* New York: Murray Hill, 1880.

Freedley, Edwin T. *Philadelphia and Its Manufacturers.* Philadelphia: Edward Young & Co., 1867.

Gaffield, Thomas. *Action of Sunlight on Glass.* New Haven: Tuttle, Morehouse and Taylor, 1867.

———. *Glass for the Studio and Dark-room.* Philadelphia: Benerman and Wilson, 1876.

Gross, Samuel D. *Autobiography of Samuel D. Gross, M.D.* Philadelphia: G. Barrie, 1887.

———. *A System of Surgery; Pathological, Diagnostic, Therapeutic, and Operative.* Philadelphia: Blanchard and Lea, 1859.

Hammond, William A. *Treatise on Hygiene with Special Reference to the Military Service.* Philadelphia: J. B. Lippincott, 1863.

Hartshorne, Henry. *Our Homes.* Philadelphia: Presley Blakiston, 1880.

Higginbottom, John. *A Practical Essay on the Use of the Nitrate of Silver, in the Treatment of Inflammation, Wounds, and Ulcers.* London: John Churchill and Sons, 1865.

Hunt, Benjamin P. *Why Colored People in Philadelphia Are Excluded from the Street Cars.* Philadelphia: Merrihew & Son, 1866.

Jefferson, Thomas. *Notes on the State of Virginia.* 1781–82. Reprint, New York: Library of America, 1984.

Laycock, Thomas. *Lectures on the Principles and Methods of Medical Observation and Research for the Use of Advanced Students and Junior Practitioners.* Edinburgh: Adam and Charles Black, 1856.

Lea, Mathew Carey. *A Manual of Photography.* Philadelphia: Benerman and Wilson, 1868.

———, ed. *Newman's Manual of Harmonious Coloring.* Philadelphia: Benerman and Wilson, 1866.

Leeds, Lewis W. *A Treatise on Ventilation: Comprising Seven Lectures Delivered Before the Franklin Institute, Philadelphia, 1866–1868.* New York: J. Wiley & Son, 1871. 2d ed., 1876.

Moore, George R. *Ventilation in Our Homes.* Philadelphia: George S. Harris and Sons, 1882.

National Photographic Association of the United States. *Manual of the National Photographic Association of the United States.* Philadelphia: Sherman & Co., 1873.

Nott, Josiah C., and George R. Gliddon. *Types of Mankind, or Ethnological Researches, Based upon the Ancient Monuments, Paintings, Sculptures, and Crania of Races, and upon Their Natural, Geographical, Philological, and Biblical History.* Philadelphia: J. B. Lippincott, Grambo, 1854.

Ormsbee, T. *The Influence of Blue and Sun-Light upon the Unbalanced Human System.* Chicago: Jameson and Morse, 1877.

Ourdan, J. P. *The Art of Retouching.* New York: E. & H. T. Anthony and Co., 1880.

Palmer, B. Franklin. *The Palmer Arm & Leg: Correspondence with the Surgeon-General U.S.A. and the Chief Bureau of Medicine and Surgery U.S.N. with Letters from Eminent Surgeons, and a Communication from B. Frank. Palmer to the Board of Surgeons Convened to Decide on the Best Patent Artificial Limbs to Be Adopted for Use by the Army and Navy of the U.S.* Philadelphia: C. Sherman and Son, 1862.

Pancoast, Seth. *Blue and Red Light, or Light and Its Rays as Medicine; Showing That Light Is the Original and Sole Source of Life, as It Is the Source of All the Physical and Vital Forces in Nature; and That Light Is Nature's Own and Only Remedy for Disease . . . Together with a Chapter on Light in the Vegetable Kingdom.* Philadelphia: J. M. Stoddard and Co., 1877.

Pleasonton, Augustus J. "Blue and Sunlights, Their Influence in Developing Animal and Vegetable Life, in Arresting Disease and Restoring Health in Acute and Chronic Disorders to Human and Domestic Animals." Four-page circular. Philadelphia: Claxton, Remsen and Haffelfinger, 1877.

———. *The Influence of the Blue Ray of the Sunlight and of the Blue Color of the Sky, in Developing Animal and Vegetable Life; in Arresting Disease, and in Restoring Health in Acute and Chronic Disorders to Human and Domestic Animals.* Philadelphia: Claxton, Remsen and Haffelfinger, 1876.

Potter, Samuel O. L. *A Compend of Materia Medica and Therapeutics, with Especial Reference to the Physiological Actions of Drugs.* Philadelphia: P. Blakiston, Son and Co., 1883.

Prince, David. *Plastics: A New Classification and a Brief Explanation of Plastic Surgery.* Philadelphia: Lindsay and Blakiston, 1868.

Rodgers, H. J. *Twenty-Three Years Under the Sky-Light, or Life and Experiences of a Photographer.* Hartford: H. J. Rodgers, 1872.

Root, Marcus Aurelius. *The Camera and the Pencil, or The Heliographic Art.* 1864. Reprint, Pawlet, Vt.: Helios, 1971.

Scharf, John Thomas, and Thompson Westcott. *History of Philadelphia, 1609–1884.* 3 vols. Philadelphia: L. H. Everts and Co., 1884.

Shove, George. *Life Under Glass, Containing Suggestions Toward the Formation of Artificial Climates.* Boston: James R. Osgood, 1874.

Snelling, Henry H. *The History and Practice of the Art of Photography, or The Production of Pictures Through the Agency of Light, Containing all the Instructions Necessary for the Complete Practice of the Daguerrean and Photogenic Art, Both on Metallic Plates and on Paper.* New York: G. P. Putnam, 1849.

The Soldiers' Guide in Philadelphia. Philadelphia: Geo. H. Ives, n.d. [ca. 1861–65].

Taft, Jonathan. *A Practical Treatise on Operative Dentistry.* Philadelphia: Lindsay and Blakiston, 1877.

Taylor, Henry S. *The Family Doctor: A Counselor in Sickness, Pain and Distress, for Childhood, Manhood, and Old Age; Containing in Plain Language, Free from Medical Terms, the Causes, Symptoms, and Cure of Disease in Every Form; with Important Rules for Preserving the Health, and Directions for the Sick Chamber, and the Proper Treatment of the Sick; the Whole Drawn from Extensive Observation and Practice.* Philadelphia: John E. Potter, 1860.

Tissandier, Gaston. *History and Handbook of Photography.* Edited and translated by John Thompson. London: S. Low, Marston, Low, and Searle, 1876.

Towler, John. *The Silver Sunbeam: A Practical and Theoretical Text-Book on Sun Drawing and Photographic Printing; Comprehending All the Wet and Dry Processes at Present Known.* New York: Joseph H. Ladd, 1864.

United States Sanitary Commission. *An Appeal to the People of Pennsylvania for the Sick and Wounded Soldiers.* Philadelphia: United States Sanitary Commission, 1861.

———. *Great Central Fair of the Sanitary Commission: To Professional and Amateur Photographers.* Philadelphia: United States Sanitary Commission, 1864.

Upham, Samuel C. *The Wonders of Blue Glass as Seen Through a Blue Glass Bluely.* Philadelphia: Samuel C. Upham, 1877.

Vogel, Hermann. *The Chemistry of Light and Photography.* New York: D. Appleton, 1875.

Wilson, Edward L. *Wilson's Photographics; A Series of Lessons, Accompanied by Notes, on All the Processes Which Are Needful in the Art of Photography.* Philadelphia: Edward L. Wilson, 1881.

Winslow, Forbes. *Light: Its Influence on Life and Health*. New York: Moorhead, Simpson and
Bond, 1868.

Woodworth, John M. "The General Subject of Quarantine, with Particular Reference to
Cholera and Yellow Fever." In *Transactions of the International Medical Congress of
Philadelphia, 1876,* ed. John Ashhurst Jr., 1059–71. Philadelphia: International Medi-
cal Congress, 1877.

PUBLICATIONS AFTER 1900

Alewitz, Sam. *"Filthy Dirty": A Social History of Unsanitary Philadelphia in the Late Nineteenth Century*. New York: Garland, 1989.

Amelunxen, Hubertus von, Stefan Iglhaut, and Florian Rötzer, eds. *Photography After
Photography: Memory and Representation in the Digital Age*. Amsterdam: G and B Arts,
1996.

Amirault, Chris. "Posing the Subject of Early Medical Photography." *Discourse* 16, no. 2
(1993–94): 51–76.

Armstrong, David. "Public Health Spaces and the Fabrication of Identity." *Sociology* 27, no. 3
(1993): 393–410.

Arnheim, Rudolf. "On the Nature of Photography." *Critical Inquiry* 1 (September 1974):
149–61.

Baker, Robert, ed. *The Codification of Medical Morality: Historical and Philosophical Studies of
the Formalization of Western Medical Morality in the Eighteenth and Nineteenth Centuries,* vol. 2, *Anglo-American Medical Ethics and Medical Jurisprudence in the Nineteenth
Century*. Dordrecht: Kluwer Academic Publishers, 1995.

Banta, Martha. "Medical Therapies and the Body Politic." *Prospects: An Annual Journal of
American Culture Studies* 8 (1983): 59–128.

Barthes, Roland. *Camera Lucida: Reflections on Photography*. Translated by Richard Howard.
New York: Hill and Wang, 1981.

———. "Rhetoric of the Image." In *Image/Music/Text,* trans. Stephen Heath, 32–51.
New York: Hill and Wang, 1977.

Batchen, Geoffrey. *Each Wild Idea: Writing, Photography, History*. Cambridge: MIT Press,
2001.

———. "The Naming of Photography: 'A Mass of Metaphor.'" *History of Photography* 17,
no. 1 (1993): 22–32.

Battani, Marshall. "Organizational Fields, Cultural Fields, and Art Worlds: The Early Effort
to Make Photographs and Make Photographers in the Nineteenth-Century United
States of America." *Media, Culture, and Society* 21, no. 5 (1999): 601–26.

Baylis, Gail. "Remediations: Or When Is a Boring Photograph Not a Boring Photograph?"
Photographies 1, no. 1 (2008): 29–48.

Bazin, André. "Ontology of the Photographic Image." In *What Is Cinema?* Vol. 1. Translated
by Hugh Gray, 9–16. Berkeley and Los Angeles: University of California Press, 1967.

Beatty, Heather Renee. "The Body Politic: Medical Metaphor in the Age of the American
Revolution." Honors thesis, College of William and Mary, 2002.

Beer, Ken. "The Secrets of Their Success: Industry Leaders Share Unique Promotions."
Digital Imaging Digest, June 1, 2002.

Behling, Laura L. *Gross Anatomies: Fictions of the Physical in American Literature*. Selinsgrove:
Susquehanna University Press, 2008.

Bengston, Bradley P., and Julian E. Kuz, eds. *Photographic Atlas of Civil War Injuries: Photographs of Surgical Cases and Specimens, Otis Historical Archives*. Grand Rapids: Medical
Staff Press, 1996.

Benjamin, Walter. "The Work of Art in the Age of Mechanical Reproduction." In *Illuminations*, ed. Hannah Arendt, 217–52. New York: Schocken Books, 1969.

Berger, Martin A. "The Anatomy of the Early Republic." *Early Popular Visual Culture* 7, no. 3 (2009): 231–52.

Bianculli, Anthony J. *Trains and Technology: The American Railroad in the Nineteenth Century.* 3 vols. Newark: University of Delaware Press, 2001.

Bjelajac, David. *Washington Allston, Secret Societies, and the Alchemy of Anglo-American Painting.* Cambridge: Cambridge University Press, 1997.

Bledstein, Burton J. *The Culture of Professionalism: The Middle Class and the Development of Higher Education in America.* New York: W. W. Norton, 1976.

Blumin, Stuart M. *The Emergence of the Middle Class: Social Experience in the American City, 1760–1900.* Cambridge: Cambridge University Press, 1985.

Bolter, Jay David, and Richard Grusin. *Remediation: Understanding New Media.* Cambridge: MIT Press, 1999.

Bourdieu, Pierre. *Distinction: A Social Critique of the Judgment of Taste.* Translated by Richard Nice. Cambridge: Harvard University Press, 1984.

———. "The Forms of Capital." In *Handbook of Theory and Research for the Sociology of Education,* ed. J. Richardson, 241–58. New York: Greenwood Press, 1986.

———. *La noblesse d'état: Grands écoles et spirit de corps.* Paris: Les Éditions de Minuit, 1989.

———. *Photography: A Middle-Brow Art.* Translated by Shaun Whiteside. Stanford: Stanford University Press, 1990.

Bourdieu, Pierre, and Loïc J. D. Wacquant. *An Invitation to Reflexive Sociology.* Chicago: University of Chicago Press, 1992.

Braddock, Alan C. "Bodies of Water: Thomas Eakins, Racial Ecology, and the Limits of Civic Realism." In *A Keener Perception: Ecocritical Studies in American Art History,* ed. Alan C. Braddock and Christoph Irmscher, 129–50. Tuscaloosa: University of Alabama Press, 2009.

Brey, William, and Marie Brey. *Philadelphia Photographers, 1840–1900: A Directory with Biographical Sketches.* Cherry Hill, N.J.: Willowdale Press, 1992.

Brieger, Gert H. "A Portrait of Surgery: Surgery in America, 1875–1889." *Surgical Clinics of North America* 67, no. 6 (1987): 1181–216.

Brown, Elspeth H. *The Corporate Eye: Photography and the Rationalization of American Commercial Culture, 1884–1929.* Baltimore: Johns Hopkins University Press, 2005.

———. "Technology, Culture, and the Body in Modern America." *American Quarterly* 56, no. 2 (2004): 449–60.

Brown, JoAnne. *The Definition of a Profession: The Authority of Metaphor in the History of Intelligence Testing, 1890–1930.* Princeton: Princeton University Press, 1992.

Brown, Julie K. *Health and Medicine on Display: International Expositions in the United States, 1876–1904.* Cambridge: MIT Press, 2009.

———. *Making Culture Visible: The Public Display of Photography at Fairs, Expositions, and Exhibitions in the United States, 1847–1900.* Amsterdam: Harwood Academic Publishers, 2001.

Bruno, Giuliana. "Spectatorial Embodiments: Anatomies of the Visible and the Female Bodyscape." *Camera Obscura* 28 (January 1992): 239–62.

Buck-Morss, Susan. "Aesthetics and Anaesthetics: Walter Benjamin's Artwork Essay Reconsidered." *October* 62 (Fall 1992): 3–42.

Burbick, Joan. *Healing the Republic: The Language of Health and the Culture of Nationalism in Nineteenth-Century America.* New York: Cambridge University Press, 1994.

Burns, Sarah. *Painting the Dark Side: Art and the Gothic Imagination in Nineteenth-Century America.* Berkeley and Los Angeles: University of California Press, 2004.

Burns, Stanley B. *Early Medical Photography in America (1839–1883).* New York: Burns Archive, 1983.

———. *A Morning's Work: Medical Photographs from the Burns Archive and Collection, 1843–1939.* Santa Fe: Twin Palms, 1998.

Bushman, Richard L., and Claudia L. Bushman. "The Early History of Cleanliness in America." *Journal of American History* 74, no. 4 (1988): 1213–38.

Caffin, Charles H. *Photography as a Fine Art: The Achievements and Possibilities of Photographic Art in America.* New York: Doubleday, Page, 1901.

Canguilhem, Georges. *The Normal and the Pathological.* Translated by Carolyn R. Fawcett. New York: Zone Books, 1989.

Cartwright, Lisa. *Screening the Body: Tracing Medicine's Visual Culture.* Minneapolis: University of Minnesota Press, 1995.

Clack, Randall A. *The Marriage of Heaven and Earth: Alchemical Regeneration in the Works of Taylor, Poe, Hawthorne, and Fuller.* Westport, Conn.: Greenwood Press, 2000.

Collins, Lauren. "Pixel Perfect: Pascal Dangin's Virtual Reality." *New Yorker,* May 12, 2008, 94–103.

Collins, Paul. *Banvard's Folly: Thirteen Tales of Renowned Obscurity, Famous Anonymity, and Rotten Luck.* New York: Picador USA, 2001.

Condran, Gretchen A., and Jennifer Murphy. "Defining and Managing Infant Mortality: A Case Study of Philadelphia, 1870–1920." *Social Science History* 32, no. 4 (2008): 473–513.

Connor, James T. H., and Michael G. Rhode. "Shooting Soldiers: Civil War Medical Images, Memory, and Identity in America." *Invisible Culture: An Electronic Journal for Visual Culture* 5 (Winter 2003). http://www.rochester.edu/in_visible_culture/Issue_5/ ConnorRhode/ConnorRhode.html (accessed January 15, 2010).

Dahlberg, Laurie. "The Material Ethereal: Photography and the Alchemical Ancestor." In *Art and Alchemy,* ed. Jacob Wamberg, 68–81. Copenhagen: Museum Tusculanum Press, 2006.

Daly, Tim, and David Asch. *Digital Photo Doctor: Simple Steps to Diagnose, Rescue, and Enhance Your Images.* Pleasantville, N.Y.: Reader's Digest Association, 2006.

Davis, Allen F., and Mark H. Haller, eds. *The Peoples of Philadelphia: A History of Ethnic Groups and Lower-Class Life, 1790–1940.* Philadelphia: Temple University Press, 1973.

Dawber, Martin. *Pixel Surgeons: Extreme Manipulation of the Figure in Photography.* London: Octopus Publishing Group, 2005.

De la Peña, Carolyn Thomas. *The Body Electric: How Strange Machines Built the Modern American.* New York: New York University Press, 2003.

———. "'Slow and Low Progress,' or Why American Studies Should Do Technology." *American Quarterly* 58, no. 3 (2006): 915–41.

Dermer, Rachelle A. "Joel-Peter Witkin and Dr. Stanley B. Burns: A Language of Body Parts." *History of Photography* 23, no. 3 (1999): 245–53.

———. "Photographic Objectivity and the Construction of the Medical Subject in the United States." PhD diss., Boston University, 2002.

Dinerstein, Joel. *Swinging the Machine: Modernity, Technology, and African American Culture Between the World Wars.* Amherst: University of Massachusetts Press, 2003.

Douglas, Mary. *How Institutions Think.* Syracuse: Syracuse University Press, 1986.

———. *Natural Symbols: Explorations in Cosmology.* New York: Pantheon Books, 1970.

———. *Purity and Danger: An Analysis of Concepts of Pollution and Taboo.* London: Routledge and Kegan Paul, 1966. Reprint, New York: Routledge, 2002.

Duffy, John. *The Sanitarians: A History of American Public Health.* Urbana: University of Illinois Press, 1990.

Dunkelman, Mark H. *Gettysburg's Unknown Soldier: The Life, Death, and Celebrity of Amos Humiston.* Westport, Conn.: Praeger, 1999.

Dyer, Richard. *White.* London: Routledge, 1997.

Earle, A. Scott, ed. *Surgery in America: From the Colonial Era to the Twentieth Century.* New York: Praeger, 1983.

Edwards, Steve. *The Making of English Photography: Allegories*. University Park: Pennsylvania State University Press, 2006.

Eisinger, Joel. *Trace and Transformation: American Criticism of Photography in the Modernist Period*. Albuquerque: University of New Mexico Press, 1995.

Feldberg, Michael. *The Philadelphia Riots of 1844: A Study of Ethnic Conflict*. Westport, Conn.: Greenwood Press, 1975.

Fellman, Anita Clair, and Michael Fellman. *Making Sense of Self: Medical Advice Literature in Late Nineteenth-Century America*. Philadelphia: University of Pennsylvania Press, 1981.

Figg, Laurann, and Jane Farrell-Beck. "Amputation in the Civil War: Physical and Social Dimensions." *Journal of the History of Medicine and Allied Sciences* 48, no. 4 (1993): 454–75.

Finkel, Kenneth. *Nineteenth-Century Photography in Philadelphia: 250 Historic Prints from the Library Company of Philadelphia*. New York: Dover Publications, 1980.

Flannery, Michael A. *Civil War Pharmacy: A History of Drugs, Drug Supply and Provision, and Therapeutics for the Union and Confederacy*. New York: Haworth Press, 2004.

Foucault, Michel. *The Archaeology of Knowledge*. Translated by A. M. Sheridan Smith. New York: Pantheon Books, 1972.

———. *The Birth of the Clinic: An Archaeology of Medical Perception*. Translated by A. M. Sheridan Smith. New York: Pantheon Books, 1973.

———. *Discipline and Punish: The Birth of the Prison*. Translated by A. M. Sheridan Smith. New York: Vintage Books, 1977.

———. *History of Sexuality: An Introduction*. Translated by Robert Hurley. New York: Vintage Books, 1978.

———. *The Order of Things: An Archeology of the Human Sciences*. New York: Pantheon Books, 1970.

Fox, Daniel M., and Christopher Lawrence. *Photographing Medicine: Images and Power in Britain and America Since 1840*. New York: Greenwood Press, 1988.

Frederickson, George M. *The Black Image in the White Mind: The Debate on Afro-American Character and Destiny, 1817–1914*. New York: Harper and Row, 1971.

Fried, Michael. *Realism, Writing, Disfiguration: On Thomas Eakins and Stephen Crane*. Chicago: University of Chicago Press, 1987.

Gallman, J. Matthew. *Mastering Wartime: A Social History of Philadelphia During the Civil War*. New York: Cambridge University Press, 1990.

Gernsheim, Alison. "Medical Photography in the Nineteenth Century." *Medical and Biological Illustration* 11 (1961): 85–92.

Gilman, Sander L. *The Face of Madness: Hugh Welch Diamond and the Origin of Psychiatric Photography*. Secaucus: Citadel Press, 1976.

———. *Making the Body Beautiful: A Cultural History of Aesthetic Surgery*. Princeton: Princeton University Press, 1999.

Glenner, Richard A., Audrey B. Davis, and Stanley B. Burns. *The American Dentist: A Pictorial History with a Presentation of Early Dental Photography in America*. Missoula: Pictorial Histories, 1990.

Goler, Robert I. "Loss and the Persistence of Memory: 'The Case of George Dedlow' and Disabled Civil War Veterans." *Literature and Medicine* 23, no. 1 (2004): 160–83.

Gould, Stephen J. *The Mismeasure of Man*. New York: W. W. Norton, 1981.

Green, Harvey. *Fit for America: Health, Fitness, Sport, and American Society*. New York: Pantheon Books, 1986.

Green-Lewis, Jennifer. *Framing the Victorians: Photography and the Culture of Realism*. Ithaca: Cornell University Press, 1996.

Grier, Katherine C. *Culture and Comfort: Parlor Making and Middle-Class Identity, 1850–1930*. Washington, D.C.: Smithsonian Institution Press, 1988.

Grosz, Elizabeth. "Inscriptions and Body Maps: Representations and the Corporeal." In *Space, Gender, Knowledge: Feminist Readings,* ed. Linda McDowell and Joanne P. Sharp, 236–46. New York: J. Wiley, 1997.

Haber, Samuel. "The Professions and Higher Education in America: A Historical View." In *Higher Education and the Labor Market,* ed. Margaret S. Gordon, 237–80. New York: McGraw-Hill, 1974.

———. *The Quest for Authority and Honor in the American Professions, 1750–1900.* Chicago: University of Chicago Press, 1991.

Hall, Courtney R. "The Rise of Professional Surgery in the United States: 1800–1865." *Bulletin of the History of Medicine* 26, no. 3 (1952): 231–62.

Halttunen, Karen. "Humanitarianism and the Pornography of Pain in Anglo-American Culture." *American Historical Review* 100, no. 2 (1995): 303–34.

Hartman, Saidiya V. *Scenes of Subjection: Terror, Slavery, and Self-Making in Nineteenth-Century America.* New York: Oxford University Press, 1997.

Hartmann, Sadakichi. *The Valiant Knights of Daguerre: Selected Critical Essays on Photography and Profiles of Photographic Pioneers.* Berkeley and Los Angeles: University of California Press, 1978.

Haskell, Thomas, ed. *The Authority of Experts: Studies in History and Theory.* Bloomington: Indiana University Press, 1984.

Helfand, William H. *Medicine and Pharmacy in American Political Prints, 1765–1870.* Madison: American Institute of the History of Pharmacy, 1978.

———. *Quack, Quack, Quack: The Sellers of Nostrums in Prints, Posters, Ephemera, and Books.* New York: Grolier Club, 2002.

Heller, Dana, ed. *The Great American Makeover: Television, History, Nation.* New York: Palgrave Macmillan, 2006.

———. *Makeover Television: Realities Remodelled.* New York: I. B. Tauris, 2007.

Henisch, Heinz K., and Bridget A. Henisch. *Positive Pleasures: Early Photography and Humor.* University Park: Pennsylvania State University Press, 1998.

Hepp, John Henry, IV. *The Middle-Class City: Transforming Space and Time in Philadelphia, 1876–1926.* Philadelphia: University of Pennsylvania Press, 2003.

Herschbach, Lisa. "Prosthetic Reconstructions: Making the Industry, Re-Making the Body, Modelling the Nation." *History Workshop Journal* 44 (Autumn 1997): 22–57.

Hershberg, Theodore, ed. *Philadelphia: Work, Space, Family, and Group Experience in the Nineteenth Century.* New York: Oxford University Press, 1981.

Hirschauer, Stefan. "The Manufacture of Bodies in Surgery." *Social Studies of Science* 21, no. 2 (1991): 279–319.

Hoy, Suellen. *Chasing Dirt: The American Pursuit of Cleanliness.* New York: Oxford University Press, 1995.

Jackson, Barry. *Photoshop Cosmetic Surgery: A Comprehensive Guide to Portrait Retouching and Body Transforming.* New York: Lark Books, 2006.

Jacobs-Huey, Lanita. *From the Kitchen to the Parlor: Language and Becoming in African American Women's Hair Care.* New York: Oxford University Press, 2006.

Jacobson, Matthew Frye. *Whiteness of a Different Color: European Immigrants and the Alchemy of Race.* Cambridge: Harvard University Press, 1998.

Jay, Bill. *Cyanide and Spirits: An Inside-Out View of Early Photography.* Munich: Nazraeli Press, 1991.

———. *Some Rollicking Bull: Light Verse, and Worse, on Victorian Poetry.* Munich: Nazraeli Press, 1996.

Jordan, Winthrop D. *White Over Black: American Attitudes Toward the Negro, 1550–1812.* Chapel Hill: University of North Carolina Press, 1968.

Julin, Leonard A. "A History of Still Photography in the Operating Room." *Journal of the Biological Photographic Association* 39 (1971): 129–43.

Kapsalis, Terri. *Public Privates: Performing Gynecology from Both Ends of the Speculum*. Durham: Duke University Press, 1997.

Katz, Michael B., and Thomas J. Sugre, eds. *W. E. B. Du Bois, Race, and the City: The Philadelphia Negro and Its Legacy*. Philadelphia: University of Pennsylvania Press, 1998.

Kaufman, Martin. *American Medical Education: The Formative Years, 1765–1910*. Westport, Conn.: Greenwood Press, 1976.

Kember, Sarah. *Virtual Anxiety: Photography, New Technologies, and Subjectivity*. Manchester: Manchester University Press, 1998.

Kramer, Howard D. "Agitation for Public Health Reform in the 1870s, Part I." *Journal of the History of Medicine and Allied Sciences* 3, no. 4 (1948): 473–88.

———. "Agitation for Public Health Reform in the 1870s, Part II." *Journal of the History of Medicine and Allied Sciences* 4, no. 1 (1949): 75–89.

Krauss, Rolf H. *Fotografie in der Karikatur*. Seebruck am Chiemsee: Heering, 1978.

Lakoff, George. "The Contemporary Theory of Metaphor." In *Metaphor and Thought*, 2d ed., ed. Andrew Ortony, 202–51. New York: Cambridge University Press, 1993.

Lakoff, George, and Mark Johnson. *Metaphors We Live By*. 2d ed. Chicago: University of Chicago Press, 2003.

Lane, Roger. *Roots of Violence in Black Philadelphia, 1860–1900*. Cambridge: Harvard University Press, 1986.

———. *William Dorsey's Philadelphia and Ours: On the Past and Future of the Black City in America*. New York: Oxford University Press, 1991.

Larson, Magali Sarfatti. *The Rise of Professionalism*. Berkeley and Los Angeles: University of California Press, 1977.

Latour, Bruno, and Steve Woolgar. *Laboratory Life: The Construction of Scientific Facts*. Princeton: Princeton University Press, 1986.

Lawrence, Christopher, and Steven Shapin, eds. *Science Incarnate: Historical Embodiments of Natural Knowledge*. Chicago: University of Chicago Press, 1998.

Lawrence, Robert Means. *Primitive Psycho-Therapy and Quackery*. New York: Houghton Mifflin, 1910.

Leavitt, Judith Walzer, and Ronald L. Numbers, eds. *Sickness and Health in America: Readings in the History of Medicine and Public Health*. Madison: University of Wisconsin Press, 1997.

Lee, Anthony W. "American Histories of Photography." *American Art* 21, no. 3 (2007): 2–9.

Lemire, Elise. *"Miscegenation": Making Race in America*. Philadelphia: University of Pennsylvania Press, 2002.

Lenoir, Timothy. *Instituting Science: The Cultural Production of Scientific Disciplines*. Stanford: Stanford University Press, 1997.

Lister, Martin, ed. *The Photographic Image in Digital Culture*. New York: Routledge, 1995.

Long, Diana E. "The Medical World of *The Agnew Clinic*: A World We Have Lost?" *Prospects: An Annual Journal of American Culture Studies* 11, section 2 (1987): 185–98.

Long, Lisa A. *Rehabilitating Bodies: Heath, History, and the American Civil War*. Philadelphia: University of Pennsylvania Press, 2004.

Ludmerer, Kenneth M. *Learning to Heal: The Development of American Medical Education*. New York: Basic Books, 1985.

Lynch, Michael. *Art and Artifact in Laboratory Science: A Study of Shop Work and Shop Talk in a Research Laboratory*. London: Routledge and Kegan Paul, 1985.

Lyons, Nathan. "History of Photographic Education, with an Emphasis on Its Development in the United States." In *The Education of a Photographer*, ed. Charles Traub and Steven Heller, 177–84. New York: Allworth Press, 2006.

Maliniak, Jacques W. "Facts and Fallacies of Cosmetic Surgery." *Hygeia* 12, no. 3 (1934): 200–202.

Manovich, Lev. *The Language of New Media.* Cambridge: MIT Press, 2001.

Martin, Charles D. *The White African American Body: A Cultural and Literary Exploration.* New Brunswick: Rutgers University Press, 2002.

Marvin, Carolyn. *When Old Technologies Were New: Thinking About Electric Communication in the Late Nineteenth Century.* New York: Oxford University Press, 1990.

McCarthy, Michael P. *Typhoid and the Politics of Public Health in Nineteenth-Century Philadelphia.* Philadelphia: American Philosophical Society, 1989.

McKee, Gary Robert. "Climate, Science, and Politics in Victorian Britain." PhD diss., Queen's University of Belfast, 2002.

McPherson, James M. *Abraham Lincoln and the Second American Revolution.* New York: Oxford University Press, 1990.

Miles, Melissa. "The Burning Mirror: Photography in an Ambivalent Light." *Journal of Visual Culture* 4, no. 3 (2005): 329–49.

Miller, Randall, and William Pencak, eds. *Pennsylvania: A History of the Commonwealth.* University Park: Pennsylvania State University Press, 2002.

Miller, Toby. *Makeover Nation: The United States of Reinvention.* Columbus: Ohio State University Press, 2008.

Mitchell, Mary Niall. "'Rosebloom and Pure White,' or So It Seemed." *American Quarterly* 54, no. 3 (2002): 369–410.

Mitchell, W. J. T. *The Reconfigured Eye: Visual Truth in the Post-Photographic Era.* Cambridge: MIT Press, 1992.

Morris, David B. *The Culture of Pain.* Berkeley and Los Angeles: University of California Press, 1991.

Nash, Gary B. *First City: Philadelphia and the Forging of Historical Memory.* Philadelphia: University of Pennsylvania Press, 2002.

———. *Forging Freedom: The Formation of Philadelphia's Black Community, 1720–1840.* Cambridge: Harvard University Press, 1988.

Newberry, Susan Annette. "Commerce and Ritual in American Daguerrean Portraiture, 1839–1859." PhD diss., Cornell University, 1999.

Newhall, Beaumont. *The History of Photography: From 1839 to the Present Day.* New York: Museum of Modern Art, 1939.

———, ed. *Photography, Essays and Images: Illustrated Readings in the History of Photography.* New York: Museum of Modern Art, 1980.

Novak, Daniel A. *Realism, Photography, and Nineteenth-Century Fiction.* Cambridge: Cambridge University Press, 2008.

Numbers, Ronald L., ed. *The Education of American Physicians: Historical Essays.* Berkeley and Los Angeles: University of California Press, 1980.

O'Connor, Erin. "Camera Medica: Towards a Morbid History of Photography." *History of Photography* 23, no. 3 (1999): 232–44.

———. *Raw Material: Producing Pathology in Victorian Culture.* Durham: Duke University Press, 2000.

Ogle, Maureen. "Domestic Reform and American Household Plumbing, 1840–1870." *Winterthur Portfolio* 28 (Spring 1993): 33–58.

O'Hara, Leo. *An Emerging Profession: Philadelphia Doctors, 1860–1900.* New York: Garland, 1989.

Ollerenshaw, Robert. "Medical Illustration: The Impact of Photography on Its History." *Journal of the Biological Photographic Association* 36 (1968): 3–12.

Olmstead, A. J. "Snelling: The Father of Photographic Journalism." *Camera* 47 (December 1933): 391–94.

Ortony, Andrew, ed. *Metaphor and Thought.* 2d ed. New York: Cambridge University Press, 1993.

Pageau, Gary. "Presidential Profile: PMA President Allen Showalter Talks About Growing Up in the Photo Industry." *PMA Magazine* 83 (March 2008): 44–45.

Panzer, Mary. "Romantic Origins of American Realism: Photography, Arts, and Letters in Philadelphia, 1850–1875." PhD diss., Boston University, 1990.

Peiss, Kathy. *Hope in a Jar: The Making of America's Beauty Culture.* New York: Henry Holt, 1998.

Pennsylvania Academy of the Fine Arts. *In This Academy: The Pennsylvania Academy of the Fine Arts, 1805–1976, a Special Bicentennial Exhibition.* Philadelphia: Pennsylvania Academy of the Fine Arts, 1976.

Pernick, Martin S. *A Calculus of Suffering: Pain, Professionalism, and Anesthesia in Nineteenth-Century America.* New York: Columbia University Press, 1985.

Philadelphia Museum of Art. *Legacy in Light: Photographic Treasures from Philadelphia Area Public Collections.* Philadelphia: Photography Sesquicentennial Project, 1990.

Pitts, Terrence R. *William Bell: Philadelphia Photographer.* Master's thesis, University of Arizona, 1987.

Poovey, Mary. "'Scenes of an Indelicate Character': The Medical 'Treatment' of Victorian Women." *Representations* 14 (Spring 1986): 137–68.

Prodger, Phillip. *Time Stands Still: Muybridge and the Instantaneous Photography Movement.* New York: Oxford University Press, 2003.

Rabinach, Anson. *The Human Motor: Energy, Fatigue, and the Origins of Modernity.* New York: Basic Books, 1990.

Rabinovitz, Lauren, and Abraham Geil, eds. *Memory Bytes: History, Technology, and Digital Culture.* Durham: Duke University Press, 2004.

Rhode, Michael G., and Blair O. Rogers. "Civil War Faces: The Wounded." Manuscript.

Ries, Linda A., and Jay W. Ruby. *Directory of Pennsylvania Photographers, 1839–1900.* Harrisburg: Pennsylvania Historical and Museum Commission, 1999.

Risse, Guenter B., Ronald L. Numbers, and Judith Walzer Leavitt, eds. *Medicine Without Doctors: Home Health Care in American History.* New York: Science History Publications, 1977.

Ritchin, Fred. *In Our Own Image: The Coming Revolution in Photography.* New York: Aperture Foundation, 1990.

Roediger, David R. *The Wages of Whiteness: Race and the Making of the American Working Class.* London: Verso, 1991.

Rogers, Blair O. "Rehabilitation of Wounded Civil War Veterans." *Aesthetic Plastic Surgery* 26, no. 10 (2002): 498–519.

Rogers, Blair O., and Michael G. Rhode. "The First Civil War Photographs of Soldiers with Facial Wounds." *Aesthetic Plastic Surgery* 19, no. 3 (1995): 269–83.

Romer, Grant B., and Brian Wallis, eds. *Young America: The Daguerreotypes of Southworth & Hawes.* New York: International Center of Photography, 2005.

Rosenberg, Charles E. *The Cholera Years: The United States in 1832, 1849, and 1866.* Chicago: University of Chicago Press, 1987.

———. *Explaining Epidemics and Other Studies in the History of Medicine.* New York: Cambridge University Press, 1992.

———. *No Other Gods: On Science and American Social Thought.* Baltimore: Johns Hopkins University Press, 1976. Rev. and exp. ed., 1997.

———. "Representing Medicine: Philadelphia, Health, and Photography, 1860–1945." In *Pictures of Health: A Photographic History of Health Care in Philadelphia, 1860–1945,* ed. Janet Golden and Charles E. Rosenberg, xxi–xxix. Philadelphia: University of Pennsylvania Press, 1991.

———. *Right Living: An Anglo-American Tradition of Self-Help Medicine and Hygiene.* Baltimore: Johns Hopkins University Press, 2003.

———. "Toward an Ecology of Knowledge: On Discipline, Context, and History." In *The Organization of Knowledge in Modern America, 1860–1920*, ed. Alexandra Oleson and John Voss, 440–55. Baltimore: Johns Hopkins University Press, 1979.

Rothstein, William G. *American Physicians in the Nineteenth Century: From Sects to Science.* Baltimore: Johns Hopkins University Press, 1972.

Rutkow, Ira M. *Bleeding Blue and Gray: Civil War Surgery and the Evolution of American Medicine.* New York: Random House, 2005.

Sandweiss, Martha A., ed. *Photography in Nineteenth-Century America.* New York: Harry N. Abrams, 1991.

Sappol, Michael. *A Traffic of Dead Bodies: Anatomy and Embodied Social Identity in Nineteenth-Century America.* Princeton: Princeton University Press, 2002.

Scarry, Elaine. *The Body in Pain: The Making and Unmaking of the World.* New York: Oxford University Press, 1985.

Seiberling, Grace. *Amateurs, Photography, and the Mid-Victorian Imagination.* Chicago: University of Chicago Press, 1986.

Sekula, Allan. "The Body and the Archive." *October* 39 (Winter 1986): 3–64.

———. "Photography Between Labour and Capital." In *Mining Photographs and Other Pictures, 1948–1968: A Selection from the Negative Archives of Shedden Studio, Glace Bay, Cape Breton*, ed. Benjamin H. D. Buchloh and Robert Wilkie, 193–268. Halifax: Press of the Nova Scotia College of Art and Design, 1983.

Shapin, Steven. *A Social History of Truth: Civility and Science in Seventeenth-Century England.* Chicago: University of Chicago Press, 1994.

Sheehan, Tanya. "African American Vernacular Photography: Selections from the Daniel Cowin Collection." *Journal of American History* 93, no. 3 (2006): 815–19.

Shortt, S. E. D. "Physicians, Science, and Status: Issues in the Professionalization of Anglo-American Medicine in the Nineteenth Century." *Medical History* 27, no. 1 (1983): 51–68.

Sinclair, Bruce. *Philadelphia's Philosopher Mechanics: A History of the Franklin Institute, 1824–1865.* Baltimore: Johns Hopkins University Press, 1974.

Smillie, Wilson G. *Public Health: Its Promise for the Future; A Chronicle of the Development of Public Health in the United States, 1607–1914.* New York: Macmillan, 1955.

Smith, Margaret Supplee. "*The Agnew Clinic:* 'Not Cheerful for Ladies to Look At.'" *Prospects: An Annual Journal of American Culture Studies* 11, section 2 (1987): 161–83.

Smith, Pamela H. *The Body of the Artisan: Art and Experience in the Scientific Revolution.* Chicago: University of Chicago Press, 2004.

Smith, Shawn Michelle. *American Archives: Gender, Race, and Class in Visual Culture.* Princeton: Princeton University Press, 1999.

Sontag, Susan. *On Photography.* New York: Farrar, Straus and Giroux, 1977.

———. *Regarding the Pain of Others.* New York: Farrar, Straus and Giroux, 2003.

Sorisio, Carolyn. *Fleshing Out America: Race, Gender, and the Politics of the Body in American Literature, 1833–1879.* Athens: University of Georgia Press, 2002.

Stallybrass, Peter, and Allon White. *The Politics and Poetics of Transgression.* Ithaca: Cornell University Press, 1986.

Stanton, William R. *The Leopard's Spots: Scientific Attitudes Toward Race in America, 1815–1859.* Chicago: University of Chicago Press, 1960.

Stark, Richard B. "Plastic Surgery During the Civil War." *Plastic and Reconstructive Surgery* 16, no. 2 (1955): 103–20.

Starr, Paul. *The Social Transformation of American Medicine: The Rise of a Sovereign Profession and the Making of a Vast Industry.* New York: Basic Books, 1982.

Sternberger, Paul Spencer. *Between Amateur and Aesthete: The Legitimization of Photography as Art in America, 1880–1900.* Albuquerque: University of New Mexico Press, 2001.

Stevens, Garry. *The Favored Circle: The Social Foundations of Architectural Distinction.* Cambridge: MIT Press, 1998.

Stewart, Mart A. "'Let Us Begin with the Weather?' Climate, Race, and Cultural Distinctiveness in the American South." In *Nature and Society in Historical Context,* ed. Mikuláš Teich, Roy Porter, and Bo Gustafsson, 240–56. New York: Cambridge University Press, 1997.

Swartz, David. *Culture and Power: The Sociology of Pierre Bourdieu.* Chicago: University of Chicago Press, 1997.

Sweet, Timothy. *Traces of War: Poetry, Photography, and the Crisis of the Union.* Baltimore: Johns Hopkins University Press, 1990.

Szarkowski, John. *Photography Until Now.* New York: Museum of Modern Art, 1989.

Tagg, John. *The Burden of Representation: Essays on Photographies and Histories.* Amherst: University of Massachusetts Press, 1988. Reprint, Minneapolis: University of Minnesota Press, 1993.

Takaki, Ronald. *Iron Cages: Race and Culture in Nineteenth-Century America.* New York: Oxford University Press, 2000.

Taylor, Frank H. *Philadelphia in the Civil War, 1861–1865.* Philadelphia: City of Philadelphia, 1913.

Thorburn, David, and Henry Jenkins, eds. *Rethinking Media Change: The Aesthetics of Transition.* Cambridge: MIT Press, 2003.

Townsend, Gavin. "Airborne Toxins and the American House, 1865–1895." *Winterthur Portfolio* 24 (Spring 1989): 29–42.

Trachtenberg, Alan. *Lincoln's Smile and Other Enigmas.* New York: Hill and Wang, 2007.

———. *Reading American Photographs: Images as History, Matthew Brady to Walker Evans.* New York: Hill and Wang, 1989.

Trotter, Joe William, Jr., and Eric Ledell Smith, eds. *African Americans in Pennsylvania: Shifting Historical Perspectives.* University Park: Pennsylvania State University Press, 1997.

Tucker, Jennifer. *Nature Exposed: Photography as Witness in Victorian Science.* Baltimore: Johns Hopkins University Press, 2005.

Volpe, Andrea. "Cartes de Visite Portrait Photographs and the Culture of Class Formation." In *The Middling Sorts: Explorations in the History of the American Middle Class,* ed. Burton J. Bledstein and Robert D. Johnston, 157–69. New York: Routledge, 2001.

Wajda, Shirley Teresa. "The Commercial Photographic Parlor." In *Shaping Communities: Perspectives in Vernacular Architecture,* ed. Carter L. Hudgins and Elizabeth Collins Cromley, 216–30. Knoxville: University of Tennessee Press, 1997.

———. *"Social Currency": Commercial Portrait Photography and the Fashioning of an American Middle Class, 1839–1889.* Philadelphia: Temple University Press, forthcoming.

Wallis, Brian, and Deborah Willis. *African American Vernacular Photography: Selections from the Daniel Cowin Collection.* New York: International Center of Photography, 2005.

Walsh, James J. *Cures: The Story of Cures That Fail.* New York: D. Appleton, 1924.

Warner, John Harley. *Against the Spirit of System: The French Impulse in Nineteenth-Century American Medicine.* Baltimore: Johns Hopkins University Press, 2003.

———. "Image-Making, Identity, and the Aesthetic Grounding of Modern American Medicine." Paper delivered at "The Art of Medicine: Image-Making and Communication" symposium, Yale University, April 15–17, 2004.

———. *The Therapeutic Perspective: Medical Practice, Knowledge, and Identity in America, 1820–1885.* Cambridge: Harvard University Press, 1986.

Warner, John Harley, and Janet A. Tighe, eds. *Major Problems in the History of American Medicine and Public Health.* Boston: Houghton Mifflin, 2001.

Warner, Sam Bass, Jr. *The Private City: Philadelphia in Three Periods of Its Growth.* Philadelphia: University of Pennsylvania Press, 1968.

Weber, Brenda R. *Makeover TV: Selfhood, Citizenship, and Celebrity.* Durham: Duke University Press, 2009.

Weigley, Russell F., Nicholas B. Wainwright, and Edwin Wolf. *Philadelphia: A 300-Year History.* New York: W. W. Norton, 1982.

Werbel, Amy. *Thomas Eakins: Art, Medicine, and Sexuality in Nineteenth-Century Philadelphia.* New Haven: Yale University Press, 2007.

Wexler, Laura. *Tender Violence: Domestic Visions in an Age of U.S. Imperialism.* Chapel Hill: University of North Carolina Press, 2000.

Wheeler, Roxann. *The Complexion of Race: Categories of Difference in Eighteenth-Century British Culture.* Philadelphia: University of Pennsylvania Press, 2000.

Wiegman, Robyn. *American Anatomies: Theorizing Race and Gender.* Durham: Duke University Press, 1995.

Wilder, Kelley. *Photography and Science.* London: Reaktion Books, 2009.

Willis, Anne-Marie. "Digitisation and the Living Death of Photography." In *Culture, Technology, and Creativity in the Late Twentieth Century,* ed. Philip Hayward, 197–208. London: John Libbey, 1990.

Willis, Deborah. *Reflections in Black: A History of Black Photographers, 1840–1999.* New York: W. W. Norton, 2000.

Winston, Brian. "A Whole Technology of Dyeing: A Note on Ideology and the Apparatus of the Chromatic Moving Image." *Daedalus* 114, no. 4 (1985): 105–23.

Witkin, Joel-Peter. *Masterpieces of Medical Photography: Selections from the Burns Archive.* Pasadena: Twelvetrees Press, 1987.

Woods, Mary N. *From Craft to Profession: The Practice of Architecture in Nineteenth-Century America.* Berkeley and Los Angeles: University of California Press, 1999.

Wrobel, Arthur, ed. *Pseudo-Science and Society in Nineteenth-Century America.* Lexington: University Press of Kentucky, 1987.

Young, James Harvey. *American Health Quackery.* Princeton: Princeton University Press, 1992.

Zeller, Bob. *The Blue and Gray in Black and White: A History of Civil War Photography.* Westport, Conn.: Praeger, 2005.

*Selected
Bibliography*

Page numbers in *italics* refer to illustrations.

The Able Doctor, or America Swallowing the Bitter Draught (Revere), 12
actinism, 81, 85, 86
Adobe Photoshop
    digital photography manuals for, 137–40, *138, 139,* 143–44, 146
    retouching photographs using, 132, 133
advertisements, 67, 75, 165 n. 17
African Americans
    calculus of suffering and photographic anesthesia, 77
    emancipation and national health metaphors, 12, *13*
    environment and health of, 89, 90, 102
    lighting, 93–94, *94,* 96–100, *98, 99, 101*
    in nineteenth-century Philadelphia, 91–92, *93*
Agnew, David Hayes, 38
alchemy, 121, 125, 178 n. 53
alcohol, 126, 127
Alewitz, Sam, 110
Allen, Samuel, 115
alternative medicine. *See* irregular medicine
amateur photographers, 4, 27, 44, 142, 164 n. 56
The American Emigrant Car, 115, *116*
American Journal of Photography, 35–36, 130, 153
American Medical Association (AMA)
    code of ethics, 162 n. 17
    formation of, 14, 28
    medical education standards, 28
    as model for photographers, 28, 29
    urban health reports, 88–89, 109–10
American Pharmaceutical Association, 130
American Photographic Almanac, 161 n. 12
American Revolution, 12
anatomical education, 39, *39–45, 41,* 71, *71*
anesthesia, 73–78, *79,* 119
Anthony, Henry T., 28
Application of Blue Light, Full Bath, 82, *83*
Arms family portrait, 98, *100*
Armstrong, David, 109
Army Medical Museum, 21, 62–66, *63, 64, 65,* 67
Arthur's Home Magazine, 23, 48–50, *49,* 51
artisans, 37, 121, 123, 124
Artot, Mlle., portrait of, 69, *70,* 144

arts, fine
    digital retouching compared to, 133
    education and medical models, 38, 40–41, *41*
    medical subjects in, 38–40, *39,* 45
    photography as, *vs.* science debates, 44–45
    professionalization of photography as, 2, 4, 34, 36, 37, 45
Asch, David, 137–38, *138,* 140
associations, professional
    medical (*see* American Medical Association)
    photographic, 21, 29–35, *31,* 114, 151

baby portraits, 100–103, *101, 102, 103*
Banta, Martha, 12
Barthes, Roland, 78, 79, 156 n .11
Batchen, Geoffrey, 9, 147
battlefield photography, 19–20, 59–60
Baxter, DeWitt Clinton, *Chestnut Street from Seventh to Eighth (South Side),* 14, *16*
Baxter's Panoramic Business Directory of Philadelphia, 14, *16,* 18
Bazin, André, 78, 156 n. 11
Beck-Goddard, Paul, 164 n. 56
Beidler, H. M., 82
Bell, William H., 62, 67
Benjamin, Walter, 78
Bigelow, Henry Jacob, 74–75
The Birth of the Clinic (Foucault), 167 n. 32
blackness, 89, 90, 91, 115–17. *See also* African Americans
Blockley Almshouse, 87
Blue Glass!, 171 n. 6
Blue Glass, A Sure Cure for the Blues (Carboy), 93
blue light/glass, 81–82, *82,* 85–86, *86. See also* phototherapy
Blumin, Stuart, 17
Bogardus, Abraham, 28, 30, *31*
Boltanski, Luc, 27
Bourdieu, Pierre, 26, 47
Bourns, J. Francis, 60
Bowditch, Henry, 111
Braddock, Alan, 112
Brady, Matthew, 20, 168 n. 51
Brey, William and Marie, 159 n. 39
Bridge, Norman, 114, 117
Broadbent, Samuel, 14

bromides, 1, 122, 126, 127
Brooks, Silas Swift, 166 n. 28
Brown, JoAnne, 10
Brownell, William, 40, 42, 45
Burbick, Joan, 19
Burns, Sarah, 68

Caffin, Charles, 4
calculus of suffering, 77–78
The Camera and the Pencil (Root), 4, 37, 46, 58
Canguilhem, Georges, 59
Carboy, John, 93–94
carte de visite
    description and popularity of, 55–56
    personifications of, 118–19
*Case of Cheiloplasty (Private Rowland Ward, Co.
    E, 4th New York Heavy Artillery)*, 62–66, 63,
    64, 65
"The Case of George Dedlow" (Mitchell), 19
Catto, Octavius V., 92
Centennial Exhibition, 21, 37, 45
Chambordeon, Jean-Claude, 27
Charcot, Jean-Martin, 145
*Charter Members of the National Photographic
    Association* (Richards), 30, 31
chemicals, photographic
    advertisements for, 127, 128
    dangers of, 113–18, 130
    personifications of, 118, 121–22, 124, 137
    as therapeutic medicines, 1–2, 109, 124–30
The Chemistry of Light and Photography (Vogel), 95
*Chestnut Street from Seventh to Eighth (South
    Side)* (Baxter), 14, 16
Chicago College of Photography, 163 n. 44
children
    cartes de visite of Civil War soldier's, 60, 61, 118–19
    hospitals for, 158n.36
    portraits and lighting, 100–103, 101, 102, 103
The Children of the Battle-Field (McClees), 60, 61
Children's Hospital of Philadelphia, 158 n. 36
Chute, Robert, 86–87, 113, 165 n. 17
Civil War
    African Americans during, 91–92
    battlefield images during, 19–20, 59–60
    battlefield tours after, 68
    medical literature during, 19
    medical metaphors during, 12–13, 13
    medical photography during, 21, 61–66, 63, 64,
        65
    military medical care, 19, 21, 62
    Philadelphian enlistees, 18
    sanitation efforts during, 110–11
    soldier portraits, 66, 66–67
    soldier's children *cartes de visite*, 60, 61, 118–19,
        124
    USSC support, 18–19, 20, 60–61
climate, and social health, 89–90
clinical gaze, 57–59
code of ethics, 30, 31–32, 48–50
College of Physicians of Philadelphia, 14
Collins, Lauren, 132–33, 142
collodion, 1–2, 122, 127, 130

Committee on Apprenticeship, 35
Committee on Photography, 61
Cornelius, Robert, 14
cosmetic surgery. *See* reconstructive surgery
Cottingham, Keith, 136
Cremer, James, 67, 98, 100
criticism, public, 6, 27–28, 43, 87–88
cyanide of potassium, 117–18, 129

daguerreotypes, 9, 14, 48–50, 49
Dahlberg, Laurie, 121
Daly, Augustin, 171 n. 6
Daly, Tim, 137–38, 138, 140
Dangin, Pascal, 132–33, 134, 142, 147
darkrooms
    chemical exposures and health in, 121
    hygiene and sanitation standards in, 106–9,
        107, 114–19
    light deprivation in, 87
    personifications of photographic materials in,
        118–23
    respectability in, 117–18
    ventilation practices, 113–14
Dawber, Martin, 137
"The Dead Soldier's Children," 60
Death's-Head Doctors.—Many Paths to the Grave
    (Keppler), 6, 7, 88
decapitation metaphors, 54–56, 57
The Definition of a Profession (Brown), 10
dentistry, 50, 51–58, 62
Dermer, Rachel, 167 n. 33
diagnosis
    of photographic materials, 119–20
    of portrait sitters, 57–59
Diamond, Hugh, 145
Digital Imaging Digest, 141
Digital Photo Doctor (Daly and Asch), 137–38, 138,
    140
digital photography
    debates about and criticism of, 135
    and makeover culture, 143–47
    medical metaphors in, 132–46, 138, 139, 141, 144
    and truth, 134
    photography's identity crisis due to, 134
dirt, 108, 119
disease
    darkrooms associated with, 87
    dirt as, 108
    due to light deprivation, 89, 90, 91, 101–2
    photographic materials with, 119–20, 122–24
    sanitation reform and, 110–11
doctoring photographs. *See* retouching
Doctor Lincoln's New Elixir of Life (Nast), 13, 12
Doctor Photo, 1, 2, 125, 127, 129
Douglas, Mary, 11
Dr. 90210, 143
Draper & Husted, 100, 102
Duchenne, Guillaume-Benjamin-Armand, 34, 164
    n. 62
Duhring, Louis Adolphus, 152
Dunglison, Robley, 89
dust, 114, 119

Eakins, Thomas
 Agnew Clinic, 38
 anatomical education and, 39–40, 41, 42, 45
 Gross Clinic, 38–39, 39, 45
 *William Rush Carving His Allegorical Figure of the
  Schuylkill River*, 112
education
 anatomical, 38–45, 39, 41, 71, 71
 medical, 27–28, 111
 photographic, 27, 28, 33–38, 163 n. 44
Edwards, Steve, 22
Elliott, J. Perry, 123
environmental issues, 109–10, 112, 113
ether, 1, 74–75, 127, 130
etiolation, 89, 90, 91, 101–2
etiquette, studio, 30, 31–32, 48–50
execution metaphors, 54–55, 55–56, 57
exhibitions, photographic, 21, 29
Extreme Makeover, 143

fashion photography, 132–34
Foucault, Michel, 11, 50, 55, 167 n. 32
Fowler Studio, 103
Fox, Joseph J., 153
Franklin Institute, 33, 34, 36, 111, 115
Fried, Michael, 38

Gallman, J. Matthew, 18
Germon, W. L., 16, 100, 101
Gihon, John L., 34, 152, 164 n. 62
Gilman, Sander, 66
Godey's Lady's Book, 77
Goddard, Paul Beck, 14
GQ, 133, 147
grave robbing, 44
Great Central Fair, 18–19, 20, 60–61
Grier, Katherine C., 52
Gross, Samuel, 36–37, 38–40, 39
Gross Clinic (Eakins), 38–40, 39, 45
gun cotton, 1, 127
Gunning, Tom, 10
Gutekunst, Frederick
 assistants of, 21
 cartes de visite produced by, 60
 Civil War photographs, 66–67
 *Group Portrait of Pennsylvania General Hospital
  Resident Physicians*, 30, 32
 Interior of the Philadelphia School of Anatomy,
  42, 43
 Portrait of an Unidentified Man, 67, 67
 Portrait of an Unidentified Soldier, 66, 66–67
 studio of, 16

H. C. Phillips & Brother, 60
Halttunen, Karen, 52
Hammond, William, 89–90
Hartman, Saidiya, 93
Hartmann, Sadakichi, 4
Henszey & Co., 57, 85, 86
Hepp, John, IV, 17
History and Handbook of Photography (Tissandier),
 107

Holmes, Oliver Wendell, 20
*Honey, Does Yer See How's I'se Bleachin' Under de
  Blue Glass?* (Worth), 94
hospitals, 19, 46–47
Hough, E. K., 35
Human Health (Dunglison), 89
Humiston, Amos, 177n.43
humor, 50, 51, 54–55
hygiene
 light associated with, 89
 as photographic concern, 108–9, 114–17
 public health and, 109–12, 113

infant mortality, 101, 110
*Influence of the Blue Ray of the Sunlight and of the
  Blue Color of the Sky* (Pleasonton), 82, 85
influenza, 110, 122
instantaneity, 76
Instinct, 135, 136
institutionalization of photography. *See* profes-
 sionalization of photography
Interior of the Philadelphia School of Anatomy
 (Gutekunst), 42, 43
International Medical Congress, 111
iodides, 1, 122, 127
irregular medicine, 6–7, 11, 172 n. 19
I Want a Famous Face, 143, 147

Jackson, Barry, 139, 139–40, 144–45
James F. Magee & Co., 60, 127, 128
Jefferson, Thomas, 12
Jefferson Medical College, 14, 28, 36, 39
Johnson, Mark, 8–9
journals, trade, 19, 21–23. *See also specific titles of
  journals*

Katz, Michael, 91
Keen, William Williams, 40–42, 41, 45
Keller, H. S., 54
Keppler, Joseph, 6, 7, 88

laboratories, 106–7. *See also* darkrooms
La Grippe, 122
Lakoff, George, 8–9
Lancaster, William I., 97–98, 98
Langenheim brothers, 14
Lazaretto, 110
Lea, Mathew Carey, 113, 114, 117, 124–25, 152
Leeds, Lewis W., 111–12, 115
legitimization of photography. *See also* photographic authority; professionalization
 education and, 27
 as fine art, 2, 4
 as medicine, 2–4, 8–13, 23, 26–-28, 87
Life Under Glass (Shove), 90–91
light. *See also* phototherapy
 agricultural experiments with, 81–82, 82
 chemical properties and effects of, 95
 in darkrooms, 87, 114
 exposure time, 85–86, 86
 health benefits of, in photographic studios,
  101–3

as public health issue, 88, 89, 90, 101–2
and race, 96–101, *98, 99, 101*
social rehabilitation and, 89–92, 104–5
Light: Its Influence on Life and Health (Winslow), 89
Lincoln, Abraham, 12, *13*
Lippincott's Magazine, 23
Lister, Martin, 135
Lutz, Louise, 140–41

magic, 170 n. 87
Magic Lantern, 153
makeover culture, 143–47
Manovich, Lev, 50, 79
Manual of Photography (Lea), 113
manuals
digital photography, 137–40, *139,* 143–45
photography, 4, 37, 46, 58, 95, 107, 113
Markoe House, 82, *84*
masculinity, as social standard, 44, 71, 114
materials, photographic, 118–25. *See also* chemicals, photographic
materia medica, 127
Maury, Frank Fontoire, 152
McAllister brothers, 14
McClees, James
The Children of the Battle-Field, 60, *61*
studio of, 14
McCollin, Thomas H., 153
McKee, J. C., 63
measles, 119, 122, 123
mechanical arts, mechanical labor, 3, 32, 34, 36, 37, 50, 53
medical models
code of ethics, 32
education standards, 27–28, 35, 36–38, 43–44
group portraits, 30, *31, 32*
overview, 2
pricing standards, 32–33
professional associations, 29–33
medical (clinical) photography
during Civil War, 21, *21,* 61–67, *63, 64, 65*
reports on value of, 46–47
medicine, overview. *See also* medical models; metaphors, medical; *related topics*
education standards, 27–28, 111
in nineteenth century, 3, 6–7, 11, 27
operative, 50, 51–58, 62 (*see also* dentistry; reconstructive surgery; surgery)
photography as, 1–3, 6–11
photography in, 21, 46–47, 61–67, *63, 64, 65*
professional associations of (*see* American Medical Association)
professional legitimacy and, 2–3, 8
trade journals of, 19, 22–23
medicine of photography metaphor, 1–3, 6–11
men
masculinity as social standard, 44, 71, 114
self-image of, 144–45
metaphors, medical
dentistry and portrait sitting comparisons, 51–57
diagnosis and clinical observation, 57–59

in digital photography, 135, 137–43, *138, 139, 141*
disease, 108, 119–20, 122–24
and establishment of professional legitimacy, 2–3, 6
function and use of, 8–13
sitters as patients, 57–58
surgery and portrait sitting, 48–50, 59, 79, 119
Metaphors We Live By (Lakoff and Johnson), 8
Miami Herald, 146
middle class
and blue-light therapy, 88
as ideal photographic subjects, 7, 18, 51
pain and, 51–53
retouching and identity of, 69
as social value, 17–18
urban health and, 87, 89, 90, 91
military medical (clinical) photography, 21, 61–66, *62, 63, 64, 65*
military medicine, 19
Milroy, Elizabeth, 18
Mitchell, S. Weir, 19, 61
Mitchell, W. J. T., 134, 135, 147
Moelling, Edward, 127
Morton, H. J., 62
Mower General Hospital, 19
museums, photographic, 159n.38

Nast, Thomas, 12, *13*
national health
individual health relationship to, 12–13
light deprivation and, 87, 89
political concept of, 12
Reconstruction and rehabilitation of, 21
wartime effects on perceptions of, 19–21
National Photographic Association (NPA)
education focus and apprenticeship committees of, 34–35
formation and purpose of, 21, 29
founding members' group portraits, 30, *31*
journals associated with, 151
and professionalization, 30–32
National Photographic Convention, 28–29
national photographic institute, 31, 35, 37, 163 n. 31
National Sanitary Convention, 112–13
neuralgia, 2, 87
neurasthenia, 87
Newell, Robert, 18–19, *20*
Newhall, Beaumont, 4
New Yorker, 132, 142
New-York Illustrated News, 12
Nip/Tuck, 147–50, *149*
The Normal and the Pathological (Canguilhem), 59
North, Walter C., 57, 58
NPA. *See* National Photographic Association

occupational hazards, 108, 109, 113, 117. *See also* chemicals, photographic; sanitation
operation (critical term), 50
operation rooms (photographic), 48–50
operative medicine, 6, 50, 51–58, 62. *See also* dentistry; reconstructive surgery; surgery
The Order of Things (Foucault), 11

orthodox *vs.* unorthodox medicine, 6–7, 11, 27
Ozier, M. Eugene, 129

PAA (Photographic Association of America), 33
PAFA (Pennsylvania Academy of the Fine Arts),
    40, 45
pain
    anesthesia and, 73–78
    calculus of suffering, 77–78
    dental compared to photographic, 54–55, 58
    photographic chemicals relieving, 129
    social class and, 51–53
painting
    photography compared to, 2
    surgery compared to, 38–40, 39, 170 n. 87
Palmer, B. Franklin, 167–68 n. 44
Parrish, Isaac, 109–10
Pennsylvania Academy of the Fine Arts (PAFA),
    40, 45
Pennsylvania Board of Health, 110, 112
Pennsylvania General Hospital (PGH), 30, 32
Pennsylvania Hospital, 14
Pennsylvania Museum and School of Industrial
    Art, 37
Pernick, Martin, 77
personifications
    of artists' materials, 119–20
    of photographic materials, 118–19, 120–25
    of photography, 1–2, 125
pharmaceuticals, 1–2, 6, 109, 124–30
Philadelphia, nineteenth-century
    African Americans in, 16, 91–92
    city center, 14–16, 15, 16
    during Civil War, 18–21, 20
    medical history, 13–14
    photographic history, 14, 16
    photographic history and community in, 21–22
    sanitation issues in, 109–12
    social challenges of, 16–18
Philadelphia College of Pharmacy, 14
Philadelphia Medical Times, 22–23, 89
Philadelphia Photographer
    educational function of, 34
    founder and editor of, 21–22 (*see also* Wilson,
        Edward L.)
    overview, 151–52
Philadelphia Photographic Society, 151
Philadelphia School of Anatomy, 40, 42, 43
Philadelphia Society for Promoting Agriculture, 81
photo doctor persona
    modern examples of, 137–43, 138, 139, 141, 143,
        145
    in the nineteenth century, 1–2, 125, 127, 129
Photographer's Friend, 21, 151
The Photographer to His Patrons (Wilson), 32
Photographic Art Journal (later *Photographic and
        Fine Art Journal*), 45
Photographic Association of America (PAA), 33
photographic authority
    definition, 6
    digital technology and modern, 137–43
    disciplining sitters and, 54

early views of, 3–4
irregular medicine and, 6–7
medical metaphors promoting, 2, 11, 54–55,
    119–20, 122–24
and modern cosmetic surgery, 147
pain as indication of, 78–79
science and, 157n.17
truth and, 147–50
types of, 4–5
The Photographic Image in Digital Culture (Lister),
    135
Photographic Journal of America (formerly *Philadel-
        phia Photographer* and *Wilson's Photographic
        Magazine*), 153
Photographic Mosaics, 152
Photographic Review of Medicine and Surgery, 152,
    164 n. 62
Photographic Society of Philadelphia, 14
Photographic World, 21, 129, 151, 152
Photography: A Middle-Brow Art (Bourdieu), 26
Photography After Photography (Amelunxen et al.),
    136
photography as medicine metaphor, 1–3, 6–11
Photoshop Cosmetic Surgery (Jackson), *139*,
    139–40, 144–46
phototherapy
    clinics for, 82, *83*, *84*
    conditions remedied by, 87, 92
    criticism and satires of, 6, 87–88, 93
    curative properties and effects, 95
    early studies supporting, 81–82, *82*, 85
    photographic studio lighting compared to,
        85–88, 95, 101–2
    popularity of, 83, 88
    as social medicine, 88–94
    and urban health, 91
phrenology, 58, 71
physiognomy, 58, 71
pixel surgeons, 137
plastic surgery. *See* reconstructive surgery
Pleasonton, Augustus J., 81–82, *82*, 85, 87–88, 92
PMA Magazine, 141
pneumonia, 123, 124
poetry, 51, 60
pollution, 109–10, 112, 113
Portrait of an Unidentified Boy (Rhoads' New Pho-
        tograph Gallery), 55, *56*
Portrait of an Unidentified Man (Gutekunst), 67, *67*
Portrait of an Unidentified Soldier (Gutekunst), *66*,
    66–67
Portrait of William I. Lancaster (unidentified pho-
        tographer), 97–98, *98*
posing apparatus
    dentistry and comparisons to, 49, *49*, 51, 52, 165
        n. 17
    pain and, 73–76, 87
    photography-surgery metaphor and, 79
    promoting social rehabilitation, 73
pricing standards, 32–33
professionalization of photography
    associations and, 29–33, *31*
    challenges to, 3–4, 6–7, 37, 44, 53, 142

chemicals and medical metaphor usage, 127
clinical photography reports and, 47
codes of ethics promoting, 31–32
early development and definitions of, 27
education standards, 27–28, 33–38, 44
group portraits and, 30, *31, 32*
hygiene and, 114–17
medical metaphor and, 10–11
pricing standards promoting, 32–33
retouching and, 70–71
public health
darkrooms and, 89, 108–9, 112–18
light deprivation and, 87, 89, 90–91, 101–2
and personifications of photography, 119–20, 122
railroad cars and, 115, *116*
sanitation reform, 109–12
standards of, 114
war and perceptions of, 19–21
Puck, 6, *7, 136*
Purity and Danger (Douglas), 108
pyroxylin (gun cotton), 1, 127

quackery
comparisons to photography, 99, 103–5
consequences of, 120
as criticism, 6–7, 11, 87
quarantine, 110

race
chemical stains and, 115–16
digital photographic manuals and, 144
environmental effects on, 89–90
perceptions of health and, 91, 102
photographic lighting and, 96–101, *98, 99, 101,*
103
photographic truth and perceptions of, 103–4
phototherapy and, 90, 93–94
railroad cars, and sanitation issues, 115, *116*
Rau, George, 16
Rau, William H., 68
reconstructive (plastic, cosmetic) surgery
clinical photography and, 61–66, *63, 64, 65*
retouching compared to, 70, 72, 132–34,
136–46, *138, 139, 141*
rehabilitation
physical, 104, 123
race and, 96–99, *98, 99*
social, 7, 11–12, 68–73, *73,* 104–5
trauma associated with, 80
virtual, and digital technology, 136
respectability. *See also* middle class; social class.
in the darkroom, 108, 114–15, 117
as health standard, 114
modern standards of, 144
nineteenth-century characteristics of, 90
pain and, 51–53
portrait sitting and, 73
race and, 96–97
professionalism and, 30–32
retouching (doctoring photographs)
as digital plastic surgery, 132–34, 136–46, *138,*
139, 141

early techniques of, 68–73, *70, 71*
frames for, 68, *69*
Revere, Paul, 12
Rhoads' New Photograph Gallery, 55, *56*
Richards, Frederick DeBourg, 30, *31*
Ritchin, Fred, 134
Robins, Kevin, 135
Robinson, H. P., 77
Rodgers, H. J., 98
Root, Marcus Aurelius
daguerreotype studio, 4, *5,* 14, 48–50, *49*
diagnosis (clinical observation) of portrait sit-
ters, 58–59
photographic school proposals, 34–37
photography as art *vs.* science debates, 45–46
photographic treatises by, 4, 14
Root Gallery, Fifth and Chestnut Streets, Philadel-
phia (Cohill), 4, *5*
Rush, Benjamin, 173n.34
Russian influenza, 122
Ryder, James, 30

Sachse, Julius F., 14, 153
sanitation, 109–15, *116,* 119, 125
Sappol, Michael, 43–44
Sarony, Napoleon, 75, 165 n. 17
Saxton, Joseph, 14, 164 n. 56
School of Photography at Chautauqua, 44
schools, photographic, 33–38, 44
Schreiber, E., 159 n. 38, 161 n. 15
science
anatomical education and, 39–40, 44–45
blue-light therapy and, 88
photographic authority and, 157 n. 17
in photographic education, 37
photography as art *vs.*, 44–45
in the retouching debates, 72
Science of Photography at Home and Abroad, 153
Scientific American, 87, 172 n. 19
segregation, photographic, 99–100
Sekula, Allan, 5
Sheridan, Philip Henry, 68
Shove, George, 85, 90–91
Showalter, Allen, *141,* 141–42
silver nitrate, 115–17, 126–27, 129
Simons, Montgomery P., 14
Simpson, G. Wharton, 34
Sipley, Louis Walton, 159 n. 38, 161 n. 15
sitters, portrait
clinical observation and diagnosis of, 58
codes of ethics for, 31–32
discipline of, 53–55
experiences of, 48–51, *49, 52,* 56, 78
pain of portraiture and, 51–55, *55, 56,* 72-8
posing of, 57–58
social rehabilitation of, 73, 95–96
Sitting for a Daguerreotype, 48–50, *49,* 56
slavery, as social health metaphor, 12, *13*
smallpox, 122
Smith, Pamela, 120–21
Snelling, Henry Hunt
Doctor Photo and, 1–2, 125, 127, 129

Snelling, Henry Hunt (*continued*)
   perception of medical models, 33
   photographic education and, 35
   photography as art *vs.* science debates, 45
   professionalization of photography and, 27
   retouching debates, 72, 133
social class. *See also* middle class; respectability
   codes of ethics and studio etiquette promoting,
     31–32, 49–50
   development of, 17–18
   education and advancement of, 35, 45
   medical metaphor and, 48–50
   modern standards of, 144
   pain and, 51–53, 73–74
   photographic lighting effects on, 95–101
   photography and advancement of, 18, 27
   pricing standards and the advancement of, 32–33
   retouching photographs and perceptions of, 72
social destabilization, 7, 99
social health and fitness
   categories of, 12
   the Civil War and, 11–13, *13*
   in the darkroom, 109, 114–18
societies, professional. *See* associations
Sontag, Susan, 78
Stephens, Charles H., 40–41, 44, *41*
Stieglitz, Alfred, 4
Studio Light, 180 n. 11
studios, photographic
   first American, 14
   lighting in, 85–88, *86*
   medical metaphors for, 48–50
   in Philadelphia, 4, *5*, 14, 16, *16*
Sugre, Thomas, 91
Summer School at Mountain Lake Park, 44
surgery. *See also* operative medicine; reconstructive (plastic, cosmetic) surgery
   anesthesia and, 74–75, 79
   medical (clinical) photography and, 69
   operation, definition, 50
   painting compared to, 38–40, *39*
   photography compared to, 48–50, 59, 68, 78, 119
Surgery, Its Principles and Practices (Keen), 163n.47
The Swan, 143
System of Surgery (Gross), 36–37
Szarkowski, John, 4

Tagg, John, 5
Taylor & Wetherbee, 126, *126*, 127
Tipton, W. H., 42–43, 44
Tissandier, Gaston, 107, 119
Towler, John, 29, 34
Trachtenberg, Alan, 9, 19
Trask, A. K. P., 34–35
Treatise on Hygiene (Hammond), 89
truth and objectivity, photographic, 6, 72, 103–5,
   134, 147–50
TV Guide, 133

United States Pharmacopoeia, 127
United States Sanitary Commission (USSC), 18,
   60–61, 111

University of Pennsylvania School of Medicine,
   14, 28
urban health. *See* public health

Vanweike, Roland, 68, 77
ventilation, 113–14
Vogel, Hermann, 37, 69, 70, 95, 104

Ward, Rowland, 62–66, *63*, *64*, *65*
Warner, John Harley, 8
Weber, Brenda, 143
Wenderoth, F. A., 16
Wenderoth, Taylor & Brown, 127, *128*
Wenderoth & Taylor, 60
West Philadelphia Hospital Register, 67
Weyde, P. H. van der, 161 n. 13
whiteness
   baby portraits and, 101
   calculus of suffering and, 77
   chemical stains and, 115–16
   as health standard, 114
   photographic rehabilitation and, 96–99
   social superiority and dominance of, 100–101
   as social value, 18, 73, 90–93, 144
*William Rush Carving His Allegorical Figure of the
   Schuylkill River* (Eakins), 112
Willis, Deborah, 97
Wills Eye Hospital, 158 n. 36
Wilson, Edward L.
   cyanide of potassium as therapeutic medicine,
     129
   on the darkroom interior, *107*, 107–8, 114
   hygiene standards of photographers, 114–15
   on the national photographic institute, 35
   pamphlet for studio sitters by, 32
   professional association founding member, 30,
     31
   promoting photographic education, 37
   trade journals founded and edited by, 14, 21–22,
     151–53 (see also *Philadelphia Mosaics*; *Phila-
     delphia Photographer*; *Wilson's Photographic
     Magazine*)
Wilson, L. W., 153
Wilson's Photographic Magazine, 21, 123, 151, 153
Wilson's Photographics (Wilson), 107, *107*
Winfrey, Oprah, 133
Winslet, Kate, 133, 146, *147*
Winslow, Forbes, 89, 90
Withers, William C., 96–97, 99
women
   as doctors of photography, 44
   exclusion of, from anatomical education, 44
   modern self-image, 144–45
   pain of portraiture and, 77
   retouching and, 71
Worth, Thomas, 94

Yellow fever, 119